Tinsley Harrison, M.D.

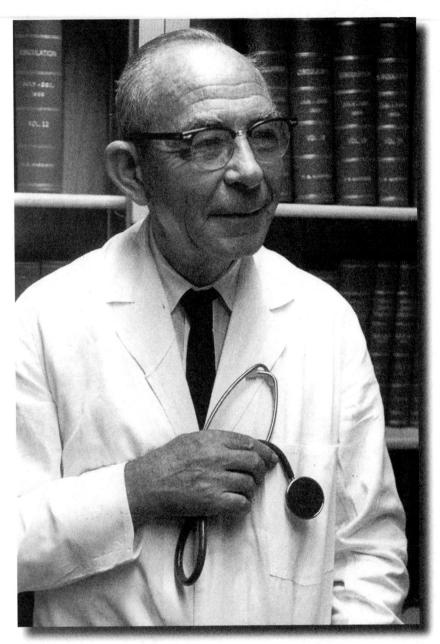

Tinsley Randolph Harrison at UAB, about 1970.

TINSLEY R. HARRISON

M.D.

Teacher of Medicine

James A. Pittman Jr., M.D.

NewSouth Books

Montgomery

NewSouth Books
105 S. Court Street
Montgomery, AL 36104

Library of Congress Cataloging-in-Publication Data

Pittman, James A. (James Allen), Jr., 1927–
Tinsley R. Harrison, M.D. : teacher of medicine / James A. Pittman Jr., M.D.
pages cm

ISBN 978-1-58838-226-9 (hardcover)
ISBN 978-1-60306-251-0 (ebook)

1. Harrison, Tinsley Randolph, 1900–1978. 2. University of Alabama at Birmingham. School
of Medicine—History. 3. Physicians—United States—Biography. 4. Medical education—
Alabama—History. I. Title.
R154.H274P58 2013
610.92—dc23
[B]

2013034245

Photos appearing in this volume are courtesy of the UAB Archives.

Design by Randall Williams
Printed in the United States of America

From the 9th Edition of *Principles of Internal Medicine*:

This edition is dedicated to the Editor-in-Chief of this text during its first five editions, Tinsley R. Harrison.

From time to time a personality scintillates across the medical firmament who dazzles all beholders. Tinsley Harrison was such a person. A delightful, vivacious, passionate physician, he stimulated everyone with whom he came in contact, and he placed an indelible stamp on the medical events of his day.

As a thoughtful physician he excelled in the care of the sick, and the words which he penned for the first edition of this book reflect the importance which he attached to his role as a physician:

No greater opportunity or obligation can fall the lot of a human being than to be a physician. In the care of the suffering he needs technical skill, scientific knowledge, and human understanding. He who uses these with courage, humility, and wisdom will provide a unique service for his fellow man and will build an enduring edifice of character within himself. The physician should ask of his destiny no more than this, and he should be content with no less.

CONTENTS

TRH Timeline

1900 Born on March 18 at the family home in Talladega, Alabama

1906 Family moves to Birmingham, Alabama

1916 Completes one year at Marion Institute, Marion, Alabama

1919 A.B., University of Michigan

1922 M.D., Johns Hopkins School of Medicine;
Begins residency at Peter Bent Brigham Hospital, Boston

1924 Begins senior residency at Johns Hopkins Hospital, Baltimore

1925 Becomes chief resident at Vanderbilt Hospital

1926 Joins Vanderbilt University School of Medicine Faculty

1940 Accepts Chair of Internal Medicine at Bowman Gray Medical School, North Carolina

1941 Moves to Winston-Salem, North Carolina

1944 Becomes Chair and Dean, Southwestern Medical School, Dallas, Texas

1950 Publishes *Principles of Internal Medicine*;
Becomes Chair of the Department of Medicine, Acting Dean, and Director of the Division of Cardiology, University of Alabama;
Moves back to Birmingham

1957 Resigns as Chair of Medicine

1964 Named Distinguished Professor by University of Alabama Board of Trustees

1965 Resigns as Cardiology Director

1968 Named Veterans Administration Distinguished Physician

1978 Dies on August 4, at his home in Birmingham

EDITOR'S NOTE

D r. Jim Pittman had worked on his biography of Tinsley Randolph Harrison for many years. Meanwhile, in 1992, the earlier iteration of our publishing company published the memoir of a Montgomery physician who was a close friend of both Drs. Pittman and Harrison. Then in 2006, we published a history of the University of Alabama Medical Alumni Association. Evidently on the strength of those two books and the recommendation of Birmingham-based medical writer Anita Smith, when Dr. Pittman felt he was ready to let go of his biography of Dr. Harrison, he brought the project to NewSouth Books. Or rather, he summoned us to come and wrest the project from him. Pacing along narrow paths between piles of papers, journals, and books towering on every surface of the attic office in his home on Ridge Drive, Dr. Pittman was still scribbling notes on the margins of his manuscript pages as we gathered his materials for taking back to our office in Montgomery.

The manuscript itself proved to be a sprawling, loopy mess of insight, passion, anecdote, and history. It ran to almost a thousand pages. He gave it to us in two different bound versions—in the front of one he had handwritten: "with many errors, omissions, and inadequacies"—another version of loose manuscript pages, and yet another version copied in digital word processor format from his home computer. Clearly, this was going to be no simple book project. Equally clearly, we would be working with a brilliant if eccentric author whose warmth and wit were as obvious as his somewhat challenged filing abilities.

Sadly, we did not get to work with that quick-witted personality long enough for him to see his book to completion. Soon after we began working with Dr. Pittman, his health began to decline and he became less and less able to participate in the editing and the considerable shaping and trimming that his book required.

Then he became unable to respond at all to our requests for clarification or to read and correct proofs.

Dr. Pittman had made it clear that although his was a biography of a great physician—and, though he might not have said it himself, was written by another great physician—and was intended primarily for other physicians, he also wanted Tinsley Harrison's story to be accessible to general audiences. He felt that Dr. Harrison was not just an important doctor but an important Alabamian and American. He felt that Tinsley Harrison's "century of medicine" was fundamentally significant and that the general public should be able to learn about and understand it.

To that end, Ben Beard, the editor assigned to assist Dr. Pittman with a complete revision of the manuscript, organized the text, moved some passages from one chapter to another to strengthen the narrative flow, corrected names, dates, and place, and cut some sections about medical history that, while interesting, were tangential to Harrison's story. Some of the cuts—long anecdotal footnotes to sections that we kept, and some documents that Dr. Pittman had intended as appendix but were too long to include—have been made available in an online supplement at www. newsouthbooks.com/tinsleyharrison/supplement. References to these supplemental materials will be found throughout the text and the notes. The doctors who have assisted in the proofreading of the text provided still more anecdotes and documents about Dr. Harrison and Dr. Pittman, and we expect to add more materials to the online supplement as they are provided to us.

Dr. Pittman's citations were perhaps the most difficult editorial challenge. The almost one thousand footnotes in the original manuscript were often cryptic and sprinkled with blanks or approximate dates or simply said "source???" or something similar.

After Dr. Pittman became unable to assist us with the editing, we did the best we could with these notes. And over time, we enlisted the aforementioned doctors who had worked with Dr. Pittman, and sometimes with Dr. Harrison, as proofreaders and fact checkers. Dr. Clifton Meador was especially helpful in the earlier chapters of the book. After Dr. Pittman's death, Dr. Joe LaRussa came forward to ask what he could do to help us get the book through its final steps before publication; he then organized a small team of additional proofreaders. UAB archivist Tim L. Pennycuff was especially helpful in verifying some sources and in providing publication-quality photographs to be used in the book.

At NewSouth Books, significant thanks are due to Joel Sanders, Blair Underwood,

Ashley Stanaland, Thomson McCorkle, Lisa Harrison, McCormick Williams, Brian Seidman, Suzanne La Rosa, and Lisa Emerson. Ben Beard, now a teacher and librarian in Chicago, continued to read proofs and to consult on footnotes and text shifts through the complete editorial process.

Notwithstanding everyone's efforts, we realized we would not catch every error in the text or the notes. Had Dr. Pittman been able, he probably could have rummaged around in his study until he came up with the piece of paper for a last errant citation. As it is, we invite readers to submit corrections and clarifications to be included in future printings or immediately in the ebook version.

In the end, we hope that we have delivered a version of Dr. Pittman's manuscript that does justice to his intentions, to the prodigious effort that went into the research and writing, and, finally, to his devotion to Tinsley R. Harrison, M.D., and to Harrison's medical school. Make that Harrison's *and Pittman's* medical school.

— HORACE RANDALL WILLIAMS

FOREWORD

JOE B. LaRUSSA, M.D.

Dean Pittman died on January 12, 2014, and his memorial service on February 6 was a somber but celebratory occasion.

He was the dean of the UAB School of Medicine for 19 years. That comes out to be about 3,000 medical students, including myself.[1] He was the quintessential dean: steely blue eyes, glasses, balding, white goatee, bowtie, and long, white, starched lab coat, with name embroidered, and pens in the pocket.

Four words come to mind that describe Dean Pittman. Wisdom. Desire. Compassion. Devotion. Desire was the most obvious, for he loved to teach, direct, guide, lead, lecture, instill, enlighten . . . mentor. But he also loved to learn himself.

Dean Pittman could walk fast, and when you went on rounds with him, it seemed they had added four more blocks to UAB. You were like a deer in the headlights, dragging behind, HR 160, diaphoretic. He never took the elevators; he flew up six flights of stairs. Then he would stand outside of a patient's room and begin quickly speaking as he reviewed the case before going in to examine the person. When you walked out of the room, you would be in awe, and you would think that Dean Pittman must be the smartest person you'd ever met.

After my chief year, we moved to Charlottesville for a fellowship, and then returned to Birmingham. We would run into Dr. Connie [Pittman's wife, Dr. Constance Ming-Chung Shen Pittman, who died in 2010] and Dean Pittman at the Alys Stephens Center, going to the symphony. Busy with medicine and young children, time passed. Early in 2012, I was going through my trusty file cabinet and my eye caught a file with a tab that said "TRH." It turned out to be an old file about the TRH Society, which was supported by an endowment by Hall Thompson and was named for Tinsley Randolph Harrison. A group of third- and fourth-year

1. UASOM, 1990.

XII

medical students met twice a month in the CAMS building and had dinner with a small group of faculty members. Following dinner, a student presented a paper. Dean Pittman had been my sponsor when I was a student and I gave a presentation on the painting *Medical Giants of Alabama*, commissioned by Dr. Pittman in 1982 and painted by Marshall Bouldin III.

Dean Pittman had long since retired and I knew he was not in good health. But, reminded by that old file, I decided to go visit him. The slides from the presentation were Kodak projector slides, so I had them put on a CD to show him. He had suffered several strokes since I had last seen him. We talked about William Crawford Gorgas and Marion Sims, two of the subjects in the painting, and before I left I asked him if he wanted me to come again. He said he would like that. So from then on we visited every other Saturday at two o'clock. We covered Hippocrates, Galen, Harvey, Pasteur, Lister, the penicillin discoverer Alexander Fleming, James Watson and Francis Crick of DNA fame, Thomas Aquinas, St. Augustine, the New York Yankees and their 27 World Series championships, Babe Ruth, Lou Gehrig, Mickey Mantle, Yogi Berra, Joltin' Joe Dimaggio, Marilyn Monroe and the list went on and on.

At a particular session I remember we were talking about the discovery of DNA, and the scientists Watson and Crick. DNA, mRNA, tRNA, amino acids, proteins. Dean Pittman said, "You're a smart fella'." I told him, "I'm not sure about that; I have a lot to learn." So many years ago, I knew how much there was for me to learn, and he was the teacher. Now he was at his kitchen table, in his comfortable flannel shirt and slippers, no bowtie, not torturing medical students, not grilling residents. If not being taught, which he was not, he was being reminded of all the things he had long known.

My take-home message that day was the realization it is more about a person's willingness to teach than about their being smart. It was Tinsley Harrison who believed and said, "Learning is more a matter of the heart than the brain," and he acted accordingly, and so did Dean Pittman.

In August 2013, Dean Pittman was moved to St. Martin's. Just before his move, he was admitted to the hospital and dermatology put him on 60 mg of Prednisone. The next day I went by to visit. I asked, "Have you had a good day?" He said, "A great day, a great day." If I had been on Prednisone, I would have felt pretty good, too. Then he surprised me and he said, "How has your day been?" I said, "Oh, pretty good. I saw a patient with Urticaria today, and they can be tough, they can be tough." He looked at me and said, "why?" I felt like a resident again, and said, "Well, 20 percent of the population will have hives, and when you look in the literature, for 70 percent of the cases you never find a cause." They are idiopathic, meaning we don't know why, but there has to be a cause. He looked at me, and said nothing. I thought I would turn the table on him. There is some controversial data with certain thyroid conditions that can be associated with hives. So I asked him, "Did you ever have a thyroid patient that had hives? He immediately went into teaching mode, and sat up, his eyes got big and bright, and he started talking. His brain was spinning, but because of the strokes he had suffered, the words were not clear. I could not understand him. He said it again, the exact same thing, then a third time. He then stopped, frustrated, and sat back in his bed. You could hear a pin drop, it was so quiet. We looked at each other and we both knew he was no longer able to teach.

Yes, medicine can be tough.

But, knowing Dean Pittman, he would want the story to have a happy ending. He had high standards; he put the bar way up there. It is up to us, because if we teach what he taught us, and then if those young doctors teach the others, then in a sense, Dean Pittman will still be teaching. It is perpetual, everlasting.

At the end of each visit I would shake Dean Pittman's hand, put my hand on his shoulder and say, "See you at grand rounds this week." He would look at me and say, "Sure." Both of us, with smiles on our faces, knew it would not happen. But it became a ritual and it made it easier to end our time together. Grand rounds is a part of the medical learning process, where attending physicians, fellows, residents, interns, and medical students are all together in an auditorium while a professor discusses his or her area of expertise. There is also a time when a case is presented and the other subspecialties join in to solve the case. It is a great medical learning environment where these attendings pass down their way of thinking and their knowledge.

At one of three sessions that Wayne Finley and Scotty McCallum visited Dean Pittman, we talked about grand rounds. I asked them what it was like to be at grand rounds with Tinsley Harrison and Champ Lyons on a Saturday morning (which Dean Pittman memorably describes in this book). Who won? Wayne said that "it was always a lively, spirited duel, but Tinsley Harrison usually won. Sorry, surgeons." But then Scotty was quick to say, "the pathologist always had the final word."

Dean Pittman is now gone, of course, but I guess if I could tell him two things, first would be to express my gratitude and to thank him for giving me the opportunity to be a physician. And second would be that "I'll see you at grand rounds, Dean Pittman. But the next time it will be the biggest grand rounds of all, His grand rounds. And if I could ask one more favor of you, Dean Pittman, it would be to save me a seat next to Galen, Harvey, or Pasteur, maybe even Lister. And maybe after lunch we could swing by and visit Tinsley Harrison."

AT THE TIME OF Dean Pittman's death, NewSouth Books was trying to wrap up his biography of Harrison, as one of the editors has explained in a preceding note. I have been privileged to work with a team who have read proofs and verified information and tried to help resolve questions about sources, citations, spellings of names, and so on. Among those who have helped in this effort are John B. Harrison, D.M.D., M.D.; Dick D. Briggs Jr., M.D.; Dr. Clifton Meador; Timothy Pennycuff, UAB archivist; and Dr. W. B. Stonecypher. Lastly, having never met Tinsley Harrison myself—he died when I was a sophomore in high school—I am also grateful to Drs. Scotty McCallum and Wayne Finley for sharing their Tinsley Harrison stories with me so that I was able to appreciate even more why he was and is a true medical giant. For it was Newton who so famously said, "If I see further than others, it is by standing on the shoulders of giants."

ACKNOWLEDGMENTS

JAMES A. PITTMAN JR., M.D.

The first thanks must go to Tinsley Harrison himself, since he patiently recounted material from past times during long evening meetings in his small apartment surrounded by his beloved books. These interviews took place between July 1973 and his death in August 1978. All were recorded on audiotapes made by a hand-held tape recorder. These are invaluable for his early memories and beyond. All these tapes are now in the UAB Archives.

Special thanks also must go to Allan Brandt, Ph.D., chair of the Department of the History of Medicine at Harvard University and professor of social medicine at Harvard Medical School; Arthur Kleinman, M.D., Ph.D., chair of the Department of Social Medicine at Harvard; Leon Eisenberg, M.D., a faculty member in that department and professor of psychiatry and chief emeritus at the Massachusetts General Hospital; and especially Daniel C. Tosteson, M.D., dean of Harvard Medical School at the time, who generously appointed me visiting professor for 1992–1993. It was during this time that the book really got started.

Dr. Eisenberg, formerly professor and chief of psychiatry at the Massachusetts General Hospital, also reviewed the patient records of Tinsley Harrison's psychotic sister, "Weeze," who was hospitalized during the last period of her life in Bryce Hospital, a state mental institution.

I am very grateful to Mr. Timothy Pennycuff, UAB Archivist, who has furnished invaluable help in assembling the photos and documents that form the basis of the story, as well as to Michael A. Flannery, author of several medical books himself and an expert on the history of pharmacy, for his advice and help. Bruce Horne, manager of the UAB Print Plant, provided the essential help of putting the physical copies of the original draft together in book form. Lloyd L. Hefner, M.D., an accomplished cardiologist and investigator who joined Harrison in the early 1950s, put together the only complete bibliography of Harrison's publications. Thanks also to my long-time secretary, Ann Harrell, to President S. Richardson Hill, M.D., one-time dean of medicine, then vice president, and then president of UAB, as well as to President Charles A. McCallum, D.M.D, M.D., and finally to President Carol Garrison, M.S.N., Ph.D., for continuing support.

FOR THE TIMES BEFORE 1992 the acknowledgments must be more general, vague, and imprecise, since I was devoted primarily to medical administration and teaching, and I kept poor and often incomplete records of sources then, as is evident.

I tried, insofar as possible, to follow the tracks of Tinsley Harrison as he made his way through his life in the developing medicine of the twentieth century.

This started as simply an attempt at a biography of a local hero in the development of our University Medical Center in Birmingham. As such it may have mainly local interest. However, since Harrison was born in 1900 and lived in the upper reaches of academic medicine in the South, with strong connections to medicine throughout the nation and world, his life also relates to the remarkable development of medicine in the twentieth century.

In following Harrison's tracks, I am indebted to many local people, such as Richard Bliss, M.D., Talladega, and Miss Willie Welch, daughter of Samuel W. Welch, M.D., state health officer of Talladega. Miss Willie taught me how to chalk the tombstones to make the printing show in photographs. As a lifelong librarian, Miss Willie knew much local lore and gossip not retrievable otherwise.

Ms. Nancy McCall, archivist at the Chesney Archives at Johns Hopkins, was especially helpful in retrieving material about Harrison's Hopkins years, but also in the wonderful collections of material on Alfred Blalock, Harrison's closest friend throughout his life, and the very complete collection of correspondence between the two.

The Harvard University Archives in Cambridge were valuable for such things as the tuition and fees in 1915 and later, and similar material, as was the Bentley Historical Library at Ann Arbor, Michigan. The Dorothy Carpenter Archives at Wake Forest University in North Carolina (formerly Bowman Gray) provided material on the early 1940s, but especially valuable was the guidance of their former dean of medicine and vice president, the late Manson Meads, M.D., and his assistant Katherine Davis. (Mrs. Carpenter, the late dean's wife, was pleasant and helpful in learning public information, but was so discreet that she was of no help at all in ferreting out gossip.) Similarly, Miss Mary Teloh of special collections in the Eskind Medical Library at Vanderbilt was essential in uncovering such details as departmental budgets in the 1920s and 1930s. Roscoe R. Robinson, M.D., nephrologist turned vice chancellor and superb administrator, guided me to all sorts of details. The time at Southwestern was well covered by Dr. John Chapman's history of the school and Jean D. Wilson's excellent review of Harrison's years at the new Southwestern Medical School, 1944–1950. Dr. Wilson gave a thorough review during a "Harrison Centennial" held at UAB in the year 2000. Ms. Christine Beal-Kaplan researched the aviation portion of Harrison's son, Lemuel Woodward Harrison, his service in naval aviation in Florida, and his death there in 1944. She also reviewed large parts of the drafts of the text.

In Germany the members of the Medizinische Fakultaet of Albert-Ludwigs-Universitaet Freiburg, in Freiburg im Breisgau, were most hospitable and helpful in running down details of Harrison's stay there in 1928. The administration of the Josephinum, a wonderful center for the history of medicine in Vienna, and the history of medicine faculty at the Allgemeines Krankenhaus, were most helpful in learning about the social climate in 1928 and postgraduate medical education at that time (and why Harrison did not like it).

FINALLY, THE HELP AND support of local people were essential, especially the Harrison family and especially John B. Harrison, D.M.D., M.D., and Dr. Charles A. McCallum, former president of UAB and the one who established the UAB Archives, where much of the material referred to is housed. S. Richardson Hill, Jr., M.D., former student and patient of Harrison at Bowman Gray and later president of UAB, Dr. Carol Z. Garrison, current president of UAB, provided continuing support for the project. Ultimately, none of this could have been done without my late wife, Constance S. Pittman, M.D. (Shen Ming-chung).

A Writer's Apologia

James A. Pittman Jr., M.D.

This is the story of Tinsley Randolph Harrison—one of the most important and pivotal medical doctors in U.S. history—but it's also the story of the practice of medicine in America in the 20th century, and more specifically about the practice of medicine in the Southern United States. Harrison was born in 1900 with the hope and fear of the new century; he died in 1978 just as the century was beginning to sense its looming end. His life affords an opportunity to look at the explosive progress that took place in medical research, education, practice, and administrative arrangements in the 20th century, which has been called the greatest period for medicine in all history.[1] The story is not only about what Tinsley Harrison made of things, but also of the things that made him. For this the story must begin farther back with his father, a physician, and that physician's father, also a physician.

This book begins and ends with a patient. In the first instance, the malady began abruptly, just as illness often is discovered suddenly and unexpectedly by a patient. In the second, old age and lifestyle dictated the terms of death. Patients are central to Tinsley's life and to the practice of medicine. For medicine is about *patients*—curing, managing, or ameliorating their diseases, disabilities, pain, and suffering—and in the last analysis that is all medicine is about. Obviously, the various aspects of prevention—vaccinations, prevention of epidemics, provision of clean and pure water, food, and air, policies concerning the macro-allocation of public resources—are necessary and historically have usually been introduced or supported (though sometimes opposed) by the physicians, who best understood the problems. But the more these community concerns take first priority, the more the effort becomes public health and the less it is the practice of medicine. Present-day

1. J. Le Fanu, *The Rise and Fall of Modern Medicine* (New York: Carroll & Graf Publishers, 2000).

2. J. Eisenberg, "Patient Centered Medicine," *AHCPR REPORT* (July 1998), 1.

3. A. Nevins, "Irving Stone," *Book of the Month Club News,* reprinted in Irving Stone, "Foreword" for *The Origin, A Biographical Novel of Charles Darwin* (New York: New American Library, 1980). Nevins quotes Marguerite Yourcenar as saying, in a note appended to her *Hadrian's Memoirs,* ". . . history has its laws, and poetry or imaginative reconstruction also has its laws; 'the two are not necessarily irreconcilable.' Irving Stone believes that in the hands of a conscientious writer they are perfectly reconcilable."

discussions trying to emphasize "patient-centered medicine" only demonstrate how far we have strayed from that fundamental concept.[2]

Which would be the more true and accurate description of a mountain in the sunset: that of a team of an engineer, a geographer, a biologist, and a geologist, or that of a solitary poet? The team of scientists might write a very accurate description of the mountain, with its exact location and geographic relations using tables, graphs, maps and a global positioning satellite fix, the mountain's dimensions, maximum height of its peak, mass, quantification of its geological constituents, the types and distribution of foliage and fauna, perhaps the economic value of the timber and mineral resources, the amount of light reaching the various parts of the mountain at sunset, and so on. The poet, on the other hand, might emphasize the massive size and increasing darkness of the mountain, its rocky outline against the sky, the clouds over it, the song of the water in the brook along its side, the whisper of the wind in its trees, the evening murmurs of birds in the lower branches, the lengthening shadows as the sun sets, the crepuscular rays from the sun and the fading tints of colors, the apparently increasingly rapid rate of descent of the sun as it nears the horizon. Whose description is more accurate, that of the scientists or that of the poet? Which is really *true*? Both are correct; they just appeal to different senses, different perspectives. One may be more detailed, but the other more intense, therefore more immediately real to the observer. Cliometrics is great for history, but it is not necessarily truer than the poet's descriptions.

The author Irving Stone divided his biographies into biographies and biographical novels. The former stick as much as possible to statements documentable in various archives and collections. The latter include imagined scenes, conversations, actions, and so on, not strictly documentable but always carefully researched so as to be highly plausible and compatible with the facts and the truth, whatever that is.[3]

THERE ARE TWO BOOKS about Tinsley Harrison in these pages. One book adheres closely to documents located in files at various universities and medical schools, oral histories documented on audiotape recordings, family letters, many secondary and tertiary sources from academic literature, and the like. This is a true biography in the usual pseudo-unambiguous sense of the professional historian.

The other book attempts to convey a sense of what it was really like to be on the forefront of practicing medicine, in this case in rural Alabama shortly after the Civil War. Back then records were often sparse or nonexistent, especially records of personal conversations between doctor and patient. A writer must use general sources and try to fill in details in the most plausible way from what data are available, such as material from contemporary medical books or journals, case reports, and individual medical records or day books from doctors' offices, and sometimes from memories of old colleagues. I am aware of the contempt professional historians heap on colleagues who, when attacked on the validity of some point, reply, "But that's just the sort of thing he *might* have said."[4]

Limited by the dearth of materials and the passage of time that dims everyone's memories, I've had to use composites, personal interviews, archival material, and my own firsthand memories to construct this narrative. I met Tinsley in 1956 when I was 29 years old, a new doctor in the widening field of internal medicine. Tinsley was already a developing legend, which is why I chose to move to Alabama—still blighted by the decimations of the Civil War, poverty, and the simmering civil rights movement—from the National Institutes of Health in Washington, D.C. Thus I knew Tinsley for 22 years, from 1956 to 1978, when he died.

The early and middle parts of the 20th century, just after the end of World War II, were a magical time for medicine. Never before (and perhaps never again) was there such an explosion of advances in medical knowledge and technology, both clinically and in medical and biological science. Although these changes had started in the latter 19th century, the real advances occurred during Tinsley's lifetime. He participated in them and was intimately involved with the leaders of the medical world. He was particularly important in the development of medicine and medical education in his native South, where he was founding chair of medicine and/or dean in three medical schools.

I was extraordinarily fortunate to have been thrown into the same post–World War II world, having been born in the South, attended college in the South (Davidson), and trained at Harvard Medical School and the Massachusetts General and other Harvard hospitals. This, with the NIH, put me in touch with various Nobel laureates (especially Marshall Nirenberg, who led the breaking of the genetic code) and other leaders in medicine. I then returned to the South solely because of Tinsley Harrison and his reputation.

This reputation was based on his abilities as a teacher of medicine, and this in turn on his famous book, *Principles of Internal Medicine,* first published in 1950, a novel approach to clinical medicine textbooks [now in its 18th edition and published in 18 languages].

4. A conversation I had with two visiting Russian scientists in 1990 was revealing. Over lunch I asked, "What do you think is going to happen in the Soviet Union and Russia?" They laughed and said, "You're asking us to predict the future? In our country we can't even predict the past!"

5. Peter Novick, *That Noble Dream—The "Objectivity Question" and the American Historical Profession* (Cambridge: Cambridge University Press, 1988).

6. I observed patients and doctors in most medical schools of the United States (as a faculty member of four), some in Canada, Mexico, several countries in Central and South America, most countries in Western and Central Europe and some in Eastern Europe, Africa, the Middle East (Israel, Iraq, Jordan, Saudi Arabia), and East Asia (Japan, People's Republic of China, Republic of China [Taiwan], Bangladesh), and have actually practiced medicine in Canada (Newfoundland/ Laborador, with John Olds), Africa (Bulape, Kasai, Belgian Congo; and Lambarene, Gabon, French Equatorial Africa, with Albert Schweitzer), and the United States.

7. Sir George Pickering to J. Pittman, August 5, 1978 (UAB Archives).

8. I. L. Bennett Jr.,"Bennett's Reminiscences," in *Harrison's Principles of Internal*

I believe the reader will enjoy and profit from descriptions of medical practice put together in this manner, consistent with the medicine and society of the times, and will gain a more intimate and intense picture of that most intimate and personal of professional activities—the practice of medicine. The practice of medicine in many ways consumed Tinsley's life, so it seems fitting to devote much of a biography about him to this purpose.[5]

Such is the material in chapters 1, 10, and 13, patient care in each quarter of the 20th century, and it is no more nor less imaginary than the patients which often appear in written or oral examinations, composed as they are from fragments of clinical observations. Chapter 4 was similarly composed from stories told by Tinsley and recorded on audiotape, supplemented by fragments from conversations with Tinsley and others of the same age and locality, sometimes events personally witnessed by me, but not documentable in any strict literary sense. In fact, the conversations and events of these particular chapters are based on 50 years of observing patients in all circumstances and many geographic locations,[6] and listening to hours and weeks of medical war stories in doctors' lounges and cafeterias of hospitals and clinics of similar variation. Many of the patients and episodes described occurred exactly as related. I contend that these chapters are not imaginary at all, but composites, or collages, which give a true picture—more immediate than those in graphs and tables of data. Medicine is first of all an interaction between warm-blooded, breathing, feeling, living people, which we forget at our peril. It is at least half poetry rather than technology, and as life progresses towards its inevitable end, the poetry must increase and the technology decrease.

SIR GEORGE PICKERING, Nuffield Professor of Medicine at Oxford, said that Tinsley's chief characteristic was *passion*.[7] He was rarely neutral on any topic, and he was usually most intense on medical topics. Dr. Ivan Bennett of Emory, Johns Hopkins, and New York University said, "His motto seemed to be that anything worth doing is worth doing in excess."[8] The editors of the ninth edition of the book—his book, *Principles of Internal Medicine*, sometimes called *PIM* for short—in press when Tinsley died in 1978, remarked as they dedicated the book to his memory, "From time to time a personality scintillates across the medical firmament who dazzles all beholders. Tinsley Harrison was such a person. A delightful, vivacious, passionate physician, he stimulated everyone with whom he came in contact, and he placed an indelible stamp on the medical events of his day."[9]

Pickering considered Tinsley an overtly emotional person when it came to medical matters, teaching, and patients. He believed that a properly calibrated emotional involvement of a doctor with his patients, and especially with his students, was absolutely essential to doing a good job for either. And no doctor better exemplified the combined qualities of goodwill and sympathy for his patients together with objective application of the best and most advanced scientific medical knowledge than did he.

Tinsley Randolph Harrison was indeed a great doctor. He was also an accomplished medical investigator, primarily a clinical investigator (president of the American Society for Clinical Investigation at the age of 39); member of the Association of American Physicians (winner of the Kober Medal of that organization, its highest honor); author of an influential text on failure of the circulation; and producer of more than 200 publications in medical research. But his greatest stature was in the teaching of medicine, which he did for some 54 years—the middle half of the 20th century.

Tinsley was unique in medicine. He was a major participant at a time when medicine in the United States was changing from the worst to the best in the world and erupting into the middle of the social scene. He was probably the only physician in America to become the first full-time regular chairman of three separate medical school departments of internal medicine, at Bowman Gray/Wake Forest in Winston-Salem, North Carolina, Southwestern Medical School in Dallas, Texas, and UAB in Birmingham, Alabama. His crowning achievement was the origination of *Principles of Internal Medicine*, which became probably the largest-selling textbook of internal medicine in all history.[10] His peak years as a clinician were around the age of 40 to 60. After that, his medical activities declined. He seemed to sense this, and he resigned his post of chairman of the Department of Medicine in Birmingham at the age of 57 to become a Distinguished Professor. He stayed active with students and writing till his last few years and died a bitter critic of the mindless overuse of the medical technology he himself had helped develop and of what he considered the disoriented nature of universities and their even more disoriented medical schools.

The course of 20th century medicine in the United States paralleled the career of Tinsley Harrison. In 1900 when he and the new century were born, the disease from which he would die was unknown to most physicians. Myocardial infarction (weakness or death of the heart muscle because of interference with the

Medicine 1950–1987, ed. Jean D. Wilson, M.D. (McGraw-Hill, Inc., 1987), 54.

9. J. D. Wilson, et al., *Harrison's Principles of Internal Medicine*, 9th ed. (New York: McGraw-Hill, Inc. 1980), dedication page. This was the first time the book was designated *Harrison's Principles of Internal Medicine*, and it was the first time the book had contained a dedication to any particular person, the first edition thirty years earlier having been dedicated to "Our students and colleagues." [See page v.]

10. The claim that Harrison's *Principles of Internal Medicine* has sold more copies than any other textbook of internal medicine is impossible to document conclusively, but it is probably true. This is discussed further in the text.

11. D. J. Weatherall, J. G. G. Ledingham, and D. A. Warrell, eds., "The Role of Medicine" in *Oxford Textbook of Medicine*, vol. 1 (1996).

flow of blood through the coronary arteries) was not a clinical entity—though it had been described in the literature of pathology—recognized by practicing physicians. The main causes of death as the century began were various kinds of pneumonias, which brought to a close the lives of many of the elderly debilitated by advanced age or chronic illness. Antibiotics were unknown; pneumonia was the old man's friend.

Tuberculosis was the second most frequent cause of death, killing the famous and wealthy as well as the unknown. The bacterium which causes tuberculosis had been discovered only 18 years before, by Robert Koch in March 1882, but medicine had nothing to offer except rest in a clean environment, good nutrition, and fresh air. And of course a more accurate and certain *diagnosis* than had been possible only 20 years earlier. Though European medicine was electrified by the discovery and by the rise of bacteriology, American medicine was slow to react, particularly in the poverty-stricken and backward rural South. Indeed, the decline of tuberculosis deaths in the industrial west had begun long before that time, calling into question the role of medicine in this improvement in the public's health.[11]

Tinsley Harrison was a practicing physician. The *first* work of the individual physician is not the health of the public or community, but rather the healing and prevention of diseases of the physician's individual patient. This is what the patient has expected of the doctor since the dawn of man.

Diarrheal diseases were the third leading cause of death, and many of those affected died in infancy. Tinsley's great-grandfather, Jared E. Groce (1810–85), who lived his life in rural Alabama some 50 miles east of Birmingham, had nine children. Five lived fewer than 20 years, and four lived seven years or less. Taking statistics into account, at least some of these died of infantile diarrhea.

In 1900, average life expectancy from birth in the United States was about 45 years, a grim statistic exaggerated by the large number of infant and early childhood deaths. Heart diseases—largely rheumatic heart disease—ranked fourth as a cause of death. Cancer ranked eighth. Diphtheria was 10th. Venereal diseases were widespread but not discussed in polite company, though they were crippling, degrading, and often fatal, there being no effective treatment and little understanding of the relation of primary infections to the late sequelae—particularly among older doctors in the rural South.

By mid-century, diseases of the heart ranked first among causes of death in the United States, accounting for more than half of all deaths. Tinsley published

Failure of the Circulation in 1935, with a second edition in 1938. He was president of the American Heart Association in 1948, the year it transformed itself from an introverted scientific club to a major fund-raising and lobbying organization. He had been on the original National Heart Council of the National Heart Institute at its founding, converting the National Institute of Health to the National Institutes of Health.[12] He was a close friend of U.S. Senator Lister Hill of Alabama, the legislative architect, builder, and ardent supporter of the NIH and its biomedical research activities in the 1950s, 1960s, and later. Tinsley's book, *Principles of Internal Medicine,* was taking the market by storm. Cardiac catheterization was beginning to make an impact in cardiac diagnosis. Experiments were underway which would lead in 1955 to reliable pump oxygenators for day-to-day use in the cardiopulmonary bypass procedures that would make extensive intracardiac surgery widespread throughout the nation and the world, including especially Tinsley's own institution in Birmingham.[13]

Nevertheless, Tinsley always denied being "a heart doctor," or a specialist. He was, he insisted, a general physician first, foremost, and always. He might have had a special interest in the heart, but his first love was *general* internal medicine.

As the century drew to a close, Tinsley despaired the passing of the old values. Not all of his perceptions would be considered laudable in the year 2014. But he was, despite his prejudices, a man of good will toward all, and a physician who tried to do his very best for each of his patients and each of his students, regardless of status. This attitude was probably lifelong and shines through in the first and last paragraphs of his introduction for the first edition of *PIM* in 1950.[14]

> No greater opportunity, responsibility, or obligation can fall to the lot of a human being than to become a physician. In the care of the suffering he needs technical skill, scientific knowledge, and human understanding. He who uses these with courage, with humility, and with wisdom will provide a unique service for his fellow man, and will build an enduring edifice of character within himself. The physician should ask of his destiny no more than this, he should be content with no less.

And later,

> Tact, sympathy, and understanding are expected of the physician, for the patient

12. Victoria Harden, *The National Institutes of Health: A History Since 1937* (forthcoming).

13. J. W. Kirklin, "The Development of Cardiac Surgery at the Mayo Clinic," *Mayo Clinic Proceedings* 55, no. 5 (1980).

14. P. B. Beeson, to J. Pittman, March 1997. (UAB Archives). There is no doubt that Harrison wrote this section of the first edition himself.

15. This estimate is complicated by the facts that although most doctors practicing in the U.S. as the century ended were young, more than 20 percent were graduates of foreign medical schools.

16. L. Garret, *Emerging Infections* (1993); J. Lederberg, R. E. Shope, and S. C. Oaks Jr., eds., *Emerging Infections: Microbial Threats to Health in the United States* (Washington, D.C.: National Academy Press, 1992).

is no mere collection of symptoms, signs, disordered functions, damaged organs, and disturbed emotions. He is human, fearful, and hopeful, seeking relief, help, and reassurance. To the physician, as to the anthropologist, nothing human is strange or repulsive. The misanthrope may become a smart diagnostician of organic disease, but he can scarcely hope to succeed as a physician. The true physician has a Shakespearean breadth of interest in the wise and the foolish, the proud and the humble, the stoic hero and the whining rogue. He cares for people.

As Tinsley's life closed, smallpox was gone—eradicated except for samples at several government labs, and there were arguments over whether to destroy those, and thus the species, or preserve them for research. Tuberculosis, once conquered, was again threatening. Cancer, only eighth in mortality causes in 1900, had risen to second rank by mid-century and was still advancing as the population aged. Heart disease remained the number one killer. Many, perhaps most, U.S. doctors at the end of the 20th century had never seen cases of lobar pneumonia, acute poliomyelitis, diphtheria, scarlet fever, rheumatic fever, glanders, scurvy, beriberi, rickets, tularemia, brucellosis, typhoid, malaria, smallpox, hookworm or most other worm diseases and other tropical diseases, or a host of other diseases common at the beginning of the century.[15] Although effective drugs were available for syphilis and gonorrhea, those were still depressingly prevalent, and other venereal infections were increasing with the clash of cultures, changing views of morality, and the sexual revolution: herpes genitalis, human papilloma virus, mycoplasma, chlamydia, and the coming onslaught of AIDS—perhaps presaging a cycling back toward the old moralities. New and often deadly viruses were discovered frequently: ebola, hanta, EMV (equine morbilliform virus), and others.[16]

Drug abuse had become as endemic in the United States as it had been in China 150 years earlier. Operations on the heart, considered impossible by the famous surgeon Theodor Billroth a century before, had become commonplace and were performed at many hospitals around the world by the time Tinsley died in 1978. Above all, medicine had become more complex technically, socially, and economically. With the struggles of M.D. physicians to maintain dominance among other providers and over popular alternative medicines in what had come to be known as healthcare; with the intrusion of third parties into the previously two-party conversation between doctor and patient; with the further addition of U.S. and state government payers to the transactions as medical care became a right of citizenship (and noncitizen residents); and with the resulting huge infusions of cash from the relatively wealthy U.S. institutions into the system of medical care primarily through the doctors and hospitals—with all this, medicine became transformed from a personal service into a business.

TINSLEY HATED THESE CHANGES, even though he himself unwittingly had helped bring them about.

With the capacities brought by 20th century technology, including medicine's ability to extend life at its beginning and end; with the aging U.S. population and the increasing political strength of the aged; with increasing numbers of patients with chronic diseases, such as severe arthritis or chronic renal disease; with the new assertiveness of non-M.D. health professionals previously considered allied health professionals; with the markedly high financial rewards for some physicians, administrators, and healthcare corporations, obvious to the public despite lack of health insurance for nearly one-fifth of the U.S. population, and the consequent resentments—with all these and other changes, entirely new questions of ethics and economics confronted medicine, and confronted each practicing doctor, as the century drew to a close. Medicine continued, as it always would, but it had changed.

As one century ended and another began, I sometimes heard complaints about lack of progress. As indicated here, the changes in medicine brought major benefits to many individual patients. A great many individuals suffered undiagnosed fatal heart attacks at the beginning of the century but could have been given additional years of productive life had they been stricken with the same disease in the late 20th century. Most sick people from 1900 would have fared better if they had lived 75 years later, or would never have become patients at all from the diseases which killed them or maimed them for life. If President Garfield had been shot in 1981 and Ronald Reagan in 1881 instead of the reverse, Reagan would surely have died, and Garfield would surely have lived. Reagan's wound was more serious and life-threatening, but his treatment was much better.[17] There has been progress!

But progress implies a goal and movement in a given direction toward the goal, or away from something undesirable. Medicine continues to move away from human disease, disability, and suffering. It is not clear today exactly what it is moving toward or what the boundaries of medicine are. Kaufmann has written that medicine is a discipline driven by means, not ends.[18] Is the goal of medicine the promotion

17. "The Gunshot Wounds of Presidents Garfield and Reagan." *JAMA*, 1981.

18. S. R. Kaufmann, *The Healer's Tale: Transforming Medicine and Culture* (Madison: University of Wisconsin Press, 1993).

19. J. A. Pittman, "Service and Significance" (address to medical school graduating class at Ben Gurion University, Beersheva, Israel, 1985). *Alabama Journal of the Medical Sciences* 24, no. 1 (1987): 79-82.

of overall happiness for the greatest number of people? Is the objective of medicine the improvement of statistical indicators of health for the population at large? Or is it more restrictive: prevention, amelioration, or cure of clearly definable organic diseases in individual patients? What is medicine for? And who is responsible for what?

NOT ALL THESE PROBLEMS are new. Tinsley was emphatically on the side of his individual patient. However, though he did not have to deal with most of these modern social issues during his active medical career, he did confront such social questions as how long a working and responsible, but poor, patient—with no insurance coverage—should remain in the hospital, when to allow a debilitated elderly patient to die, whether to tell a spouse about the venereal disease in her husband, how much time to devote to an elderly patient dying of metastatic cancer when he had a young patient with undiagnosed fever in the next room, and similar questions. That is, like other doctors of his time, he made social choices taking into consideration the allocation of resources and the needs of the family and others in the community as well as his own individual patient before him at the moment.

The challenge before the physicians and other healthcare workers in the 21st century will be how to remain faithful to the principle of the patient's welfare first in the face of not only the doctor's perception of his own professional needs and just rewards, but also growing community, industrial, governmental, and legal demands.

In meeting the modern challenges, Tinsley, without thinking much about his own compensation or perhaps even the legal problems he might precipitate, would probably have attempted to subvert the system for the benefit of his individual patient.[19]

I once accused Tinsley of being a 19th-century physician. He disagreed. "No!" he said. "I'm an *18th*-century doctor!"

Tinsley Harrison, M.D.

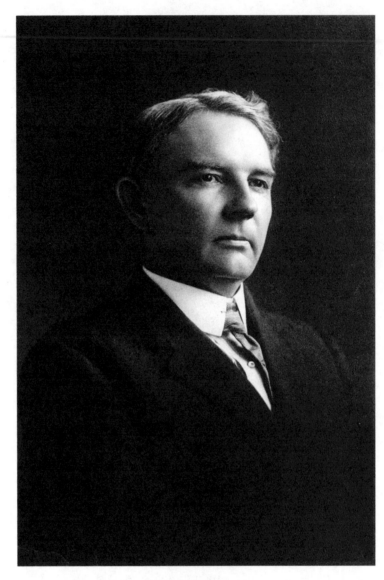

W. Groce Harrison Sr.

THE PATIENT

1900

Man also knoweth not his time: as the fishes that are taken in an evil net, and as the birds that are caught in the snare; so are the sons of men snared in an evil time, when it falleth suddenly upon them. — Ecclesiastes 9:12

It began as a small discomfort in the middle of his chest, a deep burning sensation. Over the next few minutes it quickly grew to a severe pressing ache close to his heart. The feeling of something, some weight, pressing down hard on his chest became overwhelming, and his left arm began to ache, especially around the elbow. Forty-five year-old Jesse Smith had never experienced anything like this before. He stopped chopping the cord of wood he was working on—almost finished anyhow. Now he was sweating. He felt nauseous as he walked the few yards to the elegant old house and called for his wife and 20-year-old son George. They helped him into bed, and George jumped on the fastest horse they had without bothering to saddle up and rushed to get Dr. Groce Harrison from the town of Talladega, Alabama, some five miles away to the west.

It was Sunday, the 18th of March, 1900. The morning was cool and misty along Chocolocca Creek, and a foggy cloud hung over the winding course of the stream like a great fluffy string. It was a beautiful spring morning, but George had no time to admire it as he hurried along the red clay road. He found the young doctor finishing a cup of coffee as he talked with a farmhand about the planting that spring on his father's farm, which was very near that of the Smiths. Dr. Harrison was also thinking about his wife's pregnancy and the imminent delivery of their second child. He hoped it would be a boy. Mrs. Harrison was already slightly overdue, but this pregnancy had gone well, and the previous child, Emily, had been born with no difficulty, so no problems were expected. He had enlisted the help of an excellent local black granny midwife with considerable experience delivering babies over many years.

"Dr. Harrison! Come quick! Daddy's having some kind-a spell—a real bad one."

A friend of the Smiths for the seven years he had been practicing in Talladega County, the doctor lost no time in getting the saddle and saddlebags on his own horse and starting at a gallop behind George. It would be another Sunday without church. When they arrived, Mr. Smith was lying in bed, but his head was propped up on three large pillows. He felt more comfortable that way. Dr. Harrison took a brief medical history, obtained the information about the pain—its location, onset, radiation down the left arm, quality, constancy, intensity, duration, precipitating and ameliorating factors, and time course, as well as associated symptoms such as the nausea. Having known the patient and his family well, he had no need to obtain a family history or review of past illnesses.

The pain had eased up a bit, and the aching in the arm was gone. But the chest pain was still there. Physical examination revealed nothing important. Jesse was a stocky, well-muscled redhead who had led a vigorous but proper life, though he did smoke a lot of cigarettes and chew tobacco. He attended church regularly. Unlike many of the other men in the area, he did not drink moonshine or other alcoholic beverages. Dr. Harrison had examined Jesse several years ago, and the only thing of note was that the pulse was very hard, reflecting the somewhat high blood pressure revealed by his new Riva-Rocci rubber blood pressure cuff. The pressure was 160 then, found by feeling for the pulse at the wrist or elbow while slowly releasing the pressure from the cuff. That was as much as you could tell about the blood pressure in the early 1900s, unless you wanted to put a tube into an artery and measure the pressure. The pressure did not seem to make much difference, though—probably just indicated a heart that was a little overactive. Jesse had continued to work hard on the farm and as the informal mayor of the village. His 38-year-old wife had birthed their ninth child two months before.

Dr. Harrison gave the patient a fresh nitroglycerine tablet to place under his tongue, but the pain persisted. He tried a second dose of nitroglycerine, but now the patient said his head was beginning to pound. The chest pain remained, unchanged.

The doctor took a small vial from his black bag and removed one of the small grayish tablets from it. He placed the tablet in a teaspoon, added clean well water to fill the spoon, then heated the spoon over a candle to dissolve the tablet. Next he sucked the clear fluid from the spoon into a syringe through the attached needle. He inserted the needle into Jesse's arm, giving an intramuscular injection of the entire contents of the syringe, a quarter-grain of triturated morphine sulfate.

They watched as the pain eased. The patient hadn't vomited, and now the nausea also subsided despite the morphine—or perhaps because of it. After 20 minutes, Jessie blinked his eyes at ease and dozed off to sleep. The doctor felt it would be safe to return home and perhaps visit again later that day. He did not know what had caused the attack. Maybe acute indigestion, but more likely an attack of angina pectoris. This was not good. It was not known what the cause of this angina was, but it was known that such patients had a tendency to die suddenly without warning. There was no hospital closer than Birmingham, some 50 miles to the west. And there was nothing at the hospital that could be of much help in a situation like this anyhow.

WHEN THE DOCTOR ARRIVED home, his wife announced that the abdominal pains she had been having off and on had now become regular and were coming every few minutes. "How often?" he asked. They timed them, and they were now about every two minutes. Mrs. Harrison remained in the clean sheets of the bed, the old sheets having been exchanged for new freshly boiled linen. The granny midwife was an elderly black woman named Onnie, who had "borned more than 200 babies." She stayed close by, examined the patient frequently, and when the time came for delivery arranged the patient's legs and helped her bear down, while the doctor-husband handled the delivery itself. The baby was a fine loud boy, so the name had already been chosen: Tinsley Randolph Harrison.

As soon as the placenta was delivered and it was clear there was no abnormal bleeding and the mother and child were in good condition, Dr. Harrison turned his attention to Sally Chambers, a young black woman who had arrived in an agitated state some half-hour before. Susan Chambers, her mother, was coughing up substantial quantities of bright red blood. It had started with small amounts last night, but this morning there were spoonfuls then cupfuls. Her mother had not been well since the miscarriage of a pregnancy several months ago. Would the doctor come and see her?

THIS TIME THE DOCTOR placed a horse between the traces of his buggy, threw in the large black leather bag of instruments, dressings, bandages, and medications, and left with the young messenger for the patient's house. The girl, 16, had walked the two miles to the doctor's house by herself so her father could stay with the sick woman. They soon arrived at a clapboard house on a small farm. The house was unpainted, with a foundation of fieldstones. There was also a fieldstone chimney, cemented with mortar made from the local clay. This house was better than most in that area; it had a floor made of boards rather than the raw earth. Inside, it was dark, the only illumination an oil lamp helped by glimmers from two small windows covered with oiled paper.

"She was just comin' back to the house from the privy this morning when a hard coughin' spell took her, and she started coughin' up all this here blood," Elijah Chambers explained. "Here's some I saved in this here cup." Dr. Harrison took the cup outside for a better look. Indeed, it was bright red, and there was nearly a full cup of it. He returned to the patient.

"Have you had any other symptoms—pains or aches, nausea, vomiting, diarrhea, or anything like that?" he asked.

"Nothing but feelin' weak and run down and sort of short of breath."

"How long have you felt like that?"

"Ever since I had that funny miscarriage five months ago. I's had seven babies, but never anything like that. It warn't normal, and the midwife said it was just as well it didn't go to term and get borned. But we buried it just the same."

"How far along in the pregnancy were you?"

"About two or three months, I guess. I never seemed to get over that. Just stayed weak and puny and got worse. Then today I started coughing up this blood. Do you think I's got TB?"

The doctor continued to obtain information: Anybody else in the family have tuberculosis? Anybody else in the family losing weight? Did she or anybody else in the family have night sweats or fevers? He made certain that she had actually coughed up the blood and had not vomited it. "How much weight has she lost?" he asked.

"Maybe 20 or 30 pounds." She was a large woman, but they had no means of actually weighing her.

"My clothes done got real loose on me," she said.

He examined her as closely and carefully as possible, bringing the lamp close and lighting the two others they had in the house for help. He listened to the lungs with his new binaural stethoscope; the breath sounds in the left apex were indeed abnormally loud, and there were crackling rales lower on the left side. But the sputum had not been filled with pus. He considered. Maybe it was TB. The pulse was 110 per minute and soft, suggestive of anemia or recent blood loss. There was nothing to be seen except that she had obviously lost weight and was extremely pale. The rest of the examination was unremarkable. He gave her a bottle of oil of cloves for the cough and told her to remain in bed all day. He promised to return the next morning to check her again.

Elijah Chambers followed him outside to the buggy. "I ain't got no money, Doc. But how about this here fat chicken for your trip? It's a good'un and will make a fine fryer." Dr. Harrison knew from the vicinity and the house that the man was telling the truth about his finances, so he took the chicken in a croker sack as payment, thanked him, and rode home.

He arrived at noon to find mother and baby resting well and Onnie beaming. Dolores the maid fixed some eggs, bacon, grits, red-eye gravy, and superb crumbly, hot white biscuits. It was food fit for a king, especially since he had not had a real breakfast. He ate.

HE LAY DOWN TO take a quick nap before going to his office in the south wing of the house to see the four patients who had accumulated there over the past hour since church and Sunday dinner. However, he had just dozed off when Isaac Davis rushed in with, "You've got to come right now, Doc. Susan is real bad—never been this bad before." Dr. Harrison knew what was coming. Three weeks before, Susan, a white girl age 13, had started passing large volumes of urine and drinking even larger amounts of water to assuage her seemingly unquenchable thirst. The water just seemed to run right through her. Although there was no laboratory test to confirm it, diabetes mellitus was clearly the cause of her problem. She was losing weight rapidly despite a ravenous appetite, and her lungs were quite normal to physical examination. Since then she had lost weight, gone downhill, and this morning she had become drowsy. Now she could not be awakened from her afternoon nap.

For the third time this Sunday, the doctor left for a house call, again taking the buggy. Nearly all medicine in the area was practiced in the home of either the patient or the doctor. There was no hospital nearby, nor was there any separate outpatient clinic. The doctor's home was his clinic. More affluent doctors sometimes built an extra room or wing onto or adjacent to the house for a waiting room, examination/treatment room, and office. Otherwise they just used the living room of their house for a waiting room and a converted bedroom for the examining, treating, and consulting room. One Talladega doctor, Dr. Barclay W. Toole, who had died in 1898, did have a small office on the second floor above the pharmacy in the town square. But he was the rare exception to the general pattern.

The Davis house was very near, only about a mile. When they arrived, Mrs. Davis was on the porch crying. "I think she's done gone," she wailed.

When Dr. Harrison reached Susan, he found her small withered body absolutely still. There was no breathing, no pulse, and no heartbeat audible by stethoscope. No moisture accumulated on a mirror held to her mouth, the family's test. She did not respond to strong pinching. She was dead. The diet he had prescribed for her had done essentially nothing to change the course of her juvenile diabetes. He stayed several minutes with the family, and they sent another daughter to fetch the preacher.

WHEN HE REACHED HOME, 10 patients were waiting. Some had been there since about 1 P.M., having had noon dinner right after church, and now it was nearly 4:30 in the afternoon. He quickly handled the problems of a 10-year-old boy with a sprained ankle, which he wrapped with a strong cotton gauze bandage; a five-year-old girl with enlarged red tonsils, whom he advised, "Better get those tonsils removed. You may get more bad throats," and gave some cough medicine, oil of cloves; an elderly man with a long-standing stroke who was having difficulty swallowing (reassurance and words of caution about aspiration); an 88-year-old great-grandmother with known tuberculosis, living in the same house with eight of her grandchildren and chronically coughing up small amounts of blood (10 drops of Lugol's iodine solution three times a day in a glass of water and rest in a well-ventilated room); a young man who came in with a lacerated hand (two stitches of silk suture; come back in a week to have them out); and assorted others. He was finished before 6:30.

The day had been hard and he treated himself to a short walk-around to the edge of the town not many blocks away. The fields were already planted with this year's cotton, a crop he still relied upon for most of his income. His practice was doing well, and he was less dependent on cotton than his father had been, but most of his patients still paid largely or entirely in kind rather than cash. He had himself started working at the age of six in the cotton fields of his father's farm, some six miles to the east near Munford. He had worked the fields all the time he was not in school until he finished high school. His father, Dr. John Tinsley Harrison, had saved money from the cotton crops in a special account which had permitted the son to attend medical school. Dr. Groce Harrison also wanted to provide an education for his children. And to do that he also would have to rely on the cotton crops. Practicing medicine just could not produce enough money.

THE EARLY SPRING EVENING was still cool as dusk settled to near dark. There was no Spanish moss on the trees as there was 90 miles to the south in Montgomery. Talladega County was in the northern half of the state, and Alabama, like many states, might be divided into northern and southern halves quite different from one another. Much of the southern half was typical Old South, old plantation land—flat, with black dirt and large numbers of black people, many of whom had been slaves. Much of the northern half was more like the hill country of storybooks, less typical of the Deep South, filled with the southernmost Appalachian hills—locally called mountains—the ground a red-yellow clay, very few black people in some counties, and a white population so independent that one county, Winston, attempted to secede from the State when the latter seceded from the United States to join the Confederacy.

Indeed, the northwestern corner of the state was known as "Freedom Hills," a point of origin for the Underground Railroad before the "War Between the States." Dr. Harrison's mother had long ago explained to him that it was *not* a *civil* war. A civil war occurs when a group tries to overthrow the government, and the South did not want to do this. They just wanted the sovereignty of the individual States promised by the Constitution agreed upon in 1787. So explained the mothers and grandmothers of Dr. Harrison's generation. "And it was certainly not over slavery," they said. "The South was on its way to solving that problem and could have done it peaceably, had the North just left us to work it out more gradually. It was all just economic exploitation by the North."

His own father had served in the Confederate Army as a doctor, and, curiously, also in the Grand Army of the Republic with the Yankees as a prisoner-doctor. Confederate veterans often held rallies, especially the big annual one in Birmingham.

In any case, it was a pleasant spring evening, and Dr. Harrison loved his medical work, even though he had to raise cotton to help make money for his growing family.

Mother and baby were fine. The doctor slept well that night.

ON MONDAY THE 19TH, Baby Boy Tinsley was one day old and crying loudly. So the doctor was just as happy to answer an early morning call from Sam Tidwell, a young white farmer about 24 years old with a family of three children plus his wife and her mother and grandmother. The younger two women could work well in the fields, dress out hogs, and put up preserves and the like, but the grandmother had become increasingly sluggish over the past several months. Sam had come to fetch help for her. She was just getting drowsier and drowsier. They could awaken her, but she would not get up and about. She did not want to eat and was terribly constipated, taking large amounts of herb tea to help her bowels along. Despite her lack of appetite, she did not seem to lose weight. She also complained of the cold, even when other members of the family found the room too warm. In fact, she sat so close to the fire in the potbellied wood stove last winter that she repeatedly got burns on her shins.

When they arrived at the simple but clean clapboard house, the grandmother, Mrs. Slone, a very heavy person, sat outside on the front porch in a rocking chair placed directly in the morning sun. She responded pleasantly and appropriately to questions. She did, however, have a tendency to drowse off to sleep if left alone for more than several minutes. Dr. Harrison noticed that her face appeared puffy and sallow, almost yellow. Her skin was thick and dry and scaly, especially over the elbows, which seemed discordantly dirty as compared with the rest of the skin. Her hair was dry and fine, and she had lost almost all her eyebrows. As he continued to examine her, he found that her pulse was only 58 per minute, and she had a slight but definite goiter in her neck. Her thyroid was perhaps two or three times normal size and of a thick rubbery consistency. It was not painful. But it was, she said, "a bit sensitive to the touch."

The family took her inside to complete the examination, but there was nothing more that Dr. Harrison thought important, except one thing: the ankle jerk deep tendon reflex, which was prominent but seemed extremely slow to relax. The goiter had been the clue and the slowly relaxing ankle jerk reflex the confirmation. This unusual young doctor had caught the disease just as it was about to progress to its final coma and probably the death of the patient.

Eight years prior, Groce Harrison had been studying for his second medical degree at the Baltimore Medical College, and he had befriended a prominent doctor across town at the new hospital and the medical school just opening, Johns Hopkins. He had attended some of this doctor's conferences and ward rounds, and a patient he had seen then was very similar to Mrs. Slone. The doctor, William Osler, a Canadian, had told the group of a book which had been published in 1888 in London, England, describing the disease they called "myxedema" in great detail, giving all the symptoms and signs. Harrison had found the book in the Johns Hopkins library and had studied it carefully. It was a wonderful book prepared by "The Myxedema Committee of the London Clinical Society," which collected 109 cases of patients with this disease; had analyzed these in great detail and with remarkable perspicacity; and had formed subcommittees or had assigned individual members to study the effects of surgically removing the thyroid glands of animals, to carry out autopsies or study the autopsies done by others, to review the world literature on the subject—especially that from Switzerland—and to complete a comprehensive study of the disease. The Myxedema Committee had formed itself in 1883 and had conducted its work over five years, finally publishing this book—a classic for all time. Osler had an interest in diseases of the thyroid and wrote articles on them, and young Dr. Groce Harrison remembered all this very well.

Though the disease now had a name, simply giving it a name did not imply understanding the diagnosis of hypothyroidism and myxedema. The word *diagnosis* comes from the Greek word for *through* or *thorough* plus the Greek word for *knowledge* or *understanding*. Thus, when a physician arrived at a diagnosis, he was supposed to have not just a name but a thorough knowledge and understanding of the disease.

After the problem of *naming* the disease and *understanding* it as a "disease entity" came the problems of *treatment* and *prognosis*, so the doctor could advise the patient as to what to expect. The ultimate problem then was that there had been no treatment for myxedema. It was often fatal. Just a few years before, however, in 1891, a Dr. Murray in England had described how feeding such a patient thyroid tissue from animals could restore the patient to health. All this was reviewed in detail by Dr. Osler, and absorbed in detail by the young Dr. Groce Harrison, who remembered it now in 1900 as he looked at Mrs. Slone in Talladega. He understood there were now pills made up from animal thyroids which had been ground, dried, and compressed, but it might take a week or more to obtain such thyroid pills. The animal thyroids originally used had been administered in various ways, such as lightly fried. Myxedema sometimes ended in a fatal coma, and Mrs. Slone appeared to be drifting into such a coma from which there would be no return. There was no time to wait for the uncertain arrival of thyroid pills from afar.

"Didn't you say you killed a big hog just this morning, Sam?" he asked.

"Yes, sir. Stopped the butcherin' till you'd finished your medical work here."

"Do you still have the guzzle?" asked the doctor, referring to the trachea and attached organs, including the thyroid.

"Yes, sir. Didn't throw nothin' away yet. It's all good for somethin' anyhow, even if just fertilizer."

"Let's go look at the guzzle," the doctor suggested.

When they arrived at the smokehouse, they found the hog hanging outside by the hind legs and the trachea intact, not yet removed, with the thyroid still wrapped around it just below the larynx. The doctor carefully cut the hog thyroid free from the trachea, and they walked back to the front porch.

"Sam," Dr. Harrison said, "I think Mrs. Slone has myxedema, and that this thyroid may help her."

"What's that?" asked Sam.

"Well, people need a properly functioning thyroid gland—right here in the neck—to stay healthy, and if they don't have one they sicken and eventually die. But taking thyroid by mouth can cure it. Now what I want you to do is take this hog thyroid inside right now and fry it in a skillet, just enough to get it cooked. Don't overdo it. Then serve it to Mrs. Slone with some scrambled eggs. Make sure she eats the whole thyroid. Don't let her waste it or not eat it. This is important, understand?"

Sam allowed as how he did and took the precious thyroid inside to his wife's stove. Dr. Harrison then explained that Mrs. Slone would have to take more thyroid regularly the rest of her life and that they could get some thyroid pills for her in town. But until then, she should eat half a hog thyroid three times a week, every Monday, Wednesday, and Friday.

Dr. Harrison bid them good-bye, saying that he would find some thyroid pills and check back in a few days. They should send for him immediately if Mrs. Slone got worse. As he rode along he remembered that his father had once told him about two patients who sounded like spitting images of Mrs. Slone. They were sisters, elderly, and the family complained of their gradually increasing sluggishness. Dr. John Harrison had also noticed a small goiter on one, but none on the other. They had just drifted off to sleep and death, one during an exceptionally cold winter, and her sister in the spring a few months later. He would have to ask his father what they had, though he suspected that he knew. Later, when he did ask, old Doc J. T. replied, "Well, I just marked 'em off to old age."

The way home took him close to the house of Elijah Chambers, so he detoured down the clay road lined by huge ancient oaks. He got out of the buggy, tied his horse to a post on the front porch, and went into the house to find the patient in bed. Susan looked worse, and her pulse was 120. She had continued to cough up blood during the night, though in smaller amounts. Dr. Harrison took Elijah outside for a talk. "I think we'd better get her to Birmingham so she can get an X-ray of her chest, and we'd better do it today. Can you take her?" It would not be easy, and before Mr. Chambers could answer there came a loud spasm of coughing from inside.

"Come quick!" Sally cried. "She's bleedin' real bad!"

They found Susan coughing continuously and producing a solid flow of bright red blood. Dr. Harrison administered a half-grain of morphine by deep intramuscular injection, but she kept on coughing. The blood kept coming. She had been sitting on the edge of the bed, but now she fell back, her open eyes glazed and staring.

"Oh, Mama!" Sally cried.

"Give her another shot, Doc!" Elijah yelled.

Dr. Harrison thought it was too late. He should have sent her to Birmingham yesterday for the chest X-ray. It was probably TB, though, so it wouldn't have made much difference. She took a shallow breath, then was quiet. But then there was another. They waited.

"We need to get her to Birmingham, Elijah," said the doctor. The train would not pass through on the way to Birmingham for several hours, but even so it would be faster than trying to get their buckboard wagon over the 50 miles of dirt road for the trip. The wagon was readied, with an ample supply of blankets and sheets on the floor over a mattress. Sally and Elijah, with the help of the doctor and Charley Dismukes, a neighbor, carried the patient on the mattress to the wagon, drowsy but responding. Then they were off. It was 9 in the morning. With luck they might make it by late afternoon.

The wagon rolled away, leaving the doctor and Charley, a white man about 40. As the doctor started to leave, Charley asked if Dr. Harrison would take a look at his 10-month-old infant son, who had been having diarrhea for several days now. When they arrived at the house only a few hundred yards down the road, Dr. Harrison was astonished to see how dehydrated the child appeared. He looked like an old man. The skin was deeply wrinkled and the child was listless and unresponsive. Diarrhea fluid was on the rags, and Mrs. Dismukes was boiling more diapers in a large black iron pot over a fire in the yard. On the clothesline another dozen diapers were hung out to dry.

"We give him some paregoric, Doc, but it don't stop. Just keeps right on."

They discussed the dose of paregoric, but as they talked the wizened little creature's chest stopped moving. The eyes remained opened in a fixed gaze straight ahead. Then, slowly, the eyelids drooped. Dr. Harrison felt for a pulse. Finding none, he searched the chest with his stethoscope for heart sounds—none. They held a mirror up to the mouth and nose of the infant, but no moisture appeared. The baby was dead. This was the fourth child the Dismukes had lost, one other from diarrhea, one from "croup"—probably diphtheria—and one from miliary TB.

They covered the tiny body with a blanket, and Mr. Dismukes went for the preacher. There was no discussion of compensation for the doctor, and none was expected. The doctor left.

Before he could get back home, he was met by George Smith, Jesse's son, riding fast on the same horse he had used yesterday. "Daddy's worse again, Doc. He was fine all night, but then this mornin' he started havin' the pains again, and they're real bad."

So they turned eastward and back down the clay road to the Smith farm at full speed. The maid Maizie was standing outside by the west end of the yard and waved them down as they approached. "Lordy, Lordy, the Massah's done gone home!" she cried. George urged the horse on across the broad yard and leapt down and into the front door almost in one movement. Dr. Harrison was close behind. But they were too late. Mrs. Smith was on her knees beside the bed, her hands folded and her head down, a large Bible nearby. Jesse lay still, eyes closed, facing the boarded ceiling.

For the third time in just a few hours Dr. Harrison checked for signs of life, then, finding none, pronounced the patient dead—a legal necessity as well as a biological and social reality. Mrs. Smith did well to pray. Now she was alone with a big farm and nine children. Jesse had been a bit old in 1879 when they married, 24, and she had been 17. They had this son George almost right away. Then there was a four-year dry spell when no children came. Then there were two girls, now 16 and 14, then a boy now 11. All the rest were less than 10 years old: nine, seven, four, two, and two months. George was now the male head of the household. The Smiths had good land and some animals and equipment, but very little money. While they still had some sharecroppers, Jesse had actually done much of the physical labor around the farm, and had directed the rest. This would now fall to George. The doctor left the scene, returning to his own family.

AFTER A BRIEF LUNCH in the dining room, served by Dolores, the doctor went upstairs for a 20-minute nap. Then he turned to the patients waiting downstairs.

They presented the usual problems: a 12-year-old boy with a fish hook stuck clean through his ear (Dr. Harrison cut off the barb with a wire clipper and pulled the hook out backwards, rinsing with Mercurochrome); another elderly lady coughing up blood and wasting away, her great-grandchild having just died of miliary tuberculosis (he prescribed oil of cloves for the cough, told her to keep away from the children and sleep on the screened porch out back, and he also tried a liver shot, without much faith in it); and so on.

One patient was particularly puzzling. She was 38 and complained of being very depressed and weak. On examination she had an odd sort of obesity. Her trunk appeared very fat—in fact, there were purple streaks in the skin down the sides of the abdomen. But her legs and arms were so thin they were spindly. Her face had a peculiar fat appearance, unnatural and very round, like a rising moon. She complained of being extremely weak, perhaps related to the fact that her monthly periods had become very irregular in timing and amounts. And there were bruises almost everywhere there was skin—great purple marks of blood being resorbed on the forearms, elbows, upper arms, chest and abdomen, thighs and calves, even on the back, where up at the neck there was a hump of fat like that of a buffalo. She denied having been struck by anyone or anything or having run into furniture. There was no good explanation of all these bruises. Although her family was poor, they were well-supplied with food, and the husband and children were healthy. He supposed she had some secret reason for being depressed and had been eating excessively in an attempt to overcome the sadness. So he treated her with a diet to reduce weight and some tonic water. He never saw her again, but another doctor later told him that she had died in Birmingham several months after he had seen her, apparently of a stroke.

Around noon the next day, Tuesday, as Dr. Groce Harrison was sitting down to a light lunch, there was a knock at the door. It was Sally Chambers with a letter from Birmingham. Her mother had continued to breathe for the whole trip to Birmingham, and the coughing up of blood seemed to have slowed greatly. But at the hospital, just as a roentgenogram was being taken of her chest, she had started coughing violently, had expectorated "a pail of blood," and had simply stopped breathing. The doctors wanted to do an autopsy, since they thought it might be tuberculosis which might endanger the rest of the family. So Elijah had agreed. The letter was from the doctors at the hospital who had done the autopsy.

The letter explained that this appeared to be an unusual case. There was no evidence of the cheese-like rotting of the lung tissue characteristic of tuberculosis, and they could find no tuberculosis organisms on the stained microscope slides. Instead there was a growth of some kind, extremely vascular with large pools or pockets of blood within thin walls. It was from these that the blood came when she coughed so hard. The doctors could not say for sure what it was, but they thought it was a kind of cancer called chorioepithelioma. They would study it with microscopes and bacterial cultures, and maybe that would help clarify what the problem was. In the meantime, the good news for the remaining family was that there was no evidence of tuberculosis.

The experience with Susan Chambers reinforced in Dr. Harrison's mind the need for a hospital in Talladega. There had never been one, but he had saved some money and could borrow more. Perhaps his father, now 66, could help. Any facility would have to be small and self-sufficient. No money was available elsewhere to help or to pay for patients who could not pay for themselves, so to take patients who could not pay would force the hospital into bankruptcy.

THAT SUMMER WAS ORDINARY, which is to say, hot. There were a number of medical successes, which were very satisfying. Most deliveries in the county were handled by midwives, but Dr. Harrison delivered 10 babies, including three very difficult births. Then there were the inevitable fractures of legs and arms, and the cuts that required suturing.

The doctor felt he really did some good here for patients like these. Sometimes there were medical problems he helped, like the 53-year-old lady whose breathing trouble eased after the doctor gave her digitalis to slow her heart. And he promoted public health and disease prevention, such as school vaccination programs against smallpox. In fact, the public health programs throughout the entire state were run by the state medical association, the Medical Association of the State of Alabama, and the county programs were run by the county medical societies, which promoted clean drinking water, hygienic location of privies, proper care of teeth, and the like.

But there were discouraging numbers of patients for whom little could be done. In many cases—chickenpox, mumps, measles—one just understood the disease and its prognosis then gave reassurance and waited out the illness. There were several children younger than 10 who had infantile paralysis caused by polio. Two died, one was left without any use of his legs, and the rest recovered with no apparent impairment. One hunter had skinned a rabbit and found that it had a spotted liver. He had prepared, cooked, and eaten it anyhow, only to come down with a fever a week later. The fever was of the continuous kind, and it just got worse and worse. When he called for Dr. Harrison in the afternoon, the fever was 104. Dr. Harrison felt sure that he had tularemia, but there was nothing to do for it except give him aspirin. He was a strong man and lasted another week before dying. Soon there was a large article in the local newspaper cautioning other hunters about tularemia.

Then there were those people who had intermittent fever, malaria. Since the records of the fevers were often incomplete or inaccurate, a common diagnosis in those days was "typhoid/malaria." When a doctor many years later asked a patient if he had ever had a fever, a frequent answer was, "Oh, yes. I had typhoid/malaria years ago." There were the ever-present patients with tuberculosis—nothing to do except rest and a good diet, plus hope and prayer, and try to keep the kids away from the patient. The occasional wealthy TB patient might go away to a sanitarium, but there were few wealthy patients in Talladega in 1900. Several children had scarlet fever and rheumatic fever that summer, and one developed carditis and died. There were also a number of older patients who had chronic heart disease from rheumatic fever years before—especially mitral stenosis. One of these died of an infection on a heart valve deformed by rheumatic fever, bacterial endocarditis, a diagnosis equivalent to a death warrant.

The doctor worked hard. He was surrounded by death and the dying, but he continued his profession.

So the summer went, and when the wind turned chill and the leaves turned bright yellow and red, Groce and Lula Harrison's little girl was four, and young Tinsley already had teeth and was, they were sure, making sage comments about the world around him.

2

The Harrisons and the Early Practice of Medicine

What was the practice of medicine in the rural areas of the U.S. South like at the end of the 19th century? And what was the South itself like? The temptation is to depict the Southern states as primitive, poor, and uninformed, lagging far behind the advances seen in the large cities of the Northeast. This is in many ways true. But the lag was uneven. Indoor plumbing was introduced in parts of the South around the same time as in large parts of major cities farther north. Poor as they might have been, the children of the rural South often had more resources for play and learning in the fields and farm than did their tenement-bound counterparts in the teeming inner cities of the North such as New York. Throughout the Old South, pockets of education and wealth could be found both in the cities and in the countryside. However, severe poverty was widespread, especially in rural areas, and this contributed in some areas to general health concerns and abbreviated life spans.

Although self-designated doctors were sometimes around, people in farming communities everywhere experienced logistical difficulties obtaining medical care from physicians trained in European-style medical schools. Getting the patient to a doctor or a doctor to the patient, or getting patients to a distant hospital by horse and buggy over unpaved, often muddy or frozen roads was difficult, sometimes impossible. In the rural South these problems were aggravated by the severe lack of money, residual destruction of the Civil War, and the lingering effects of the old slave system. Things were different in the South, poorer.

Facilities and equipment were sparse. There was no hospital in Talladega, Alabama, as the new century opened, though there had been a private hospital of about four beds in the home of Dr. Arthur R. Toole, a local practitioner.[1] No X-ray machine was available until the 1920s. Physicians relied on their senses as aided

1. Arthur F. Toole, M.D. (Talladega, AL, June 1993).

18

by stethoscopes, thermometers, laryngoscopes, otoscopes, and ophthalmoscopes.[2]

Some Southern physicians, through family guidance, native intelligence, and drive, were as well-educated as most physicians in the North. Dr. Clarence Salter, for example, who entered practice in Talladega in 1912, traveled to the Mayo Clinic for a month every summer to review the latest advances in medicine.[3]

TINSLEY CAME FROM A family of medicine. He claimed to be a seventh-generation physician. His great-great-great-great-grandfather was a physician, as were all the males up to Tinsley. His mother's uncle was a physician. His wife was a nurse. One of his sons is a physician, dentist, and oral surgeon, who has a son who in turn became a physician—a ninth-generation physician. Another of his sons became a dentist. His brother was a physician. Each of his sisters married physicians. A nephew was a physician. But most important of all, his father was a physician and wanted intensely for Tinsley to become not just a physician, but an outstanding doctor. His was thus a medical destiny in a medical family, and medicine permeated their lives. Medicine was their reason for being, their guiding star. [A "Harrison Medical Family Tree" is available at www.newsouthbooks.com/tinsleyharrison/supplement and a shortened version is on page 93 herein.]

Tinsley liked to trace his family history in biblical fashion at least as far back as King Henry VIII of England on his father's side and Henry IV of France on his mother's side—a sort of double Harrison, he joked. He also claimed to be related to Thomas Jefferson through the lineage of both his father's and his mother's families as well as to Robert E. Lee and Stonewall Jackson. One ancestor, Benjamin Harrison, signed the Declaration of Independence.

He traced the more immediate background of the Harrison side of his family to his paternal great-grandfather, who was from the elite James River Harrisons of Virginia. This great-grandfather, whose name was John Tinsley Harrison, is said by family tradition to have attended the University of Virginia medical school in Charlottesville.[4] He became enamored of a young lady named Melinda Stone, of whose family his own family disapproved. He announced that he was marrying her anyhow, did so, and left for Tennessee where both families had relatives. In Tennessee, he began practicing medicine. No credentials were required. He soon found that the Harrisons in Tennessee were a disreputable lot, "bartenders or people of such ilk, big-time hunters and carousers," while the former Miss Stone's Tennessee relatives were the pillars of the community.[5]

2. Stanley Reiser, *Medicine and the Reign of Technology* (Cambridge: Cambridge University Press, 1981).

3. C. L. Salter, taped interview, 1975 (UAB Archives).

4. Review of the names of all students for the University of Virginia School of Medicine from its opening in 1825 to the time of the Civil War failed to disclose the name of John T. Harrison, or a similar name (though there are several Harrisons listed). The lists were kindly supplied by Robert M. Carey, M.D., dean of the school, in 1992. However, this does not preclude this J. T. Harrison's having been a doctor, or perhaps even having attended some classes at the school on an informal basis in its first years.

5. Tinsley Harrison, interview by author.

6. *History of Alabama and Dictionary of Alabama Biography* (Chicago: The S. J. Clarke Publishing Company, 1921).

7. The graves of John Tinsley Harrison Sr. and his wife, Melinda Stone Harrison, have been located by Dr. John Bondurant Harrison. The graves are in Madison County, Alabama, some three miles west of the community of New Hope, just north of the Tennessee River. The tombstone in the New Hope cemetery gives the dates of birth and death for J. T. Harrison Sr. as 1799–1875, and the *Huntsville Weekly-Independent* of December 2, 1875, includes an obituary: "Died at his residence 3 miles west of New Hope, Alabama on the 8th. Mr. John T. Harrison aged 76." The dates are also given in *Alabama Records* 235, Madison Co., Gandrud: "J. T. Harrison/born Aug. 21, 1799/died Nov. 8, 1875/Our Father. Melinda Harrison/born July 28, 1796/died March 26, 1868/Our Mother." Also listed is W. B. Harrison, born April 17, 1824, died July 9, 1866—John T. Harrison Jr.'s older

After a short time in Tennessee, Dr. J. T. Harrison Sr. moved to a small farm in Alabama on the north bank of the Tennessee River just across and downstream from Guntersville, in Madison County.[6] Both J. T. and his wife had some ties with the state. J. T. was "a former soldier in the War of 1812 and in the Indian War, who took part in the skirmish which drove the Indians across the Coosa River" in central-east Alabama. He had returned to the state in 1818, when he participated in surveying the lands around Huntsville, the first state capital in 1819. Melinda Stone Harrison had a cousin who later became a chief justice of Alabama. When Dr. J. T. Harrison and his wife Melinda arrived sometime before 1830, Alabama was a brand new state still transitioning from Indian territory.[7]

This man, Dr. John Tinsley Harrison Sr., the great-grandfather of Tinsley, considered himself a doctor and apparently loved medicine, but he could not earn a livelihood from it. The economy was still based on subsistence: people lived on the plants and animals they grew.[8] His patients were poor farmers who lived off the land, or slaves, or a few black freedmen, and cash was in short supply. Only a few families had much money. So, to support himself and his family, he was also a cotton farmer.

In mid-19th century America, cotton farmers were more highly respected than doctors anyhow. Regular doctors—physicians following European traditions and developments—used therapeutic methods which were held in suspicion by the general populace as well as by many of the leading doctors themselves. In those years probably half or fewer of the doctors in the region of Alabama were regular doctors. The rest were either self-educated or herbalists or Thomsonians[9]; most were homeopaths, who believed that most diseases could be cured through small doses of drugs or other substances. The regular doctors—struggling to suppress their competitors, many of whom were uneducated and dangerous—formed the American Medical Association in 1847. These uncertainties, the lack of agreement on the nature of diseases and how best to treat them, and the political machinations of the various groups for recognition and influence, together with the spirit of Jacksonian democracy of the time, so discouraged the New York legislature that they simply abolished medical licensure in 1844. A similar spirit prevailed around the entire country. Anybody who wished could practice medicine.

Then, as Lincoln said, the war came.

JUST HOW POOR THE South was relative to the rest of the nation is debated. Fogel and

Engerman, authors of *Time on the Cross: The Economics of American Negro Slavery*, believe that just before the Civil War the South was generally as prosperous as some other parts of the U.S. and more so than such civilized areas as Italy.[10] Their data do show that even in the era just before the Civil War the per capita income was lower in the Southeast than in other parts of the U.S., but these income figures include the slaves, and they change significantly when confined to the free population.[11] Per capita income in the East South Central states for free residents was similar to other parts of the nation before the war, but after the war incomes for all Southerners sank to a much lower proportion of the national average and remained there until well into the 20th century. The wealth in the United States at the turn of the 20th century was concentrated mostly in the Northeast.

After the Civil War, there was not only the destruction of property and some of the most productive lives of the region, but also continuing disputes about who owned what, with former slaves claiming parts of their former masters' lands.[12] The depression of the 1870s hurt the South far worse than the rest of the nation. The South saw the value of cotton fall by nearly 50 percent between 1872 and 1877, to a selling price of about what it cost to produce. This depression plunged into poverty farmers already living on the economic margin, bankrupted merchants, closed businesses, and reduced chances for employment among all citizens, especially former slaves.

And it got worse. By 1880 the South was economically worse off than it was in 1870, with a per capita income only one-third that of the rest of the nation.[13] Outside the former Confederacy, the U.S. economy was booming. Fueled by railroad expansion, the steel mills were operating full tilt. Most of the steel produced in the United States during the last decades of the 19th century went to manufacture steel rails for the nation's westward-reaching railroad system. In the South, however, railroads failed. Not a single Southern road that fell into receivership escaped Northern financial influence. The entire regional economy slid into a colonial model. Northern banking interests and businessmen controlled much of the economy in the South.[14]

Alabama was a poor state before the war and an even poorer one afterwards. The scars of the war could be seen well into the 20th century and are still felt today. In 1920, for example, per capita income in Alabama ranked 44th among the states (by 1935, 46th; in 2000, 44th). All its counties were poor. The average annual income for Cleburne County was $156.

brother and also a physician. The *Deed Record Book G* for adjacent Marshall County, in the courthouse in Guntersville, lists land transactions between W. B. Harrison and J. T. Harrison in 1863, 1866 (two weeks before W. B. died), and 1870. John T. Harrison Jr. had a brother about six years his elder, James A., who became a teacher. (*Gandrud's Madison County Records* 85, 1830, Huntsville Library, and 1850 Federal Census, Madison County, Alabama, M432 Roll 9, 407. If the 1799 birth date for J. T. Harrison Sr. is correct, he would have been only 13 to 16 years old when he "fought in the Indian wars with Andrew Jackson." However, the 1799 date appears well established.

8. Charles Sellers, *The Market Revolution—Jacksonian America 1815–1846* (New York/Oxford: Oxford Univ. Press, 1991).

9. See discussion on 28–29.

10. R. W. Fogel and S. L. Engerman, *Time on the Cross: The Economics of American Negro Slavery*, vol. 1, (Boston: Little, Brown

and Co., 1974), 232–57. This two-volume work is an example of "cliometrics," a word derived from combining the word "Clio," the Greek muse of history, with "metrics," measurement. It was attacked at the time of its publication as biased against the American black population. Then a review published photos of both authors and their wives; Fogel's wife was black. The authors have published other cliometric studies, including *Railroads and American Economic Growth: Essays in Econometric History* and *Race and Slavery in the Western Hemisphere: Quantitative Studies, The Dimensions of Quantitative Research in History.*

11. Ibid., 248. See also Eric Foner, *Reconstruction: America's Unfinished Revolution, 1863–1877* (New York: Harper & Row, 1988).

12. Foner, *Reconstruction*, 104–.

13. Ibid., 525.

14. John F. Stover, *The Railroads of the South, 1865–1900* (Chapel Hill, 1955) xv–xviii, 66–7, 125–54, 282. Also Robert L. Brandfon, etc., of Foner,

Poverty translates into poor health statistics. Comparisons of leading indicators of health status of the populace in Alabama with those of other states for the late 19th century are difficult to collect because of lack of data. But the health status was low. We know that. Other indicators provide evidence. In 1900 only 54 percent of the Alabama population between ages 10 and 14 even attended high school (66 percent of this number were labeled "native whites"); only a few percent of the state's population had achieved a high school diploma, and fewer still a college degree. Alabama ranked fourth in the nation in illiteracy—after New Mexico, North Carolina, and Louisiana. More than half the total Alabama population over 10 years of age was illiterate, including 25 percent of the "native white population."

Despite all of the negative facts, after the war, the South had a proud tradition. How much of this tradition and attitude of aristocracy was based on historical facts and how much was wishful mythology has been questioned.[15] There was, however, some basis for pride. The first permanent English settlement in North America was in the South in 1607, and the British surrender concluding the Revolutionary War occurred in the South. One Southern state, Texas, had actually been an independent country for a time. Nine of the first dozen United States presidents came from the South. During the early years of the Civil War, the rural South's armies, often outnumbered and out-equipped, had achieved spectacular accomplishments against the armies of the industrial North. The South had shown initiative and cunning in their imaginative campaigns. A functional and effective submarine was built and operated by the South—*The Hunley*, now in a museum in Charleston, S.C., perhaps symbolic of the South's whole failed efforts, since the vessel itself sank with its successful attack, killing all its crew.

In the 1890s and later, biographies of physicians who grew up in northern states sometimes hardly even mention the war. For those children it was past, and that was that. The North was in transition to a full industrial economy. They looked only to the future.[16]

Not so in the South.

THE SOUTH, RICHLY ENDOWED with physical resources such as water, timber, coal, gas, and oil, as well as the natural beauty of the land, had provided a productive and rewarding life for most of its white residents and gave the nation some of its most distinguished leaders. Of course, the South had also been the location of most of the slavery in the U.S.

The Civil War and its aftermath constituted a catastrophe that ruined the South's countryside, destroyed its cities, and left its inhabitants in a shambles. The four years of warfare resulted in destitution, as well as resentment and inferiority that smolder to this day; a similar attitude of condescension and pity, at best, or derisive hostility at worst, lingers in the North. The scars of war were very visible during Tinsley Harrison's lifetime.

Physical embodiments of the difficulties remain even today: empty fields, lines of gravestones, abandoned fortresses. At a crossroad in the village of Munford, Alabama, some 2.5 miles east of John Tinsley Harrison's farm of the 1870s–'90s, stands a stone marker, which reads:

Reconstruction, 536.

15. Virginia Van der Veer Hamilton, *Alabama, A Bicentennial History* (New York: W. W. Norton Company, 1977).

16. C. Barger, S. Bennison, and Elin Wolf, *Walter B. Cannon, A Life* (Cambridge: Harvard-Belknap Press, 1998).

A. J. BUTTRAM
CONFEDERATE SOLDIER
KILLED HERE APR 23, 1865
DURING CROXTON'S RAID
ERECTED BY VETERANS
AND THEIR DESCENDANTS

Lee surrendered to Grant at Appomattox on the 9th of April in 1865, two full weeks before Croxton's boys killed Buttram, locally claimed to be the last Confederate soldier killed east of the Mississippi.

Most Southern towns of any size also had a park with a statue of a Confederate soldier atop a tall column. The soldier was young, often with cap in one hand and rifle in the other, his gaze downcast. In the past, these served as a convenient meeting place for the community. In the late 20th century many have been removed or altered. But there were always the cemeteries, with row upon row of simple, small identical headstones. And the Confederate veterans themselves with their reunions and rallies. Healing would take time. Tinsley Harrison grew up with the war still present.

History is written by the winners. The South was demoralized in word and song. The wounds and associated traditions did not serve the South well. Most people in the South lived their lives productively, in peace. But the region was looked down on by people in other places for more than a century after the war. In the late 1940s, teachers of tropical medicine and diseases such as hookworm in northern medical schools like Harvard patronized, "The people of the South aren't lazy; they're

17. Including his
lifelong friend Dr.
James Craik, whose
descendants became
interwoven with two
other families of Ala-
bama physicians, the
Baldwins and Pollards
of Montgomery. See
Deep Family by Nicho-
las Cabell Read and
Dallas Read (Mont-
gomery: NewSouth
Books, 2005).

sick." As late as the 1950s in a lounge near Kenmore Square in Boston, the young Harvard mathematician Tom Lehrer sang derogatory songs about Alabama to his own rollicking piano score:

> *Take me back to dear ol' Dixie; / Won't ya' come with me to Alabamy, / I wanna' talk with Southern gentlemen / An' put my white sheet on again. / I ain't seen one good lynchin' in years. / The land of the boll weevil, / Where the laws are medieval, / Be it ever so decadent, / there's no place like home.*

The South, weakened by warfare and the crumbling economy, was poor—viewed with pity laced with scorn—but not just monetarily. The South's level of education, health statistics, and prestige in the rest of the country and world became the butt of jokes, ridicule, and songs of derision. In such a situation, it was difficult to attract outstanding scholars and scientists from the world's leading institutions to build similarly excellent institutions of widespread renown, though individual scholarship and academic excellence thrived here as well as elsewhere.

It was into such a rural environment that Tinsley Harrison was born on Sunday, March 18, 1900. Not only was he born into the traditions of his native South, good and bad, but he also was born into an environment already infused with a strong family tradition of medicine and academic excellence, attributable to both paternal and maternal influences. In many ways he grew up and was formed more by the practice of medicine than by other aspects of his youth. His family was not only his biological family, but also his medical heritage.

HERE A BRIEF REVIEW of the history of medicine and diseases might be helpful. In the nation's early years, therapies for the treatment of diseases were usually ineffective or even harmful, and on occasion killed the patient. President George Washington was certainly helped along to death by the repeated blood-lettings by his well-meaning physicians.[17] Not only the medical profession but also the public questioned the value of typical medical practices. Regular medicine was propelled by a complex mix of motives which included both self-serving aspects of the guild system and a more altruistic adherence to the developing scientific medicine in Europe. However, the theories of the regulars had not yet passed much beyond the primitive stage, and therapies were only beginning to emerge from the medical middle ages. Thus, regular medicine was under siege by the homeopaths, the Thomsonians, and other herbalists.

For the healing arts in America, the 19th century was a time of philosophical uncertainty and shifting sands, but of medical progress all the same. Until about 1850, the physician had made his diagnoses mainly by talking with the patient and observing him or her, perhaps examining the urine in a glass container. It was only as the 19th century neared its end that physicians began to take the perspective of the surgeons, which related a patient's symptoms and diseases to specific anatomic abnormalities. Only then had the physicians begun to add the specificity of a careful physical examination to focus on specific organs or areas and clarify their previously vague, general ideas of what was wrong with the patient and what to do about it.

Medical advancement was a worldwide pursuit. Doctors the world over burned the midnight oil looking for answers to health problems.

Auenbrugger had published in 1761 his discovery of percussion of the chest, which showed "that an abnormal tone in the thorax is, in every disease, a certain sign of the existence of serious danger." However, his brief book attracted little attention even within his own Vienna, where it was controversial. His explanations were too brief and too vague to encourage widespread emulation. Though Auenbrugger apparently related the physical findings to observations at autopsy, he neglected to describe these well. Many physicians in his time were still biased against engaging in physical activities. "The physical intimacy required by percussion threatened to undermine the professional and social standing of the physician, whose philosophical bent and intellectual training often made the application of a manual method of diagnosis beneath his dignity, or placed him in a class with the surgeon." Though Auenbrugger's study was translated into French in 1770, it was only after Napoleon's physician Corvisart made a second French translation, enriched with his own observations and commentaries, increased the explanations to 440 pages, and published it again in 1808, that physicians began to notice. It was translated into English in 1824.

The other major advance in physical diagnosis was auscultation—listening to a patient's chest and abdomen, usually with a stethoscope—popularized in 1819 by Laennec. Overuse and over-interpretation by some of his pupils, and other difficulties, made acceptance slow; though Josef Skoda, a leading medical figure in Vienna, published his classic book on percussion and auscultation in 1839, it was only during the 1850s that these methods came to be widely accepted in Britain and America.

THE MODERN SCIENTIFIC DISCIPLINES such as pathology and physiology were just

18. Thomas Weller, Harvard Medical School course in Tropical Medicine (1949). Weller, along with John F. Enders and Frederick C. Robbins, was awarded a Nobel Prize for cultivating poliomyelitis virus in non-nervous tissue. This advance made it possible for scientists to study the virus in the laboratory, which in turn led to the development of polio vaccines. Weller was a notable figure in the world of tropical medicine and at the time of his death was Richard Pearson Strong Professor of Tropical Medicine Emeritus at the Harvard School of Public Health.

developing. Bacteriology had yet to arrive. Tuberculosis was widespread and well recognized, though the cause was misunderstood. Malaria was so named because it was thought to be the result of "bad air." Most diseases (fever, for example) were not even sufficiently well-defined for what we would call a diagnosis, and there was much less any understanding of pathogenesis, etiology, or effective therapy. No one knew what caused diseases but many guessed.[18]

This was a time when scientists were attempting to organize knowledge of biology, especially the new specimens arriving back in Europe from exploration of the new world. The groupings varied according to the propensities of the individual scientist, and there was little agreement among them, much less an international standard. Carolus Linnaeus, back in Sweden after studying botany in Holland, invented the binomial system of naming individual kinds of organisms, all in Latin, of course. The first name was the *genus*, the second the *species*. Though the word *species* goes back at least to the 16th century, Linnaeus used it in this particular meaning. He understood that clarity of nomenclature and restriction of use of the terms to extremely well-defined items is crucial to the understanding of Nature itself. The importance of accuracy and clarity in communication in science continues to be of primary importance today.

Linnaeus published the first edition of his work in 1735. By the time it had reached its 16th edition, the three volumes contained 2,300 pages, and his system was recognized as a major advance for biology. He was limited, however, by the bounds of knowledge at the time. Modern ornithologists sometimes discuss with amusement what they now call the BFF—beak, foot, and feather—method of classification, since we now use not only behavioral peculiarities, but also DNA sequences. Linnaeus, for example, included the shrikes (Lanidae) with "Ordo Accipitres," chiefly hawks, in his 10th edition of *Systema Naturae* because they have somewhat hooked beaks, and he initially mistook the male and female mallard as separate species. But his was progress, and would-be scientists everywhere tried to apply such a system to their fields.

The reputation of William Cullen, a Scottish professor of medicine in both Glasgow and Edinburgh, was made by a similar publication. His attempted great leap forward in our understanding of diseases was discussed by William Smellie, editor of the first edition of the *Encyclopedia Britannica* (1768). Smellie discusses the disagreements among Cullen, Linnaeus, Vogel, and others, highlighting their focus on characteristics as opposed to cures. Smellie then "lays before our readers the last and shortest distribution, published [in 1769] by Dr. Cullen, one of the professors of medicine in the University of Edinburgh, under the title *Synopsis Nosologiae Methodicae*, or rather, *Genera Morborum Praecipua*."

Four classes of disease follow: *Pyrexiae*, or fevers; *Neuroses*, known as nervous disorders; *Cachexiae*, afebrile diseases without a nervous component; and *Locales*, local problems affecting only a part of the body.

Pyrexiae, for example, are then divided into seven orders, the first being "Febres, or fevers," in turn into 1. Intermittent, and 2. Continued (known as families in biology terminology). The first of these contains three genera: tertian, quartan, and quotidian. The last also contains three genera: synocha, typhus, and synochus. "Hemorrhagiae" and "profluvia" are also classified within the class Pyrexiae.

The second class, *Neuroses*, includes not only comas, apoplexy, paralysis, catalepsy, hysteria, melancholia, mania, and tetanus, but also dyspepsia, chlorosis, diabetes, diarrhea, pertussis, and asthma.

Cachexiae includes tabes, atrophia, rachitis, hydrothorax, anasarca, tympanites, ascites, and hydrocele, among others. Order III within this class is Impetigines and includes scrophula, syphilis, and scorbutus (now known as scurvy).

THESE OVERSIMPLIFIED CLASSIFICATIONS MAY be amusing to us today, but they were some sign of progress. However, they also make it obvious that lack of understanding of the basic mechanisms of disease precluded a more rational classification which could lead to rational diagnosis and treatment. And for the individual patient, medicine *is* chiefly diagnosis and treatment, just as a proper understanding of the causes of diseases is required for society at large and the practice of public health.

Smellie notes the discrepancies between the different classifications and is skeptical that any is free from major defects and misunderstandings. He points out that one must be familiar with the theories of causation of diseases of a particular proponent to understand the rationale for his proposed classification. "However," he says, "notwithstanding these defects arising from the theoretical distribution of diseases, we cannot hesitate for a moment in preferring even a bad method of classing to none at all. Every attempt towards a just and natural arrangement of diseases is laudable, and has a direct tendency to introduce science into the medical art; an object greatly wished for, but which still appears to be very distant."

Smellie goes on to point out the dangers in erroneous classifications peculiar to medicine, since each theory leads to particular forms of treatment, and it may be many years before major errors are discovered. In the meantime, bad treatments were used enthusiastically, perhaps to the detriment of the patient. "The theories of diseases," Smellie bemoans, "as well as the mode of prescription, are as variable as the fashions of a lady's headdress."

One of the leading figures in theories of diseases and their treatment was Samuel A. Thomson of New England. Born in 1769 in rural New Hampshire, Thomson as a boy became familiar with local folk remedies using plants. He was unimpressed by the results of treatments by "book doctors," as he later called them, especially after one failed to help his own family member, who then recovered under the herbal ministrations of young Thomson. This generated the twofold thesis which guided Thomson through his career: herbal treatments and self-help rather than calling professionals. We can still see his vast influence today.

There was also a pecuniary interest. Thomson published a book, *Brief Sketch of the Causes and Treatment of Disease*. It was "addressed to the people of the United States, pointing out to them the pernicious consequences of using *poisons* as medicine, such as mercury, arsenic, nitre, antimony, and opium, and the advantages of using such only as are the produce of our own country." This 1821 book was "designed as an introduction to a full explanation to be published hereafter of the System of Practice discovered by the author, which has been secured to him by patent." It contains testimonials, the report of a religious vision in support of the system, and the names and addresses of agents from whom Thomson's patented medicines could be obtained. He has harsh words for the traditional doctors, especially those of "the faculty," and sounds like a 19th-century Ivan Illich. His system was for sale, through his agents, for $20 to a family, a "reasonable" sum for a layman who would use the system to practice. However, Thomson had a different price for doctors. "To a physician," he said, "the price of a right to use my medicine and practice is Five Hundred Dollars."

Thomson's system seemed reasonable to many of the time, and in some particulars, he was correct. He railed against bleeding patients: "Nature never furnishes the body with more blood than is necessary for the maintenance of health; to take away part of the blood, therefore, is taking away just so much of their life, and is as contrary to nature, as it would be to take away part of their flesh." He had many examples to use as an argument for his system. For one, the famous English physician and botanist William Withering in 1785 had cured dropsy with foxglove. (Which wasn't actually the case. Foxglove did not cure all dropsy, since there was little or no understanding of the underlying pathogenesis and it was used for renal and hepatic dropsy as well as cardiac edema.)

The 12th edition of Samuel Thomson's book published by his son in 1841 gives an extensive and generally accurate review of gross anatomy of the human body and a discussion of the physiology of the internal organs, limited, however, by the understanding that "the human system is composed of 'Matter,' or earth, water, air, and fire, and their constituents." Disease was apparently caused by an imbalance in the heat of the body, caused by malfunction of the gastrointestinal tract. The aim of therapy, therefore, was to restore normal function and the balance of heat. The author of this popular mid-century medical book states at the outset: "To assist us in the progression of this work, upon animal and vegetable life, we have consulted Hippocrates, Galen, Bacon, Boerhaave, Sylvius, Cullen, Brown, Hunter, Goldsmith, Darwin, Thomson, Waterhouse, Blane, Mitchell, Hearsey, Robinson, Ingalls, Eaton, Tully, Barton, Rush, and various other authors; for the theory and practice or the adaptation of animal and vegetable substances to sustain life, or vitality in animal matter, Samuel Thomson."

It is interesting that Fielding H. Garrison's classic book, *An Introduction to the History of Medicine*, first published in 1913, subject of four editions and many reprintings well into the latter part of the 20th century, makes no mention of Thomson. Garrison does discuss Cullen, quoting approvingly Hamilton's comment that "Cullen did not add a single new fact to medical science."

UNTIL X-RAYS APPEARED ON the scene in 1896, following Rontgen's announcement in December 1895, the physician had only his own senses to rely upon to understand the normal and abnormal structures and functions of his patient's body. His sight, hearing, and touch were increasingly aided by such devices as the stethoscope, ophthalmoscope, and laryngoscope. Occasionally the physician even resorted to taste, as in tasting patients' urine to detect the sweetness indicative of diabetes mellitus. Some instruments available prior to X-rays did not so much reveal new information as they made existing information more precise. Fever was well-known from ancient times, but the thermometer made its measurement more exact and came into widespread clinical use in America in the decades after the Civil War, having become popularized by the classic and exhaustive work of Wunderlich in Germany. Similarly, good quantitative estimation of the patient's blood pressure could be easily made after Riva-Rocci's 1896 introduction of the sphygmomanometer—which measured arterial blood pressure, but only the systolic pressure; easy measuring of the diastolic as well awaited the Korotkoff sounds in 1905.

Until the latter part of the 19th century, since only the most obvious abnormalities, such as major fractures or massive bleeding, could be identified, other ailments were treated by traditional methods. These were chiefly herbal (purging and puking—giving herbs or extracts which caused diarrhea and vomiting), supplemented by bleeding, cupping, moxibustion, and similar activities. Although these treatments were applied with solemnity by the doctors, many people remained skeptical.

WE DO NOT KNOW the kind of medicine the doctors John Tinsley Harrison and his sons J. T. Jr., and W. B. Harrison practiced around the time of the Civil War. But it must have been respected and considered useful by their contemporaries, as patients continued to seek them out for help.

Many doctors, or people who called themselves doctors, formed friendly botanical medical societies, such as Thomson had advocated. The first medical school in Alabama was an herbal medical school. It was formed by a group of disgruntled faculty from a similar school in Macon, Georgia, who moved in 1844 to Wetumpka, Alabama, in the east-central part of the state just north of Montgomery. The school operated for one year then moved to Tennessee.

In 1835 the governor of Mississippi estimated that about half the medical doctors in the South were herbal doctors. However, as the last quarter of the 19th century advanced, educated Americans became aware of the medical progress occurring in Europe and searched for ways to bring these benefits to their own communities. The South, alongside the rest of the world, was of two minds about medicine, still holding to superstitions and suspicious of technology and medical advances, yet progressing towards a better understanding of medicine and the human body.

Thus was the scientific status of medicine and the environment into which John Tinsley Harrison Sr. came when he entered Alabama in the 1820s. And here at the farm on the north bank of the Tennessee River near New Hope, Dr. John Tinsley Harrison Jr. was born on April 28, 1834. The area was near the site identified on recent maps as "Harrison's Gap."

This younger John Tinsley Harrison, Tinsley's grandfather, grew up in that farming region. In 1852 at age 18 he began the study of medicine with his brother, Dr. W. B. Harrison of Guntersville, who was 10 years older. In 1855, after three years as his brother's apprentice, he entered the Nashville Medical College, forerunner of the Vanderbilt medical school. His medical schooling required less than a year, so he entered the practice of medicine himself in the shadow of the oncoming war. Two years later he married Belinda Collins of Tennessee.

John Harrison joined the Confederate forces as a physician at the outset of the Civil War; he was captured within a year by Union forces. The Yankees offered to give him a commission in the Union army as a physician. He refused. They then asked if he would practice medicine without a commission. Since he wanted to practice medicine, he agreed, but he insisted on wearing a Confederate uniform. His Union captors refused that request on the grounds that he would probably be shot by a Union sentry or soldier. They negotiated a compromise by which he was permitted to wear gray trousers with a civilian coat and hat. He also obtained their agreement that he could care first for the wounded Confederates after a battle, then

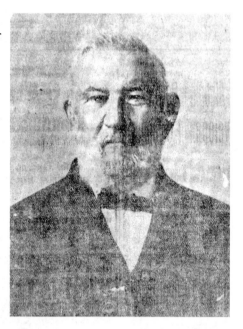

John T. Harrison Jr., M.D., at his farm near Talladega on his 76th birthday. He still looks like a man who might get into a scrap.

wounded Union soldiers. Family tradition has it that he did his very best for all the wounded, Confederate and Union alike, stanching rapid bleeding, splinting fractures, cleaning wounds, transporting all to safety behind Union lines. He was said to have made many close friends among northern physicians serving in the Union army, to have learned from them, and to have remained friends with them all his life. No letters of exchange, however, have been found.

In 1864, while he was a prisoner, Harrison's young wife died.

DURING THE EARLY PERIOD of Reconstruction when the federal government stationed troops in the South, Dr. John T. Harrison Jr. had a startling experience. A warm personal friend of his, a cotton farmer who owned adjoining land, was walking down a village street with his wife. The cotton farmer was a large, powerful man. According to the family story, a federal soldier passed them and in passing made a slurring comment to the wife, something like, "Hi, Baby. How about spending the weekend with me?" Enraged, her husband struck the federal soldier in the jaw with his fist. The soldier went down, reaching for his pistol. The cotton farmer kicked the soldier in the jaw, whereupon his head snapped back and he died instantly. This was a federal soldier of the occupying troops, and the cotton farmer knew he was in trouble and fled.

He rode his horse 15 or 20 miles to Dr. Harrison's farm where he changed to a fresh horse Harrison gave him. He then rode the fresh horse across the Tennessee River, planning to contact his wife later after he had fled southward. It was a remarkable feat, considering the width and depth of the river and the swiftness of the current. We do not know the name of the cotton farmer or what became of him.

Dr. John Harrison was in a difficult situation. Word spread that he had helped the murderer of a federal soldier escape. With a sense of foreboding he felt that he too must flee. So he took a good horse and also swam it across the river and fled southward. (Another version of this story has Harrison, and not the cotton farmer, as the murderer.)

Harrison traveled for days, keeping to himself. He stayed at several inns and private residences using different names. Finally he came to rest in a rural county where there were no federal troops or obvious dangers. The people there were cordial, and after a time, he told the story to the man in whose home he was living. This man was Jared E. Groce, who had come to Alabama from South Carolina by wagon train in the 1820s and obtained land in Talladega County in the 1830s. He now owned and operated a general store at a country crossroad near the villages of Eastaboga and Munford. The store was a friendly gathering place for the local citizenry, who came to warm their outsides by the potbellied wood stove and their insides with a drink of white lightning dipped from the ever present tub of home-brewed liquor near the stove.

Just when Dr. Harrison openly resumed his real name is uncertain. However, he started practicing medicine again and became a respected member of the community. He was later president of the Board of Censors of the Talladega County Medical Society, which also made him president of the county's Board of Health. Mr. Groce's multiple sons had moved on to Texas, but his youngest child, a girl born

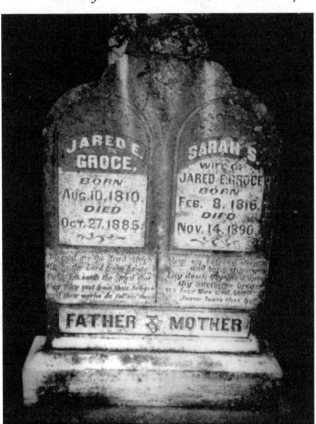

Groce tombstones in the family cemetery.

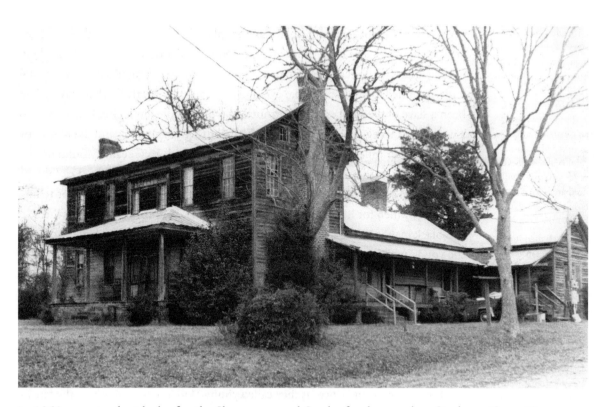

Groce Home, Eastaboga, Alabama.

in 1850, remained with the family. She was named Sarah after her mother, Sarah Simmons Groce, but because she was young and diminutive, she was known as Chick; even in her later years she was called Miss Chick. Harrison married Chick in 1869, and they obtained some farmland from Mr. Groce.[19] John Harrison became better known in the community, but he kept a low profile, fearing repercussions from the federal government.

In 1868 Andrew Johnson stepped down and Grant became president. The eight years of the Grant administration were difficult in the Old South—the period of "the bloody shirts," the symbol the Republicans and carpetbaggers waved at election time representing the blood of the Northern youth killed during the war by Southerners. Secret societies dedicated to continuing the Confederate cause cropped up. The country seemed on the brink of another disaster. The horrors of the Civil War, and the strict military presence of the Union, maintained a relative peace.

TINSLEY'S FATHER: IN 1871, Chick and John Harrison had a baby boy and named him William Groce Harrison. One day when the child was six months old, word

19. The house of J. E. Groce existed as of 2014. It is a two-story wooden frame house unoccupied for some years, owned by Elizabeth Montgomery Strange, a descendant of the Montgomery family, which intermarried with the Groce family. The lot on which the house stands, 0.5 mile south of Eastaboga, contains the J. E.

Groce Family Cemetery. The then-current owner stated that the house was built about 1832. It is large even by current standards and must have been an outstanding home in mid-19th century rural Alabama. Several of Jared Groce's children are buried in the family cemetery just behind the house.

20. Chick died in 1919, and Tinsley R. Harrison remembered this grandmother well, as well as his grandfather. She, in turn, remembered the Civil War and its aftermath vividly. "She spoke about the war a lot. We can almost hear her still, saying: 'After the war . . .'"

spread that carpetbaggers and scalawags were planning a government takeover in the area the next day. The local white men, to counter what they felt was expropriation of their affairs without an election or authorization by any recognized governmental entity, planned to fight back. That evening after dark, an elderly black man who had been a slave of the Groces and continued to work for the family hitched a horse to a wagon and threw in some blankets. He then drove Miss Chick and the new baby some 10 or 15 miles in the dark over narrow clay roads to Cheaha Mountain, the highest point in the state, where he hid them in a cave for the night. Dr. John T. Harrison remained behind to fight. Many years later, Tinsley was fond of telling this story, which for him exemplified the degree to which his grandfather relied on this black man, and the strong trusting personal relationship between the two men, the young white doctor and the elderly former slave.[20]

The takeover plans were thwarted by a tremendous storm that night, which included at least one tornado. For two weeks, things quieted down. One morning, people awoke to a horrifying sight. From the large oaks and tulip poplars hung thick ropes around the necks of dead men. They had been hanged by vigilantes for plotting the coup. Both blacks and whites were hanged. After that the community remained quiet and orderly. The veracity of the charges was never questioned.

The early years of Groce, as they called young William, were spent on the family cotton farm of some 300 acres near Chocolocca and Cheaha creeks. These creeks are fairly sizeable and might be termed rivers elsewhere. Harrison's medical practice was conducted in private homes exclusively—the doctor's or the patient's, there being no clinic or hospital in the vicinity, nor any money to construct one. Since most patients could not pay the doctor with cash, they paid with chickens, hog meat, vegetables, and the like. Nearly all the cash John Harrison could accumulate had to come from the cotton farm. In 1877 when he was six years old, Groce was put to work in the cotton fields of his father. He learned to plant, chop, and pick cotton, and he became quite proficient at it despite his young age and small size. What Groce did not know was that his father put money into a separate account in the local bank for every day Groce worked, twice the amount a regular laborer would earn. During his childhood Groce was either in school or working in the cotton fields with other farm hands, mostly freed black women and men.

There were no public schools in the area, so Groce attended a private school. The schoolmaster at this school was excellent—"a tremendous person" very attentive to each child and himself an educated man, probably self-educated. He seemed to know everything and to love knowledge and the process of learning. And he clearly loved his young pupils. This was really a teacher, for he inspired in his students a resonant passion to learn, a sort of *furor scholasticus*. In Tinsley's words, "He was the kind of man described in Oliver Goldsmith's poem, "The Deserted Village":

> *And still they gazed, and still the wonder grew,*
> *That one small head could carry all he knew.*

Groce did well under such tutelage and completed his grade school education at the age of 16. During this time, his father asked him what his hopes were for the future. Groce answered that he would like to go to college and become a doctor but that he was sure his father did not have enough money. It was only now that his father told Groce of the special savings account which he had been building over the years, largely from the set-asides for Groce's work in the cotton fields. This fund would pay for his college education.[21]

There was a new land grant college in the state, the Agricultural and Mechanical College of Alabama, at Auburn, established under the Morrill Act of 1862. In accordance with that law, it was also a military school when Groce attended it. Today it is one of the three major senior universities of Alabama, located some 70 miles southeast of Eastaboga. At a time when students at Oxford were being served in their rooms by carefully groomed servants, and students at Harvard lived in spacious dormitories called "houses," each with its own well-tended small grassy park in the middle, Auburn had no dormitories at all. The professors' salaries were so low that they supplemented their incomes by running boarding houses.

Groce roomed with Charles Glenn at the residence of Professor Anderson and his wife.[22] Groce made an excellent academic record at Auburn from 1887 through the spring of 1891, when he graduated, convinced that he should become a doctor. He finished with no demerits from the military department.

Money was tight, but Dr. John Harrison helped as he could, and Groce worked on the side. In the fall of 1891 he enrolled in the University of Nashville Medical School. He completed the course of study in less than a year and was awarded the M.D. degree in the spring of 1892. Groce's entire medical education consisted of lectures from local practitioners and a few simple written examinations. There were no anatomical dissections, laboratory exercises, microscopes, or clinical experiences with or without supervision. There was no preceptorial training. Groce was better

21. Chick and John Harrison lived on their farm for the rest of their lives. The house still existed in 1992 about 2.5 miles east of Munford amid wide fields of soybeans just south of the highway near Munford. For some years after World War II it functioned as a restaurant and lounge, The Pilgrimage Inn, under the patronage of a cousin, "Tiny" Harrison. Since 1981 when the current owners, Mr. and Mrs. Earl Allred Jr. purchased it, it has again been used as a dwelling place. The current deed for this house and the surrounding land includes a single acre, and none of the surrounding fields.

22. Glenn later became supervisor of the Birmingham system of public schools and was grandfather of Dr. Charles Glenn Cobbs, a future professor of medicine at the medical school in Birmingham.

23. One county in the Midwest, as the story goes, had a law requiring the employment of a county health officer who was a physician holding the M.D. degree. However, there was no physician to be found. Therefore, the citizens located an individual who would accept the position, established a local medical school (probably with an itinerant faculty from nearby larger towns), put their candidate through it, then closed the school and appointed its only graduate the county health officer.

educated than most medical students and doctors of the time, but he felt medically uneducated after completing this course. Tinsley later said that the professors in this school "didn't even know that bacteriology existed," even in 1892. Perhaps Groce was independently aware of the advances occurring in Europe—the discovery of the tubercle bacillus by Koch in 1882, and the discussions then occurring in major U.S. medical centers about the new discipline of bacteriology.

Most American medical schools were commercial businesses and had such low requirements that men, and a very few women, could be admitted with no college education and often without a high school diploma. It was said that some medical schools did not even require that their students know how to read and write. The course of study was commonly four to eight months. There were no laboratory exercises, no physiology experiments or demonstrations with animals, no bedside clinical teaching, and no gradation of curriculum or clinical responsibility. In fact, there was no patient-care responsibility at all. Some schools technically required two years before awarding the degree, but the second year was typically just the first year repeated. There were perhaps 200 medical schools in the country, though nobody really knows the exact number. Abraham Flexner's 1910 critical book-length study of medical education in the United States and Canada, published under the auspices of the Carnegie Foundation, covers 155.[23]

In 1892, Groce was not satisfied with the medical education he had obtained in Nashville, so he enrolled in a second medical school, the Baltimore Medical College in Maryland. During that year he learned of a new medical school, part of the Johns Hopkins University, opening across town the following fall, which was to emphasize high academic quality. This new school was establishing a curriculum along the best European lines and required the highest medical standards of the time.

Groce visited the Johns Hopkins Hospital, established in 1889 near the advent of the clinical bedside teaching which was to become one of the hallmarks of the new breed of medical school then developing in the United States. There Groce met and came to know William Osler, who was to set the course of his life and thence the life course and medical career of Tinsley Randolph Harrison.

Johns Hopkins occupied a central position in the reformation of American medical education and practice that occurred during the first decades of the new 20th century. Kenneth M. Ludmerer, the award-winning medical education historian, called Hopkins "the single most potent influence ever for the dissemination

of scientific medical education in America." It was
the first American medical school to require a college
diploma and a reading knowledge of both French and
German for admission. As is often the case, a completely new school such as Hopkins found it easier
to make changes than older schools with encrusted
faculties and traditions. For some years Harvard, the
University of Michigan medical school, the University
of Pennsylvania School of Medicine, the Northwestern
University School of Medicine under Nathan Davis
Smith, and others had been working to upgrade medical education and had instituted graded curricula with
laboratory work during the early phases and bedside
clinical teaching by senior doctors during the late
phases. But progress was slow, despite champions such
as Charles W. Eliot, Harvard's young—age 35—new
president in 1869.

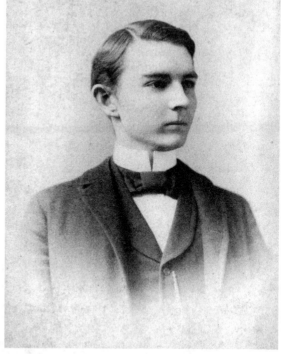

*W. Groce
Harrison Sr.,
Baltimore, 1892.*

When he could find time, Groce attended ward
rounds at the Johns Hopkins Hospital, especially with Osler, whom he greatly admired and respected. This was what he had been looking for in medical education.
He discussed the possibilities with Dr. Henry M. Hurd, first superintendent of the
new Johns Hopkins Hospital. Dr. Hurd advised him to simply start over and not
try to use his other degrees for advanced standing. Just go ahead and take the four-
year course. Despite the financial strain, Groce felt he could obtain odd jobs and
somehow make ends meet. So he applied and was accepted into the original class
of the school. At last he would be able to obtain the excellent medical education
he had sought.

But it was not to be. Having completed medical school a second time and having
obtained his second M.D. degree in the spring of 1893, Groce returned home to
his father's farm in east Alabama for the summer before returning to Baltimore to
enter the Hopkins medical school that fall. He took the opportunity to visit with
friends at the second reunion of his graduating class at Auburn. He caught the
train to Montgomery, changed, and took another train east to Auburn. He stayed
with his friends the Andersons, who on Sunday morning took him with them to
the local Presbyterian church. There he heard the most wonderful voice from the

most attractive woman he could ever imagine. He requested that the Andersons introduce him to her. They did that afternoon and thoughts of continuing his medical education evaporated. Louisa Marcia Bondurant had come into his life, and whatever doubts had lingered about continuing years three through six of his medical education were resolved: he would have to go to work, establish himself, and secure a stable income so that he could marry her. He wrote to Hopkins and withdrew from the class of 15 people, the class which included Opie, McCallum, and others destined for greatness. Thus did Groce Harrison return to Talladega County, where he entered practice as a country doctor in 1894. He had, after all, told his father years before that this is what he wanted to do.

He did not enter practice with his father, but in the town of Talladega, about seven miles west of his father's farm. His practice went well, and after two years his father moved from the farm into a house in Talladega across the street from Groce's and joined him in practice. It took Groce three years to win Miss Bondurant's hand. She was a popular young lady and harbored suspicions about Groce as a Methodist.

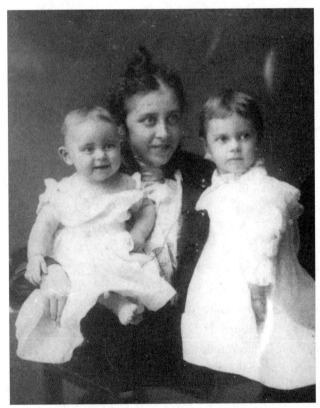

Infant Tinsley (left) with his mother Louisa Bondurant Harrison and his older sister Emily, circa 1902.

TINSLEY'S MOTHER: Louisa Bondurant, the object of Groce's affection, was at the Agricultural and Mechanical College of Alabama (now Auburn University) because her father was the first dean of the School of Agriculture there. He had attracted the university's attention by his remarkable success growing tobacco in Virginia, as well as by his education. The authorities hoped he could stimulate better tobacco crops in Alabama. Later he was invited by the government of Australia to help its farmers grow tobacco and spent several years there.

Louisa, or Lula, was a product of the old Southern aristocracy. Her father's family derived from Jean Pierre Bondurant (1677–1734), the American progenitor who was baptized into the Huguenot church at Genolhac, then rebaptized into the Catholic Church at Genolhac after revocation of the Edict of Nantes in 1685.

Jean Pierre became the first ward of his paternal uncle Andre, an apothecary, and fled from France to Aarau, Switzerland, in 1697, where he joined his uncle Pastor Guillaume Barjon and recanted his Catholicism. In 1700 Jean Pierre took a ship, *Ye Peter and Anthony*, along with about 200 other Huguenots, "aided by British charity," and settled with them in Virginia near Jamestown. He must have done well; in 1708 he sold 200 acres of land.

A descendant was Thomas Moseley Bondurant (1797–1862), who married his cousin Marcia Louisa, also *nee* Moseley (1799–1879), through whose family he obtained a large amount of Virginia farmland. The amount of land must have been vast; an 1850 assessment put its value at $77,400.

Thomas Moseley Bondurant's farm was some 40 miles south of Charlottesville, 80 miles west of Richmond, and 50 miles east of Lynchburg. Though he lived a considerable distance from Richmond, Thomas was owner, editor, and publisher of the conservative *Richmond Whig* and a bitter opponent of Southern secession. Once a week he would catch a boat down the James River to Richmond to spend a day or so there managing his newspaper and guiding its policies. He said, "Virginia must be the peacemaking state. Virginia must make peace between our brothers to the south and our cousins to the north." He was opposed to slavery but wanted to abolish it gradually to avoid major economic dislocations.

Thomas Bondurant had three sons, the eldest of whom became a physician, Dr. Lee Bondurant. (Visiting his mother's family farm as a child, Tinsley came to know Dr. Lee Bondurant, but even at an early age formed a negative opinion of him. "He was a very poorly educated doctor," he later said.) Lee Bondurant never married and produced no offspring. Thomas M. Bondurant's second son was Alexander Joseph Bondurant, nicknamed "Sandy"; he was Lula's father, Tinsley's maternal grandfather. There was a third son, George Bondurant, who married but had no children. Thus, the family farm, about 20,000 acres in Buckingham County, passed to Tinsley's maternal grandfather.

Sandy Bondurant, the one-time Auburn dean, was a tobacco grower and died on the farm in Virginia, but he was also an educated man. Tinsley knew this grandfather well and was proud of his educational heritage. He attended Hampden-Sydney College where he obtained a bachelor's degree. He then obtained a master's degree from the University of Virginia in Charlottesville. Next he obtained a third degree from Oxford, following which he went to Heidelberg and earned his fourth and final degree.

A wedding in the Bondurant family, 1903. The bride and groom are Clifford Hare and Dabney Bondurant, Tinsley's maternal aunt. Tinsley's parents, Groce Harrison Sr. and "Lula" Bondurant, are to the right of the bride looking at one another. The bride's mother, Emily Morrison Bondurant—Tinsley's maternal grandmother—is back row, far left. (Auburn fans may recognize the name Cliff Hare, as in Jordan-Hare Stadium and the Cliff Hare Award for the best Auburn athlete.) [Note: The description above is different from that in the 1997 MASA Review *article by Pittman and is based upon notations on the original photograph in the collection of the UAB Archives.]*

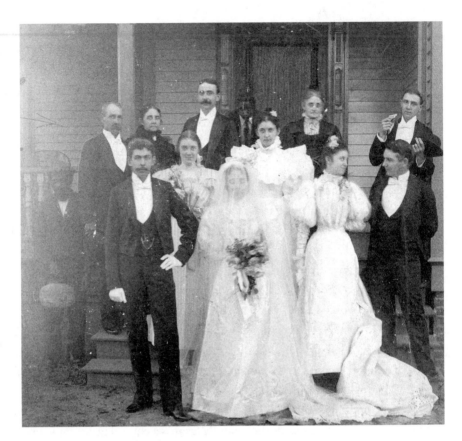

Somewhere along the line Sandy went to the Morrison School in New Market, a small town in the Shenandoah Valley of western Virginia. The school was owned and operated by James Morrison, one in a long line of Presbyterian ministers. In his school, Cyrus McCormack, Sam Houston, and the father of Woodrow Wilson all learned. James Morrison had a daughter, Emily, born in 1837 the same day Queen Victoria was crowned. Emily met Alexander Joseph "Sandy" Bondurant at the school, and they were married in 1859. One of the groomsmen, then teaching at the Virginia Military Institute, would become known as "Stonewall" Jackson; he had married Emily's first cousin. Two of Emily's brothers were also to be killed in the Civil War.

In 1872, on the family farm in Virginia, a daughter was born to Sandy and Emily Bondurant. They named her Louisa Marcia Bondurant, but called her Lula. She was to become the wife of Groce Harrison and the mother of Tinsley Randolph Harrison.

The young Groce courted this young lady of Southern aristocracy for three years, and they were finally married in Auburn on August 19, 1896. The young doctor's practice continued to grow, but even after Groce's father moved to the house across South Street in Talladega in the late '90s, they kept the family farm for income.

The newlyweds' house had been built by Mr. Seyborne Johnson in expectation of his forthcoming marriage to Miss August Brewer. However, Miss Brewer had other ideas and married Mr. J. K. Dixon from farther south in Talladega County, whereupon Mr. Johnson sold the house to Groce, who added to the south side of the house to make it a combination outpatient clinic and small hospital, with four to eight beds. A skylight was installed over a large well-lighted room (with both gas and electric lamps) for surgical procedures. The room was also well ventilated, but it is not known whether ether was used as an anesthesia there. Knowing the times, it probably was.

The Harrison Home in Talladega, Alabama, where Tinsley was born March 18, 1900. It was also the doctor's office for Groce Harrison Sr. from 1896 until the family moved to Birmingham in 1906.

Talladega in the late 1890s was a town of about 5,000 population. As such it offered immediate amenities not readily available on the Harrison farm. For

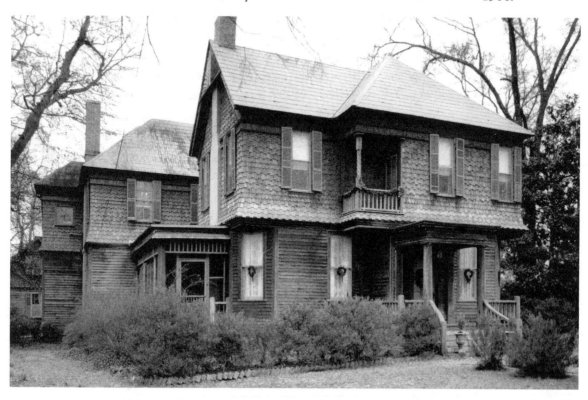

24. Tinsley's parents named their first child for the mother's mother, Emily; their second for the father's father, Tinsley (choosing for Tinsley a middle name from the mother's well-known Virginia ancestors, the Randolphs); their next son for the father, William Groce Jr.; their next daughter for the mother, Louisa Marcia; their fifth child and third son for the mother's father, Alexander Bondurant; and their sixth and last child for the father's mother, Sarah. It was a remarkably systematic and symmetrical naming of the children, commemorating both parents and all four grandparents.

example, Mayor Skaggs had installed a city water supply in 1886 and many of the newer houses had indoor flush toilets rather than the outdoor privies which remained for years longer at the farms and the outskirts of town. The cagey mayor, not wishing to stimulate resistance, did not immediately install a sewage system. Rather, he waited for the citizens to ask for one, then floated a bond issue to pay for it. The city had a working sewage system by the time Mayor Skaggs stepped down in 1891. He also managed to have the city square near the courthouse fitted with gas street lamps. And many of the houses built around that time, including the one Groce purchased from Mr. Johnson, were fitted with both pipes and wiring in the chandeliers and walls, so that the more reliable gas lighting could be used when the electricity failed. Gas lighting was gradually phased out as the electrical supply became more dependable.

The first railroad came through Talladega in 1859 and rail service continued to grow as the South began to climb out of the postwar desolation. By 1905, 16 daily passenger trains passed through the city's four railway stations. The travel time to Birmingham was at least an hour. Telephones came into use before 1900 but did not become widespread until after the Groce Harrison family moved away in 1906. Very few roads were paved; most were rutted dirt paths without even gravel. One local gentleman owned an automobile around 1900, a small electric car which ran smoothly and quietly over the dirt streets. However, he moved away around the time Queen Victoria died in 1902, leaving Talladega with no cars.

On October 22, 1897, Emily Bondurant Harrison was born. On March 18, 1900, a son was born—Tinsley Randolph Harrison. Two years later, William Groce Harrison Jr. was born (he attended Johns Hopkins and became a physician). Groce and Louisa ultimately had three more children: Louisa Dabney Harrison (1907); Alexander Bondurant Harrison (whom they called Bondurant, 1909); and Sarah Elizabeth Harrison (1912). All three of the girls later married physicians.[24]

At the turn of the century there were three other doctors among Talladega's 5,056 residents: E. P. Cason, N. R. Newman, and W. R. Bishop. The town and the surrounding areas provided enough business for all and practice went well for Groce. In 1901 he was selected to be Annual Orator for the Medical Association of the State of Alabama.

In 1900 Drs. Groce and John T. Harrison rented the J. M. Lewis home in the Highlands and opened a private hospital, Talladega's first, later known as the Nurses Home of Citizens Hospital. The other local doctors used it for occasional patients who needed it and could afford to pay. The hospital had one nurse and an average daily census of four patients. The hospital remained open until March 1, 1905. When it closed, J. T. Harrison returned to private practice.

During this time Groce continued to practice chiefly in his office at home and by making house calls. He enjoyed medicine, but it was a demanding mistress. His father was 70 years old, and although he was healthy, Groce was on call a grueling 24 hours a day, seven days a week. Further, between 1894 and 1902 he experienced four severe bouts of lobar pneumonia, each episode worse than the last. This was a time when lobar pneumonia was a very serious illness with a mortality rate of 10 percent or more. During the fourth attack, Groce very nearly died. The family was worried, but it was clear that Groce did not have tuberculosis. Each of these episodes of pneumonia followed exposure to cold, rain, and sleet while making house calls. This was a time when such exposure was believed to precipitate bouts of pneumonia. After the fourth attack, Groce became concerned about his ability to continue his current mode of practice and began thinking of other options.

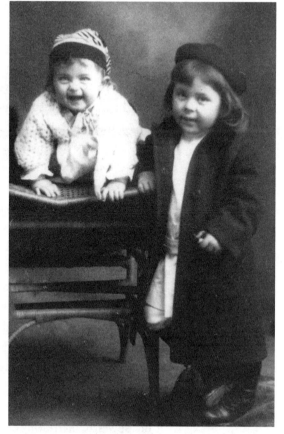

Tinsley (right) with his younger brother, Groce Jr., circa 1904.

In 1904 Groce was invited by the authorities at the Medical College of Alabama in Mobile to become chief of medicine there.[25] This was a welcome recognition, reflecting his local renown as one of the best-educated and able physicians in the state and region. He consulted his mentor, William Osler.

Osler knew Groce's wife and admired her, jibing, "Harrison, you're that fellow who outmarried himself." Groce took a train to Baltimore and met again with Osler in person. Osler advised Groce strongly to give up general practice and asked, "Harrison, how many children do you have now?"

Groce answered, "Three."

"Harrison, how much money do you have?" Osler asked.

"Not much."

"Can you afford three years in Germany for study?"

"I can afford one," Groce said.

25. Attempts in Mobile, Talladega, and Birmingham to find documentation of this offer have thus far been unproductive.

"Harrison, are any of these children boys?"

"Two," Groce said.

Osler considered before saying, "Harrison, get into a small subspecialty that does not involve exposure to all kinds of weather. Go abroad and get a year's training, if that is all you can afford. And train those boys to be teachers of medicine!"

The question was answered.

At that time, the world's most advanced medicine existed in Germany and Austria. Groce followed Osler's advice. During his childhood Tinsley was tutored in German by a young woman, Fraulein Schepke, from Konigsberg, Germany. Schepke was hired by his father for the purpose of making young Tinsley and the other children fluent in German. Tinsley recalled that she shocked the family one evening not long after she had arrived when, at the end of the meal while still at the table, she took out and lit a cigarette.

"My mother was something close to a saint," Tinsley later recalled. "My father was a man of tremendous character and intellect. But he was very rigid and inflexible. He was bitterly opposed to alcohol, since so many of his relatives were alcoholics. He also opposed smoking." In fact, Groce was an ardent prohibitionist, which led him to lose much of his practice during the prohibition era and "caused some strain between himself and a number of his most intimate friends." Groce was a man of principle, rigid and uncompromising on things he considered right and wrong. Tinsley later often emphasized his father's principled stance on work and life. It was an interesting emphasis for a doctor who would later esteem "principles" as the most important thing in medicine and who would title his text *Principles of Internal Medicine*.

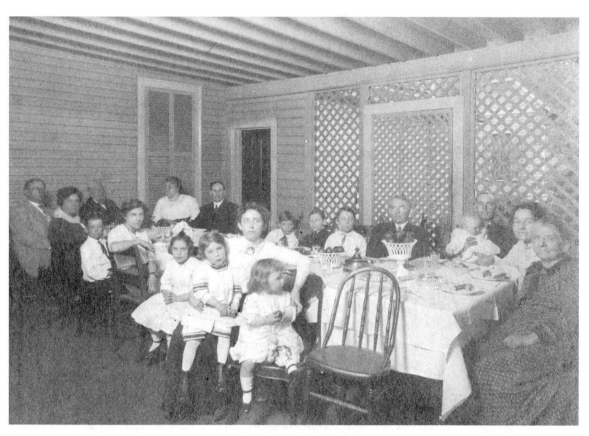

The Harrison family celebrates the 76th birthday of patriarch Dr. John Tinsley Harrison Jr., Munford, Alabama, 1910. Seated far left at the head of the table (next to the house) is the patriarch and seated far right at the other end is his wife, Sarah Groce Harrison. Facing the camera across the table is (the man in glasses) their son Dr. W. Groce Harrison Sr. To the left are his sons, next to him is William Groce Jr., and next to him, in the dark shirt, is the eldest son, Tinsley.

3

Growing Up in Alabama

1900–1916

Tinsley's earliest memory revolved around the many names of God. "I believe that learning to distinguish between the synonyms God, Jehovah, Adonai, the Lord, and Dr. Osler are my earliest memories," he said. It sounds like a joke, but he explained that all those terms were used with equal reverence around the house and at the supper table. Maybe Harrison really did think that Dr. Osler was another name for God.[1]

When he was about four years old, he had a severe case of scarlet fever, during which he was treated at home by his father. He remembered being told to stay in bed despite the fact that he felt fairly well, and he remembered the severe sore throat, the strawberry tongue, and later the extensive cutaneous exfoliation that dotted so many children in crimson, typical of scarlet fever. His only difficulty during this illness was a severe crick in the neck. His head was drawn so severely to the right that his mother and father had to help him turn over in bed. He had a high fever. To ease his boredom and discomfort, his mother read the story about the horse Black Beauty, which he loved so much that she read it over and over. They finished four complete readings before he was able to be up and about.

The studious side of young Tinsley's life was closely interwoven with his family's religious life. Every Sunday morning the family embarked for the 9:30 Sunday School classes at the Presbyterian Church, one class for the men, one for the women, one for the older children, and one for Tinsley and his friends. These were completed around 10:30, leaving a half-hour to prepare for the major church service of the week starting at 11. Tinsley tried to concentrate, but he sometimes ended up entertaining himself by counting the number of pieces in the stained glass of each window

1. Osler remained a spiritual presence with Tinsley throughout his life. His youngest son, Dr. John Bondurant Harrison, kept a letter from Osler to Groce dated January 10, 1910. Osler enjoyed his association with doctors far and wide, and his salutation "Dear Alabama

46

in the church—an early indication of quantitative interests. This temptation to quantify was particularly strong during the long pastoral prayer by the preacher, a very Presbyterian tradition consuming five minutes or more. Despite these lapses of attention, Tinsley was deeply impressed by the Bible and its wonderful stories and lessons. Later in life he said that his mother taught him from two sources: the Christian Bible and the works of Shakespeare.

After church the family had the most elaborate meal of the week, and they always ate together at a large table. Tinsley remembered these as times of excellent family fellowship—a bit formal, perhaps, but always in good spirits. The food was superb, served in large bowls filled with a great variety of sweet potatoes, ham, corn, cooked wild turkey or venison, cauliflower, and a host of other dishes that kept coming round and round the table.

After the meal, Tinsley was required to go to his room and memorize an assignment. The assignments were one or two lines of scripture, until he was about five years old. His mother or Grandmother Bondurant would read the verses to him, and he would repeat them over and over until he got them right. By age seven, he would memorize several verses from the Bible. Around age nine or 10, he would be required to memorize whole chapters from the Bible, such as the 23rd Psalm, the 100th Psalm, the 121st Psalm, and later longer chapters—First Corinthians 13, the 19th Psalm, John 14, or multiple chapters, such as the Sermon on the Mount. His mother would also review old assignments at random and require Tinsley to repeat them or write them down. He was not permitted to go out to play on Sunday afternoons until this task had been satisfactorily completed. In later years Tinsley said that he sometimes awoke at night with the old verses rumbling through his head. Seventy years later, Tinsley considered these segments from the Christian Bible "a guiding point in my life." He frequently read the Bible in bed at night just before going to sleep, even through by then he claimed to be an agnostic, perhaps even an atheist.

His mother's other intellectual orientation gave him an appreciation of Shakespeare. After Groce moved the family moved to Birmingham, Lula was president of the Shakespeare Club for many years, and she imbued in Tinsley a lifelong interest in the Bard. In his later years he could quote long passages from Shakespeare flawlessly.

TWO GREAT DIFFERENCES BETWEEN the late 19th and late 20th centuries were light and sound. In rural areas, when it was dark, it was pitch black except for the lights

Student" is a reference to his earlier essay on Dr. Samuel Bassett, an obscure but bright physician in rural Alabama whose examination and exposition of fevers in the South attracted Osler's attention. In January 1895 Osler presented one of "his best biographical essays to the Historical Society of the [Johns Hopkins] Hospital." How he came to be interested in this obscure Alabama physician is recounted by Harvey Cushing in his biography *The Life of Sir William Osler*, vol. I (London: Oxford Univ. Press, 1941) 411–12. The Bassett essay was among a series published as a book in 1896 and a copy was given by Osler to Canby Robinson at Hopkins in December 1902. Robinson was later chief of medicine at Vanderbilt, and in this capacity hired Tinsley as chief medical resident. In 1928 Robinson gave the book to another member of Vanderbilt's Department of Medicine, C. Sidney Burwell (later dean at Harvard Medical School), who gave it to Tinsley in 1958, who passed it on to his son in 1971.

2. There were no highways, in fact; as late as 1895 there was not a single mile of paved road in Alabama.

3. The episode of the boy with the broken leg is recorded on an audiotape, now in the UAB Archives, of Harrison with the author.

of nature—the pale moon, the flickering stars, and the seasonal glow of the fireflies. Sometimes large wood fires would reflect off low-lying clouds and shed a ghostly pallor over the countryside, but this was rare. There were no electric lights or other lights, except oil lamps in houses or fires in the fields or woods. The land held a creeping quiet. There were few sounds except those of nature—no airplanes, cars, or humming power lines. Sounds were owls, whip-poor-wills, or chuck will's widows— no trucks on highways,[2] no automobiles, no electric or other motors—only a rare horse or buggy, and even more rarely a distant train with its lonely, piercing whistle.

Tinsley did not remember making house calls with his father in Birmingham, though he did watch him perform tonsillectomies and adenoidectomies. In Talladega, he had sometimes accompanied his father or grandfather. He once went with his father on a house call to see a boy who had fallen out of a tree and sustained a comminuted fracture of the leg. It took perhaps half-an-hour to get to the boy's house with the horse and buggy. The break was obvious, with the leg distorted at an angle and bones sticking through the skin. The boy was writhing in great pain, but just a few minutes after Dr. Harrison gave him a shot of morphine, the boy became calm and rested quietly as they took him home and put him on the kitchen table. They cleaned the area thoroughly with soap and water, dried it carefully, then the boy's father stood at one end of the kitchen table and held him by the shoulders, arms under the boy's armpits, and Dr. Groce stood at the other end and pulled carefully but firmly until the bones were again within the skin and aligned. Dr. Harrison applied a simple splint and wrapped the leg. There were no X-rays, laboratory tests, antibiotics, special drugs, or ancillary technologies to assist—just the obvious diagnosis, and the just as obvious treatment. Tinsley later saw the boy, who had recovered without a limp, with no deformity or malfunction, without antibiotics or other modern drugs or instruments.[3] On the way back after setting the boy's leg, it was dark, quiet. "Morphine is a wonderful drug," his father had told him. "Without it I wouldn't practice medicine." Then his father began to quiz him about the stars. There were no cities or other lights to dim the stars scattered like a thick shower of sparks across the bright night. The father and son talked about the celestial bodies in the clear moonless winter sky. It remained a vivid memory.

Osler's advice to Groce to study abroad was probably motivated by a desire to see his young friend's career and family reach a higher peak than would have been possible if Groce had simply gone to join the medical faculty at Mobile. Even before the Flexner study and report, Osler would have been aware of the irreversible upgrading and improvements occurring in medical education (Ludmerer), as well as the agitation in organized medicine (such as the American Medical Association), the problems at the Mobile school as related by Groce, and the coming crackdown on poor medical schools. Osler was certainly connected well enough to know that in 1904 the newly formed AMA Council on Medical Education under Dr. Arthur Dean Bevan was planning a major assault on low-quality medical schools, with the goal of a sharp upgrading of the few schools capable of being improved and the closing of the others. He was also sufficiently perspicacious to see that the Mobile school was likely to fall into the latter category.

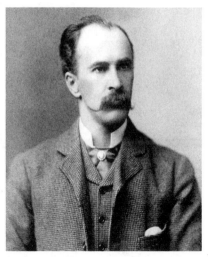

Sir William Osler, about 1880.

Groce's health—recurrent pneumonias aggravated by making house calls by primitive transportation in all sorts of weather—was also a factor in the move. His continuing in general rural medical practice was not an option. Osler liked Harrison, "his Alabama student," and these may have been Osler's thoughts when he advised his young physician friend to enter a smaller specialty with less rigorous personal demands and to try to make superior physicians of his sons. Osler also mentioned that his sons should be superior teachers; Tinsley always remembered and emphasized this.

In the summer of 1904 Groce and Lula Harrison traveled by railroad and steamship to Vienna, then the capital of the Austro-Hungarian Empire and a major center for the new scientific medicine. There Groce studied EENT, the specialty of eye, ear, nose, and throat. Tinsley later commented that his father always disliked this specialty, because it was not particularly oriented toward scholarship and reading, but toward action and operating on patients. In later years, when Tinsley wanted to make fun of a specialty, he always picked on EENT, and his sarcasm and vitriol sometimes amazed his listeners. He probably felt inured to criticism for this by his father's being in the specialty.

WHILE THEIR PARENTS WERE abroad, Young Emily, Tinsley, and the baby Groce Jr. were left at Variety Shade, the Virginia plantation owned by Louisa's father, Alexander J. Bondurant. The baby was cared for by the domestic help, especially a motherly black woman, as was customary there and then.

During their year on the Bondurant farm, the two older children were taught privately by their grandmother, Emily Morrison Bondurant, whose father, the Presbyterian minister Reverend James Morrison, had operated the Morrison School in New Market, Virginia. Emily Bondurant was a scholar and an excellent teacher. "My grandmother was one of the most cultured individuals I have ever known," Tinsley later said, "the daughter of an impecunious Presbyterian minister who learned Greek, Latin, and a good deal more in her father's home. . . . An example of her general culture was her manner of death." She had moved to Birmingham when her husband died and lived then with the Groce Harrisons at their house on Cliff Road (which Tinsley later inherited). She loved to read the Bible, and in 1926, when Emily Bondurant was 89, she died one night and was found the next morning with a New Testament on her chest—in the original Greek. Tinsley always revered this special teacher who so inspired him with her learning and love while his parents were overseas between the summers of 1904 and 1905, and forever after that.

Life on grandfather's farm was pleasant. Tinsley was given a horse for his fifth birthday. He also had as a companion a black youngster named Oscar Bondurant, three years older than Tinsley, the son of one of the farm laborers. The two boys were constant companions that year, and they maintained contact as long as Oscar lived; when he grew up, Oscar went to work in the West Virginia coal mines and died of black lung in the late 1930s.

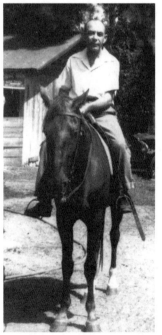

Tinsley at a "dude ranch," 1948.

For the rest of his life Tinsley loved horses, though he did not ride much in later years. His mother, Louisa, was an avid horsewoman, usually riding side-saddle. She was also active in golf and other sports and stimulated young Tinsley's interest in these. She pushed Tinsley to play golf, but tennis was his main sport, also largely attributable to maternal encouragement. His father Groce was not very interested in sports.

IN 1905 THE ELDER Harrisons returned from abroad and spent most of the next year winding up the practice in Talladega. In April 1906, one month after Tinsley's sixth birthday, the family left the country with its primitive beauty and moved to Birmingham, into the house on the high side of Cliff Road. Another house was being built across the street, and Groce negotiated with the builder to modify the plan and add an upper room. He then bought it and occupied it a few months after moving to Birmingham. The address of this second house, on the lower side of the road, was 3818 Cliff Road. The house now bears a historical marker: "The Harrison House." It was to this house on Cliff Road (now numbered 4142) that Tinsley would return in 1950 to help build the UAB Medical Center. (The house remained in the family until 1962, when it was given to the University of Alabama and Tinsley and Betty moved to the Plaza Apartments on Country Club Road.)

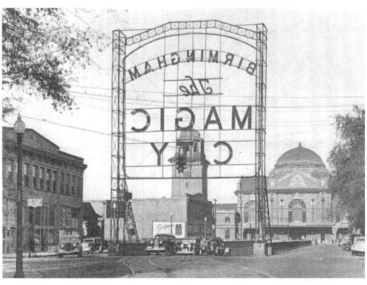

The 1906 move to Birmingham was part of a larger investment into the world of medicine by Groce, for himself and for his family. Why did Groce choose Birmingham as the place to move his family and change the arc of his and their lives? No records remain to settle this question.

Birmingham, the "Magic City," in the early 1920s.

In 1850, Jefferson County had a population around 9,000, only half that of Talladega County. But by 1900, Birmingham, the largest city in Jefferson County, had become one of the biggest in the South, with the population of the county expanding to around 140,000. More people, more business, more opportunity. Birmingham was a postwar city founded in 1871 because of the confluence there of the three critical ingredients for making iron: ore, coal, and limestone. Groce saw that the new iron and steel mills in Birmingham were making the city a major industrial center likely to grow and prosper for years to come. He could see the population of Jefferson County growing rapidly on visits to the city, a trajectory which would take it to more than 226,000 residents in 1910, 310,000 by 1920, and 431,000 by 1930—a time when the population of the entire state of Florida had just passed one million.

Birmingham's growing steel industry was the major economic and social force in the region. The city's abrupt growth and relative prosperity in the last two decades of the 19th and the early decades of the 20th century were so dramatic they prompted the nickname "The Magic City." Opportunities for practice in a specialty were much greater in such a location than in a small rural town like Talladega, pleasant as life was there.

Their first year in Birmingham, Groce participated in the founding of the

4. E. B. Carmichael, Personal communication, 1974. Recent attempts to find records of a "Dr. Bliss" working in Birmingham at that time have been unsuccessful. However, it is quite possible that he never obtained a license or joined any medical society, but simply "practiced medicine" unattached to the rest of the profession.

Protective Life Insurance Company and was its first physician. He was also on the finance committee, where he learned a great deal about making investments. He never bought stocks or bonds, however. Instead he bought second mortgages, which paid 8 percent.

Groce Harrison became prominent in Birmingham medical circles. Sometime around 1912 a conversation occurred which Tinsley remembered well. His father was speaking on the phone. "We should close it before somebody else forces us to close it. No, we need to take the initiative and close it ourselves." They were talking about their medical school, and it really was *their* medical school. This was the Birmingham Medical College, a stock company paying its shareholders 6 percent annual dividends. The *Flexner Report* had been published in 1910, and this school had been recommended for closure and termination. Flexner had recommended that the other significant medical school in the state at Mobile be converted to a two-year pre-clinical school and moved to Tuscaloosa to become an integral part of the University of Alabama. In 1919 a prominent pediatrician at Mobile, Dr. Daniel McCall, was made dean of the Medical College of Alabama, a post he held for one year. He resigned after accomplishing the school's move to Tuscaloosa in 1920. A Dr. Montgomery was on the chemistry faculty at Tuscaloosa at the time, and he was dispatched to Mobile to pack the medical school's equipment, pathology specimens, museum pieces, and other material brought years before from France by Dr. Josiah Nott. Montgomery later told Dr. Emmett B. Carmichael, who joined the biochemistry department in 1927, that the local citizenry in Mobile had been so hostile about the move of "their medical school" to Tuscaloosa that they refused to help, and he was at times even concerned about his own safety.

In 1915, the old Birmingham Medical College, with its control of the Hillman Hospital as its teaching hospital guaranteed for 99 years (until 2007), closed. There was one final party at the time the members of the class of 1915 finished school and were given their M.D. degrees—the actual certificates. It was a convivial time, and the dean sat at a table signing each of the certificates as the clerk handed them to him one by one. As the dean conversed with others and absentmindedly signed the certificates, the clerk, a Mr. Bliss, handed him one inscribed with his own name, though he had never formally matriculated in the school. The dean blithely signed, the clerk removed the certificate, and he practiced medicine in the Birmingham area the rest of his life. Apparently he was a reasonably good doctor.[4]

During their new life in Birmingham, Lula and Groce had three more children: Louisa Dabney Harrison, Alexander Bondurant Harrison, and Sarah Elizabeth Harrison. All seemed quite normal except the son, whom they called Bondurant. He had a distinctly blue hue to his skin, lips, finger and toe nail beds, and his eyes. He also had some cardiac murmurs which the doctors did not understand; he probably had some heart disorder.

Thus, Groce's family, in the naming of their children, repeated the symmetry characteristic of his own generation. First there was the mother's mother, Emily. Then there was the father's father, Tinsley. Next came the father Groce and the mother Louisa, followed by the mother's father Bondurant, and finally the father's mother Sarah—to complete the pattern, the families were forced to have at least six children.

In the fall of 1906 Tinsley started grammar school at Lakeview School. He started at age six despite the fact that the official starting age was seven. "My father pulled some strings," he explained. Tinsley was fond of his teachers and remembered their names throughout life. His first-grade teacher was Miss Carelton, an attractive lady in her late forties. Like most of the teachers, Miss Carelton was a spinster. There were about 40 pupils in the class. He remembered, "She simply loved her students, and they loved her." He was the youngest and smallest member of the class. She noticed his young age and at one time his agitation. She came to his desk and asked him in a whisper, "Do you want to go to the bathroom?"

"Yes, ma'am."

"Then hold up one finger. If you want to go for a longer time, hold up two fingers."

He also remembered how solicitous she was for his intellectual development. One day in the middle of his first year she said, "Tinsley, we are going to move you to another room for the rest of the year. You can learn more there." With this announcement his books were taken from his desk and moved to the room next door, where a more advanced class was being taught. Unbeknownst to him, she had discussed this with his parents, told them he was ahead of the class and bored, and recommended that he be moved up. They agreed to the move. This happened four times during Tinsley's grade school career, enabling him to complete the 11 grades in nine years. He started grade school in September 1906 and finished in May 1915. He finished the seventh grade in January 1912, the mid-year completion the result of his multiple advances. So for six months he attended an intermediate school, the Paul Hayne School at the corner of Fifth Avenue and 20th Street South, many years later the location of the Kirklin Clinic, the main outpatient facility for the medical faculty at UAB.

As much as Tinsley admired and loved Miss Carelton, he did not consider her his best teacher. This was Miss Thornton, his high school Latin teacher. Miss Thornton was a beautiful woman more than 70 years old, tall and dignified, stern but gentle with her pupils. At 18 she had been engaged when the war broke out. Her fiance joined the Confederate army and was killed in the fighting. Miss Thornton remained faithful to him the rest of her life and never married. She always wore black, with high black collars on her neck. "She was really a beautiful woman, beautifully groomed always. She made Latin the most thrilling subject I ever studied." He was told later that he made the highest scores in Latin in the history of the school. She loved her subject and knew the literature of the Latin authors intimately. She loved her young students as well, Tinsley remembered.

Every morning, the first activity was Bible reading and prayer. The Jewish and Catholic children were not required to participate, but were occasionally invited to lead the class in prayer themselves. Harrison said later that this was not important to him, since he had this at his home anyhow. But he thought it represented a democratic approach, which invited tolerance and participation.

During the first seven grades one teacher taught all subjects. From the eighth grade until graduation at the end of the eleventh grade, the teachers specialized, each teaching a few related subjects. Tinsley was worst in music, drawing, and handwriting, but especially in conduct. He loved to talk and seemed unable to stop, even in the face of reprimands. He never recalled receiving anything other than A's in other subjects: English, mathematics, geography, history, composition, and so on.

In grade school in Birmingham, Tinsley played baseball, basketball, and football, though in a peculiarly Harrisonian way. Because of his young age (two to four or more full years younger than most of his classmates) and his small size, he played backfield on the football team of the Lakeview Grammar School while he was in his last year of high school; he was about the same size as his sixth-grade teammates. He was proud of having drop-kicked four field goals in one game while a ringer on the grammar school team.

The school years progressed happily, and Tinsley always brought home excellent grades. Usually they were the top in the class. However, there were a few occasions when another boy beat him out for the top grade. When report card time came, each month, his father would ask, "Son, how were the grades?"

"Well," Tinsley often answered, "I had the highest in the class in all subjects except for one other boy."

"Who was that?"

"Julian Sachs."

"Well," he remembered his father's saying, "Don't worry about that. Those Jewish boys are just smart and well-organized and hard-working, and if you're up there with them, you'll be okay." Tinsley and Julian were friends as children and throughout their lives. In later years Julian lived in Florida and frequently invited Tinsley down for visits.

His family tried to keep him in the company of the best people in high school. He attended Lakeview School until another school closed and students from the textile mill section of town started attending. His parents, however, did not want him associating with uncouth people uninterested in education. For the following two years, Tinsley attended South Highlands School until a new school was built in Avondale for the millworkers' families, whereupon he returned to Lakeview. His classmates at South Highlands School included Yutch McClellan (later CEO of St. Regis paper company), Rucker Agee, Bob Wilkerson, the Barrons, and others.

Although he was with "the better people," as his parents called them, in school he had to defend himself. Once he was threatened by John Terry Badham, a larger and stronger classmate. Badham's older brothers had been on the boxing team at Yale and had taught him the rudiments of boxing. Badham used his boxing technique to good effect; he had a method of rising suddenly from a crouch and swinging, an attack the smaller Tinsley could not withstand. So Tinsley lost. Immediately after the fight, however, Badham announced, "Anybody who wants to fight Tinsley will have to lick me first!" From that time on Tinsley and Badham were friends, even 60 years later. As Terry was the largest and toughest boy in the class, Tinsley was free to return to his studies. The other toughs avoided him.

Tinsley's early plans for his future leaned toward law. There were several literary societies in Tinsley's next school, Phillips High, and Tinsley belonged to the Yancey Society, named for William Lowndes Yancey, an Alabama politician and one of the most ardent of the Southern secessionists before the war. This steered Tinsley to the debating society, and he enjoyed debating. Also, several of his relatives were lawyers.

TINSLEY FELT THAT HIS mother exerted the major influence on his life until he was about seven. After that, his father took over.

While Tinsley was a youth growing up in Birmingham, and perhaps earlier in Talladega, Groce made a habit of taking the children for walks every Sunday afternoon. Usually they went from the house on Cliff Road down a mile on Highland Avenue, or into more wooded areas. When Tinsley was about eight, Groce initiated an annual hike lasting a week or more in the late spring or early summer. They would camp out or stay at inns along the way. There were other short family hikes during the year, but this was the big one, and Tinsley looked forward to it with eager anticipation.

The general objective was to walk east from Birmingham to the farm near Munford, more than 50 miles away. Sometimes they walked all the way to Atlanta, 150 miles away. Groce, whom they always called Father, took his two older sons, Tinsley and Groce Jr. on these walks (in that era, it would have been unseemly for a young lady like Emily to go on such a prolonged hike, and the youngest son, Bondurant, was not physically able).

These long walks went on for six or seven years, and Tinsley came to look forward to them. During these walks his father would pick some subject, usually biology, but sometimes geology, astronomy, or some other area. On one walk Groce would concentrate on trees and plants. On another, birds. On still another, he might discuss mammals, reptiles and amphibians, or insects, and other animals. Years later Tinsley learned that his father spent months preparing for these walks, steeping himself in the knowledge and lore of the intended subject, so that he could be an adequate teacher for his children.

Groce's practice in Birmingham was thriving. He was sent patients not only by Dr. Thigpen, his mentor in Montgomery, but by other doctors in the Birmingham area who had come to appreciate his medical expertise and his winning but dignified ways with patients. He could also leave his practice in the hands of colleagues for a week or so without fear of losing his patients.

Groce wanted his children to learn about nature, or "Nature with a capital N," as he called it and had come to appreciate it, the source of our understanding of the universe and our place in it. Groce was well-read and skeptical of what he considered narrow, dogmatic, unscientific views of these subjects. Impressed by the rapid advances being made in medicine, he believed that progress depended on a scientific approach to understanding and applying the Laws of Nature.[5] Groce read all the time. We do not know exactly which books he read, but he was well-versed in the current science and biology texts. So, it is likely that Groce was familiar with the two-volume work *Diseases of the Interior Valley of North America* and the great reception given its physician-naturalist author, Daniel Drake, by the American Medical Association in the mid-1850s. Drake's was one of many works detailing how man is intimately a part of Nature and subject to its glories and problems. Medicine, therefore, must take into account this fact of man's being part of the natural universe. Given Groce's later interest in the history of medicine, he was probably also familiar with *A Century of American Medicine*, a book published in 1876 by John Shaw Billings, who helped develop the new Hopkins medical school. Billings's book emphasized Drake's importance in the development of medicine in America. But in addition to the science, Groce wanted his children to appreciate the beauty and simple complexities of nature as well as the serenity of the forests and streams away from the bustle of the burgeoning city.[6]

The family nature walks were some of Tinsley's fondest memories of his childhood.

6. Daniel Drake, *Diseases of the Interior Valley of North America* (1854). J. S. Billings and E. H. Clarke, *A Century of American Medicine* (Philadelphia: Lea Publications, 1876) 314.

4

Nature Study in the South

1912

It was spring 1912 as Tinsley turned 12 and it was time for the annual Harrison trek for the study of natural history. The excitement grew as the boys and their father gathered around the camping list on the kitchen table. "Tinsley, you check off the things we already have in the stack," Groce said.

Tinsley handled the various items as he said their names out loud. "Baked beans, Vienna sausages, a jar of beets, smoked ham, fishing lines, hooks, sinkers, and corks, matches in a rubber case, hunting knife for each, pocket knife, frying pan with folding handle, forks and spoons, and the other food you have over there." He paused. "What about the blankets and tent?"

"They're already in my knapsack with the heavy tins of beans," Groce responded. They were ready.

On Friday morning, Lula drove them in a buggy over to the Atlanta Highway, which was a dirt/clay road until it was paved in the 1930s. There they bid her goodbye, threw on their canvas knapsacks, and headed east on foot. As they trudged along there was not too much dust, since it had rained a good deal the previous week. Tinsley loved the tall trees lining the narrow road, making it dark and shady. He was impressed that his father seemed to know all their names: tulip poplars with interesting blossoms high above the ground, white oaks, red oaks, dogwoods, sweet gums, all the kinds of pines, junipers, and groves of pecan trees as they passed a farm. His father pointed out how to distinguish the trees by differences in the bark and the shapes of the leaves and flowers or the terrain where they were growing. On the ground Tinsley was particularly fascinated by the pitcher plants, which actually ate insects, and by the ferns on the sides of creeks, with their seeds under the leaves.[1]

1. Groce probably also read the writings of William Bartram, which described much of the plant and animal life of southeast America of those times. Perhaps later he also read of John Bartram and John Muir's 1,000-mile walk to the Gulf.

They walked for an hour before coming to a creek. They sat down to eat an apple and to drink water from their canteens. The canteen water was already a little warm, so Groce said it would be fine to drink from the cool stream. At home or in most other circumstances this strict physician would have insisted on boiling the water before drinking it, but he knew the area; this particular creek originated from a spring on a farm several miles north, with no farms or villages upstream between the farm and where they were sitting. Most of the water in Alabama was safe to drink then, and there was plenty of it. Alabama had more miles of navigable waterways than any other state.

As they drank there was a nearby squawk, and a huge bird rose majestically. Tinsley rushed toward it, but the bird wheeled and flew upstream with slow flaps of its wings.

"What was it?" asked Father.

"A heron, I think. I've seen a couple out in ponds near the farm, but never so close as that!" Tinsley said.

"Do you know what kind of heron it is?"

"Well, it was sorta blue, so maybe it was a blue heron—a big blue heron."

"Very good," his father said. "The books call it a great blue heron, and there is a picture of it in a book we have at home. It's the biggest around here, but there are lots of other kinds of herons as well. All those birds have two names in Latin—one for the genus or general sort of heron, and one for the species, or the very specific kind of heron this particular one is. Scientists need those Latin names because different people in different places may have their own local names for a particular kind of bird, and the scientists want to be sure of what they are talking about. For example, this heron was a sort of bluish gray, so some people might call it a 'gray heron,' and you called it a 'big blue heron.' But the Latin name *Ardea herodias* is something carefully thought out then agreed upon by committees of experts, so that when it is used, it is very clear to all concerned exactly what they mean." All this seemed quite reasonable to Tinsley, and he trusted everything Father told him as absolutely accurate. So he stowed it all in the back of his young but retentive and active brain.

As they walked, with frequent stops at copses to look at bushes and flowers, his father seemed to know more about birds than anyone Tinsley or Groce Jr. had ever heard. Birds seemed the main emphasis on this walk, but Father knew nearly as much about plants, insects, rocks, frogs and salamanders, spiders, worms, weather, and clouds. They saw several deer, one fox, some muskrats, beaver dams, and some small mammals. There were lots of squirrels, and Tinsley found the large, dark fox squirrels particularly interesting. They watched one afternoon as a bald eagle high in the sky dived repeatedly at an osprey carrying a fish until at last the osprey dropped the fish, whereupon the eagle swooped below the osprey and caught the fish in midair—an amazing but not rare occurrence.

THEY WANDERED THROUGH A lush world already diminishing due to the encroachment of man. Many of the species they saw were dying out as they watched.

Tinsley already knew the obvious birds of the garden: robins, mockingbirds, cardinals, towhees, the few English sparrows, and others frequent in the city, as well as the many bluebirds and shrikes of the fields. His father had told him of the passenger pigeons, which had been so numerous that when they roosted at night, the combined weight of a flock was sometimes so heavy that it broke the limbs of the trees. They were not yet extinct—the last one died in the Cincinnati Zoo in 1914—but for practical purposes they were already gone. Old "Doctor T" Harrison, Groce's father, had told Tinsley of seeing Carolina parakeets—the only parrot native to the eastern United States—as a young man once in South Carolina. These, too, were now gone. On these trips they often saw "English sparrows" (which were neither English nor sparrows) around farm houses, but they never saw a European bird called the starling, said to be increasingly common in the urban North, nor any small white herons washed with buffy brown on their backs, known as the cattle egrets. These came many years later and were common by the century's end.

They were walking through a particularly wet and shady forest of huge trees when they heard a loud high call like a musical instrument that said in a nasal tone, "Pait . . . pait . . . pait!" Almost immediately a huge form crossed the narrow slit in the forest above the road—black with white wings and a black stripe running out across the middle of the underside of each wing, and a prominent tail and bright red crest. Tinsley thought it must have been two feet long! His father became quite excited. "Do you know what that was?" he asked.

At that moment an elderly black man passed traveling in the opposite direction. "That was a Lord God-A'mighty bird, tha's what that was." And it was, for a "Lord God-A'mighty bird" was the local name for the ivory-billed woodpecker (as well as the similar pileated woodpecker), sometimes eaten for its excellent flesh and now in the new century drifting into oblivion, dependent on the large tracts of untended Southern forests and swamps, now disappearing. By the 1950s it would be gone forever.[2]

As they topped the crest of a hill late in the morning, the dirt road narrowed, and a field of rocks and sand lay on one side. Near one of the large rocks was a snake warming himself in the morning sun—a very, very large snake. His father whispered to the boys to keep absolutely quiet and still. They watched as he picked up a pine limb lying nearby and crept up on the snake from behind the two-foot-high boulder. He suddenly pounced and brought the limb down across the back of the snake with a strong blow, which broke the limb into several pieces. The snake writhed and wriggled, its back broken. It could not slither away. Groce grabbed another limb and struck the snake again near the head, then he quickly slipped his hand to the snake's neck immediately behind its head, where he was safe from its bite. He held up his kill. "It's a rattler," he said, which was apparent from the buzzing noise coming from the dying beast's tail. As he squeezed just behind the head, the snake opened its mouth wide, exposing the now unsheathed fangs that deliver the poison. Later Tinsley would learn that such poison, being biologically active, was the source of many valuable enzymes, and could perhaps even be the source of useful drugs.

They sat down in a more shady spot a few yards down the road, and Groce took out his hunting knife and slit the snake's skin from its chin to the end of its tail. He proceeded to remove the skin from the carcass. The meat looked clean, white. He put salt on the skin, which, still moist, he rolled up and placed in his knapsack, explaining to the boys that when they returned home he would give it to a taxidermist, who would put arsenic or some other better preservative on it, since this was a nice specimen nearly six feet long. Groce took a few pieces of the meat and wrapped them in oiled paper to cook later that day. He wanted to show the boys that the snake was, in fact, edible. However, when he tried to give the rest to a farmer at the next house they passed, the old gentleman declined with the statement that it wasn't fit food for humans.

"Besides," the old farmer said, "didn't the Bible say you shouldn't eat snakes?"

LATER THEY STOPPED AGAIN at a stream for lunch. Mother had fixed sandwiches and milk, which were still fresh despite the heat. As they sat, the warblers played in the trees across the water, and bream plied their way upstream.

2. There were non-definitive reports of sightings in 2004 in Arkansas and 2006 in Florida. There is a very good recording of the Ivory-billed Woodpecker on the CD-ROM *North American Birds* of the famous R. T. Peterson series, published by Houghton Mifflin Interactive, 120 Beacon Street, Somerville, MA 02143, in the 1990s. Audubon thought the Ivory-bill's call resembled "pait, pait, pait." Peterson thought it was more like "kent, kent, kent, kent." The last secure sightings were in the early 1950s in Louisiana.

After lunch they lay back to rest for a short nap. Looking up at the sky Tinsley imagined animals from the shapes of the cumulus clouds. He even knew the etymology: named "cumulus" by the Englishman Luke Howard, from the less imaginative but more descriptive Latin word for something gathered into an accumulated bundle. As the clouds drifted past, the day seemed without time, and buzzards wheeled high as they searched for dead or sick animals. Their flight seemed effortless. Father explained that this wasn't true. The buzzards were actually vultures, two kinds: turkey vultures and black vultures. Recently two bicycle mechanics from Ohio had studied vultures very carefully, noticing that they warped their wings as they circled in the rising air of the vertical thermal currents to obtain lateral guidance in their flight. These young men, Wilbur and Orville Wright, had copied this wing-warping system from nature and had used it on their new flying machine. Father observed that you have to know nature to understand it. You have to know nature to deal effectively with the practical things of life. Tinsley was impressed with this argument. Father seemed to have a great deal of faith in science. Even so, Tinsley had his doubts about this machine, something like a horse-drawn threshing machine on the farm, he imagined, that could fly all by itself. After all, there had been Santa Claus, and maybe this was just another of those made-up stories grown-ups tell children.

They resumed their walk along the road, now getting more dusty in the afternoon sun. Even this early in the late spring it was hot—no refrigeration, no ice, no air conditioning of any kind. The only respite from the heat was the caves, which they sometimes visited. There are many beautiful large caves in Alabama with magnificent underground rooms filled with stalactites and stalagmites that Father loved to discourse on. And they were cool in the summer!

They sat down again to rest at the edge of a large field surrounded by small pines and oaks. As they drank warm water from their canteens, they heard then saw a group of small birds in the branches of the brush 10 to 15 feet above the ground. Father suggested that they sneak down to see if they could identify them, and so they did. When they were about 50 feet from the little flock, he told them to sit in a comfortable position near or under a bush and be as inconspicuous as possible. "Just like an Indian on a hunt," he said. Toward the east, just across the small clearing where they were sitting, was another arrangement of trees and bushes similar to the one where the birds were playing and feeding in the late summer sun. When they were seated, Father began making a sort of hissing sound, "Pshshsh, pshshshsh,

pshshshsh, pshshshsh," then after a brief pause repeated. It was miraculous! Tinsley had never seen anything like it. First came a curious towhee flitting up into the very bush he was hiding under. Then a cardinal and some sparrows. Then the little flock of warblers, chickadees, and kinglets moved steadily along the bank of trees until they were just in front of the trio, not more than 10 feet away. They were fascinated.

A huge hawk was suddenly splayed against the bushes, his wings spread wide as his talons grasped the body of an already lifeless yellow warbler. He had swooped in on a stoop from the sun as it descended in the west. Tinsley jumped up to help the warbler, but the hawk darted away with his prey, to alight on the limb of a dead pine some 50 yards distant. A few bright yellow feathers were all that remained. Tinsley picked up a few of the yellow feathers and kept them many years. His father put a hand on his shoulder, telling him not to be sad. "All life except plants live on other life," he said, "and you have to be aggressive to survive in this world, but try to be as kind, gentle, and humane as possible as you go about your business. Otherwise you are no different from some primitive animal." Living, to Groce and later to Tinsley, was a competitive process. Life demanded life. These walks were more than private tutorials in natural history; they were courses in philosophy. They were lessons passed down from father to sons.

They talked about the episode as they continued down the road. "What kind of hawk was it, Father?" Groce Jr. asked.

"A Red-shouldered Hawk," Father replied. "It is similar to a Red-tailed Hawk, but a little smaller."

"You mean there's a hawk even bigger than that one we just saw!" Tinsley asked.

His father nodded. "Yes, and there are others bigger than the Red-tailed Hawk."

IT WAS GROWING LATE in the afternoon, and Groce, having grown up on the farm, had learned to judge the amount of daylight remaining in the day from the height of the sun above the horizon. He estimated they had a good hour's light left. They discussed why the days were longer and warmer in the summer than the winter as they searched for a good place to camp for the night.

They found a small meadow, cleared years before but now abandoned and covered with grass and flowers—an ideal place for the night. They got out the blankets but did not set up the tent. The red sunset and the clear sky allowed for sleeping under the stars. "Groce, you clear away a place for a fire and arrange the blankets. Tinsley, you go find some dried pine wood for a fire. It's been a little wet, but find the driest you can. I'm going over to that little swamp we just passed to see if I can find a bass while we still have a little light." And indeed he did. In just a few minutes he was back with a large bass weighing perhaps five or six pounds. He gutted and scaled the fish, which he then placed in the small, light frying pan they had brought. Tinsley had gathered wood, and young Groce had prepared a smooth fire bed with earth turned up by his trowel. There they stacked the wood with some dry pine straw as a starter. Soon they had a cheerful fire, and then fried fresh bass for supper, together with some baked beans heated in the can held over the fire by a branch and wire, and some sassafras tea made by boiling some roots of the plant in swamp water. The few pieces of snake were fried in the skillet after the fish, and it was good—rather like the fish. They leaned against their soft earth in the meadow, sated. It was one of the best suppers Tinsley ever had.

They were not bothered by the hooting. Young Groce had asked long ago back in Birmingham, "What's that, a ghost?" when a Barred Owl, or eight hooter, announced its presence one evening near the house on Cliff Road. Eight hooters remained prominent in the Birmingham suburbs well into the last decades of the century. They, as well as horned owls, or "five hooters," and screech owls, were well known to all the Harrisons.

The problem during the night was choosing whether to snuggle down under the blanket so as to avoid the mosquitoes but burn up with the heat, or to throw off the blanket for a more comfortable temperature but put yourself at the insects' mercy. Around midnight a soft breeze arose and the buzzing ceased. The temperature was considerably cooler, so Tinsley could remain under the blanket without roasting, and the mosquitoes were swept away by the breeze. Tinsley was drowsing with his eyes closed, but he must have made a noise as he squirmed to adjust his blanket. "Are you awake, son?" his father whispered.

"Yes, Father," he whispered back. As Tinsley opened his eyes, it was another spectacle. The sky was crystal clear, and stars were everywhere—no clouds, no smoke, no light pollution from any source except one very dim coal glowing in the dead fire. It was very dark, but very bright. There must have been a hundred million stars splayed before him.

"Which way is north?" Father asked in a soft voice. Tinsley had heard this question before, and he knew he must find the Big Dipper to locate the North Star. So he arose from the blanket, which also woke young Groce, and the three stood in the little meadow as Father pointed out how Draco the Dragon was draped around the North Star, how that star also formed the tail of the Little Dipper, the small bear, how Cygnus the Swan formed the Northern Cross, and how you could find Aquilla the Eagle and Lyra from there. On and on for maybe an hour they studied and memorized the stars. Tinsley seemed to have a peculiar affinity for stars, though in later life he showed little interest in them. They had a long-term feel, an eternal serenity far beyond our daily petty strivings. He remembered how to find north, and his father complimented him on that. They watched a while longer, as their eyes grew accustomed to the endless shimmer, then returned to sleep.

AT SUNRISE THE NEXT morning, they arose. They made another fire, and cooked their last eggs—scrambled, with pieces of smoked sausage. Even though they had a small fire, the meadow filled with large flocks of goldfinches migrating north for the summer. The ground was yellow with the huge numbers of goldfinches. Tinsley felt in awe of their numbers, there were so many!

They packed their belongings and started off along the road. Father knew of a little store a few miles further where they could purchase fresh eggs and milk. Soon they were there. Mr. Brown, the owner, offered them cups of hot coffee, which all accepted, including young Groce, who had never drunk coffee before. They thanked Mr. Brown and set out toward the east again, trudging along with their knapsacks and the eggs and milk, which they would consume for lunch, since there was no way to prevent spoilage.

The following days and nights were similar, except that on Thursday evening it was cloudy, and they put up the tent. Sometime after midnight they were awakened by a clap of thunder, and Tinsley rolled over. When his hand fell to the side of the blanket it landed in a pool of water, as the rain pattered on the canvas roof over them. His father insisted that they go out and dig a trench around the tent, which they had neglected to do earlier. This kept most of the water outside. By sunrise the rain had stopped, and they were able to start a fire for breakfast. Their things were not too wet and they squeezed out what water they could to reduce the weight of their packs. This done, they started again on the road, now muddy from the night's rain.

They took a shortcut across some fields and around a mountain, since Groce knew the road circled back into their projected route. As they made their way along a path through the forest, it began to rain again, hard at first, then more lightly. Their canvas knapsacks would keep most of their belongings fairly dry, but they themselves were soaked to the skin. As they walked along in the drizzle, Tinsley

3. "How gloriously Nature smiles to me! How the sun gleams! How the flowers laugh! / It draws the flowers from every twig, and a thousand voices from the bush, / and joy and bliss to every breast. Oh earth, oh sun! Oh happiness, oh yearning!" From Goethe's "Mailied."

thought he heard his father singing, even though Groce could hardly carry a tune and rarely sang above a whisper in church. He soon realized that it was not a real song, but a poem his father was humming in a semi-musical fashion:

> *Wie herrlich leuchtet*
> *Mir die Natur!*
> *Wie glaenzt die Sonne!*
> *Wie lacht die Flur!*
>
> *Es dringen Blueten*
> *Aus jedem Zweig,*
> *Und tausend Stimmen*
> *Aus dem Gestrauch,*
>
> *Und Freud' und Wonne*
> *Aus jeder Brust.*
> *O Erd', O Sonne!*
> *O Glueck, O Lust!* [3]

"Why are you singing, Father?" Tinsley asked.

"Because I am happy," he said. "I'm singing a poem to Nature."

"Happy? Getting soaked out here in the rain?" Tinsley said. He felt miserable. This is a mess, he thought.

But his father persisted. "There is nothing more friendly than a warm spring rain early in a day," he said. They stopped for a breather as they climbed a steep hill, and Tinsley leaned back against a huge pine, the water streaming down his face. He began to see his father's point. The water was warm. He felt no distress. They were in familiar, friendly territory, close to home. The woods seemed friendly rather than frightening. Even the snakes and frogs seemed friends, once you got to know them. The rain continued. As his father said, "Let's get going," young Tinsley thought, yes, there is nothing more friendly than a light spring rain, even—or maybe especially—when you're in it in a great forest.

On Saturday afternoon, eight days after leaving Birmingham, they reached Talladega. Tinsley felt he was the world's expert (except, of course, for his father) on trees and birds and that soon he would have all of nature mastered, or at least memorized. They found the home of Dr. Samuel W. Welch, a prominent Talladega physician and long-standing friend. Groce had written several weeks earlier telling them he would probably arrive with his boys on that Sunday, and he had received a letter in response. He felt confident of getting a supper there then a ride back to Birmingham in a wagon on Monday. Dr. Welch's house was just a few doors down from the old Harrison house on South Street where Tinsley had been born. Dr. Welch had been expecting them and said that he had room for them in the house; they would not have to sleep in the stable. So that night they all had hot tub baths. They slept for the first time in a week on cots rather than the ground.

Sunday morning they got up late, around 6:30 A.M., had a good kitchen-fixed breakfast of eggs, bacon, muffins, milk, and jam, then dressed for church in clothes that had been sent ahead. Old Grandfather "Doctor T" Harrison rode in from the farm near Munford and accompanied them. First Sunday school at 9, then the main service from 11 until after 12, all at the First Presbyterian Church they had attended after Methodist Groce had married Presbyterian Lula. Then they returned to Dr. Welch's house, where they had the traditional large Sunday noon dinner. After lunch everyone took a nap, then "Doctor T" loaded them into his buggy for the ride out to the old Harrison farm six and a half miles east of town.

On Monday they were carried back to Birmingham by George, the elderly black man and former slave who had been a family friend and farmhand for many years. Their journey was over. Tinsley cherished the memories of it for the rest of his life.

5

Michigan, Hopkins, and the Brigham

1916–1925

1. Attempts to confirm this with the admissions office of Harvard College were unfruitful. In past years the Harvard University Archives did keep records of college applicants who were accepted but never matriculated. However, a few years ago these were destroyed, as noted in the current index of those archives.

2. The tuition at Harvard the fall of 1916, as set forth in the catalogue for the year 1915–1916, apparently also used for 1916–17, was "one hundred and fifty dollars; but if a student in the College takes work in excess of the amount required of members

At Tinsley's high school graduation festivities in May 1915 the class presented a play, Shakespeare's *A Midsummer Night's Dream*. Tinsley had a minor part in the play of a young man who was accused of being nothing more than a boy. The response was, "I'm a man! I have a beard!" to be said with a gesture of stroking the beard. Tinsley ad libbed, "I have a beard—coming!" and stroked the imaginary beard. The audience laughed.

As he completed high school, his father wanted the very best education possible for him. To this end Tinsley only applied to Harvard College. And he was accepted![1] This was indeed good news, as he was interested in becoming a lawyer, and Harvard seemed to offer the best opportunities for obtaining an excellent background for law.

But there were problems, notably Tinsley's age—he was only 15—and the family finances. Groce Harrison had anticipated earning money from the cotton farm east of Talladega, which they still owned and on which they depended for income, even in 1915. In those days, much of the cotton crop was sold to Britain for a good profit. During that year so many ships were sunk in the war with Germany that Americans slowed the shipping of cotton abroad. There was a sharp decline in cotton prices in Alabama. "People didn't have enough money to pay their bills," Tinsley said. "My father's income dropped by half or more." With the decline in sales, his father simply did not have enough money to fund the college education at Harvard. So Tinsley attended a local junior college—Marion Institute, a military academy in Marion, Alabama.

This was Tinsley's side of the story and his belief more than half a century later. If he had gone to Harvard, he probably would have pursued law. So perhaps Groce's determination to see his son in medicine did not play a role in these decisions, especially since a year later Tinsley enrolled in the University of Michigan. But it's hard to say.

Tinsley had a good year at the Marion Institute. He made excellent grades, graduated fourth in his class of 29, and achieved two years' work in one. He was 16. His work so impressed the school authorities that they awarded him a degree, which he remembered as a B.S. degree, as was the custom at completion even though it was only a two-year school.

The things he most remembered about Marion, in addition to the fact that the teaching seemed to be of good quality, were the military training—especially close order drill—and his youth relative to the other boys. While the older boys bragged about their sexual exploits, real or imagined, Tinsley was protected by his youth, as well as by his Biblical upbringing.

IN THE SPRING OF 1916 Tinsley and his father concluded their discussions of his continuing in college. Harvard figured prominently in these discussions, but for three reasons the University of Michigan was preferable. It was less expensive, and money was still scarce. At Harvard the tuition would be $200 a year—it had been raised from $150 the year before—with no guarantee it might not rise again the following year. There were also additional charges: infirmary fee, $4; room, $50 to $200; board, $120 to $300; plus additional charges if he took other courses, as he would like to.[2] The annual fee at Michigan was less, and Michigan living expenses would be about $3.50 to $4.50 a week for food and $1 to $3 a week for lodgings.[3] Second, the curriculum and management of the University of Michigan was reputed to be sufficiently flexible to permit a particularly good student to move ahead at his own pace, shortening the attendance time by up to a year.[4] Three years' study was generally required for a law degree, but Michigan had allowed his Uncle Ben to obtain a law degree there in only one year. That uncle was later appointed a federal judge in Alabama. Third, the University of Michigan was known to be an excellent school, probably the leading state university in the country at the time.

Tinsley gained entrance to the University of Michigan without difficulty, helped by his excellent record in high school and at the Marion Institute. During the summer before departing for Ann Arbor, he traveled with his older sister Emily to Boulder, Colorado, to take additional courses at the University of Colorado. He

of his Class . . . or if a Freshman takes work in addition to the amount prescribed in his individual case, he is charged a supplementary fee of $20 per course for each Additional Course so taken." (Harvard University Catalogue 1915–16), 490. This catalogue also indicated (147) that during the following year the tuition would be increased to $200 per year. Archives of Harvard University, Houghton Library, Harvard Yard, Cambridge, Massachusetts (Harley P. Holden, Curator, 1993).

3. The University of Michigan charged an "annual fee" of $62 for out-of-state students ($42 for Michigan residents), plus a one-time matriculation fee of $25 ($10 for Michigan residents). Board was $3.50 to $4.50 per week, and a single room was $1 to $3 per week. (General Catalogue of the University of Michigan, 1916–17, Section on College of Literature, Science, and the Arts, 99). The annual fee for students in the medical school in 1918–19, Harrison's year of medical school at Michigan, was $127

for out-of-state male students and $122 for out-of-state female students (also 99).

4. Ibid., 26: "Students desiring to obtain the degree of Bachelor of Arts in the College of Literature, Science and the Arts, and Doctor of Medicine in the Medical School, may, by enrolling on the combined Curriculum of Letters and Medicine, shorten from eight years to seven the time required to earn the two degrees. This privilege is open only to students who throughout their course maintain a uniform record of good scholarship." The program was open to students with at least one year's work in the College of Literature, Science, and the Arts. Thus, Tinsley Harrison would not have been eligible to double-enroll until the spring of 1917 at the earliest.

5. Ibid., 24: "The academic year extends from the Tuesday preceding the first Thursday in October to the last Thursday in June, except in years preceding leap years, when it begins upon the Tuesday preceding the first Wednesday in October." Since 1916

took science courses, chemistry, and mathematics, since these would be helpful in college; he felt he could read literature, poetry, and history on his own. The studies were not excessively demanding, and they spent much of the time wandering with classmates through the local wilderness and mountains. On weekends, Emily and Tinsley would take bus trips with classmates to Long's Peak, Pike's Peak, and the beautiful valleys and rivers of the region. Despite the war raging in Europe between the crumbling royal dynasties, it was a very happy and carefree time for them.

The financial situation for Birmingham and for the Harrison family was improving. So Tinsley left the South, the only world he'd known, to go to college in the cold north of Ann Arbor, Michigan.

The war in Europe continued, far away.

IN SEPTEMBER OF 1916 Tinsley took the train from Birmingham for Ann Arbor and entered the university on Tuesday, October third.[5] Despite his earlier predisposition to law, he majored in biology. His father placed a premium on an education in hard sciences, extolling the virtues of knowing biology and chemistry for any field, including law. Tinsley received only one year's credit at Michigan for his two years' work at Marion. Although he majored in biological science, Tinsley's real love was letters and the humanities. In this preference, at this stage of his development, he was like William H. Welch, whom he would come to know and admire at Hopkins.[6]

His approach to his studies was to attend a few of the classes early in the course to learn whether the teacher took roll, then, if not, he would work chiefly on his humanities studies and spend lots of extra time memorizing poetry, especially English poetry. As the term neared its end, he would schedule study periods for himself during which he would cram on the material in the science courses in order to do well on the final examinations. The teaching of the sciences at Michigan, he said, was "the worst teaching I was ever exposed to." For the most part it was uninspired and dull with rote memorizing of poorly connected facts and no demonstration of any great interest in their subjects by the faculty. Tinsley often skipped classes.

There were a few inspiring exceptions. A "Harvard man named Bigelow" taught physical chemistry, which Tinsley loved. It may have been the topic itself in this case, but the teaching did seem a cut above the rest.

During the latter half of his first year at Michigan, on Friday, April 6, 1917, the United States declared war on Germany. Tinsley felt the call to duty. He was a month past his 17th birthday, so he immediately telephoned his father, even though long distance telephone calls then were expensive by the standards of the time. "Father," he said, "I'm going to enlist tomorrow!"

"You will not!" his father replied. "You are only 17 years old, and I have the right to control what you do. You are to remain in college and continue your studies. I admire your attitude, but not your judgment."

"The French will take me in the ambulance corps," Tinsley replied.

"I'll block that," his father said. "Nobody knows how long this war will last. If it lasts a long time, the allies will need doctors more than low-level sailors and soldiers." There was further discussion of the Harrison family's dedication to service to the nation and Tinsley's need to maintain that tradition, but Groce was adamant. They argued and argued, but Groce did not budge.

Tinsley finally accepted the inevitable, since he would need his father's permission and signature to enlist. He returned to his studies. He studied more diligently than before. The war made Tinsley and the world and everything in it more serious and mature.

He completed the year's studies. During the summer of 1917 he obtained a job from a Birmingham neighbor who was an official of the water company. This job consisted of reading the water meters over much of the city. He walked from meter to meter across the rapidly growing city. He estimated that he walked at least 10 miles every day he worked, and some days as much as 17 miles, from Ensley in the western part of the city to East Lake on the opposite side. The job also required that he act as agent to warn customers that they were delinquent in paying their water bills. Tinsley never liked this aspect. "If you don't pay your bill promptly," he would say, "we're going to cut your water off." It was difficult, uncomfortable, and awkward. It was good training, however, for his later years in medical administration.

Despite his disappointment with much of the teaching, he studied enough to make A's and B's in most subjects during his first two years at Michigan. In his third year at Michigan and first year in medical school, 1918–19, he took 90 hours of histology and of organology and embryology, 40 hours of neurology, and 96 hours of topographical anatomy supplemented by 40 hours of lectures. In addition, he took "Dissection," which consisted of 354 hours in the lab and 85 hours of associated lectures. He also took a course in bacteriology consisting of 240 hours of laboratory work plus 80 hours of lectures. Interestingly, his first-year course in physiology consisted entirely of 65 hours of lectures.[7]

When Tinsley turned 18, on March 18, 1918, he enlisted in the Navy. He again

was a leap year, this would have been Tuesday, October third. Bentley Historical Library, Ann Arbor.

6. Donald Fleming, *William Welch and the Rise of Modern Medicine* (1954; repr., Baltimore: The Johns Hopkins University Press, 1987) 20–12.

7. *Bulletin* of the University of Michigan, Bentley Historical Library, Ann Arbor.

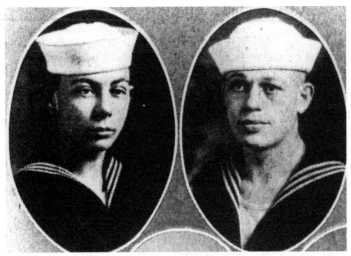

Two first-year medical students from the University of Michigan 1918 yearbook. Tinsley Harrison, left, and Walter Bauer, who later became chief of medicine at the Massachusetts General Hospital in Boston and Jackson Professor of Medicine at Harvard.

telephoned his father.

"At what rank?" his father asked.

"Apprentice Seaman, the lowest rank possible," Tinsley replied.

"I admire what you're doing, Son," his father said. "But the greater need in the armed forces is for doctors, not apprentice seamen." His father was now a prominent citizen of Alabama and he had some influence. "I'm going to pull strings and do everything possible to see that you remain in medical school."

Tinsley was not activated right away. He was told to continue his medical studies at Michigan. The official reason was that "he was studying medicine and the authorities in Washington felt it was more important to have him available as a physician later than as a apprentice seaman right away." Activation came only in the late summer or early fall of 1918, but even then he still remained at the University of Michigan working toward a career in medicine. He later wondered whether his father could have been responsible for delaying his entry into the regular Navy.

He was the youngest and smallest member of the University of Michigan Navy contingent, and he had the lowest rank possible. He had received military training at Marion, however, and he was the only one in the group with such experience. He was placed in charge of the group for purposes of drilling and similar military activities. All would rise early in response to reveille as the leader would shout, "Hit the deck!" and the group would fall in for assembly. The leader of the group would call them to attention, roll call would be taken, and then the reveille leader would turn to Tinsley: "Harrison, you take over. I'm going back to bed." The smallest and youngest member of the group would then drill the men for an hour. "I loved this," he said later. Having authority gave him added confidence in dealing with others.

One classmate through those three years was Walter Bauer, a young man from Crystal Falls, Michigan. Bauer later became a famous rheumatologist and chief of medicine at the Massachusetts General Hospital. The two served in the University of Michigan naval unit and became fast friends for the rest of their lives, their paths crossing often through their careers in internal medicine.

Tinsley was technically in the armed forces a total of only 83 days, seven days short of the number needed to qualify for U.S. veterans' benefits under the federal law. He always felt he did not deserve such benefits, since all he ever really did was continue his medical studies, as he would have otherwise.

His story about skipping classes was probably an exaggeration, but in 1918 he tried his non-attendance system in organic chemistry and it did not work. He neglected to attend the required laboratory sessions and flunked despite making an A on the final exam. He was given an opportunity to make it up without loss of time by taking a summer course at the University of Chicago. So he spent the summer of 1918 in the Windy City, retaking the organic chemistry course and this time doing well. Julius Stieglitz taught this course and Tinsley found him fascinating. Stieglitz was stimulating and compatible with Tinsley's own love of organic chemistry which grew greater and greater the more he studied it—a common phenomenon generally under-appreciated by young students. The problem is somehow obtaining that initial burst of enthusiastic interest in the student, then maintaining it. In this, Tinsley would become a master teacher.

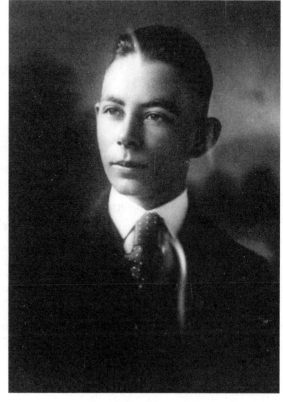

Tinsley Randolph Harrison, about the time of his graduation from the University of Michigan in 1919.

During that summer in Chicago, Tinsley continued to play tennis and in the U.S. Open tournament met Bill Tilden, the national men's singles champion from 1920–25 and again in 1929. He played Tilden and lost but felt he had acquitted himself well.

In the spring of 1918 Tinsley had finally made up his mind about medicine: he would try for the double enrollment and attempt to use his senior year of college as a simultaneous first year of medical school. Thus he was able to enter medical school at age 18, the age which was becoming the standard for completion of high school and starting college. He was four years ahead of his peers.

He achieved good grades at Michigan and in 1919 was awarded the A.B. degree.

Tinsley did not like the details of gross anatomy studies and the dissection of cadavers. He considered both a waste of time. He felt that all doctors needed to know "organology"—the gross relations of internal organs to one another and to surface anatomy—for clinical purposes. There was such a course in the Michigan medical school curriculum at the time. He knew that even internists must be thoroughly familiar with many details of the circulation of the blood and which vessels supply which organs. He just didn't enjoy cutting into cadavers. He enjoyed neuroanatomy and the related circulatory anatomy. He often delighted in showing students and fellow faculty members how much he remembered of which artery or nerve supplied which organ or part of an organ. In the end he learned anatomy then and relearned and taught it the rest of his life.

His aggravations with gross anatomy were minor, and some of his courses were fascinating. This was the year he had the histology and neuroanatomy courses from "the best teacher at Michigan": G. Carl Huber, professor of anatomy and director of the anatomical laboratories. Tinsley considered Huber his best teacher since grade school, erudite and enthusiastic. Huber had graduated from Michigan with an M.D. in 1887 and had joined the faculty of medicine soon after that. Huber's academic career followed the orthodox lines of teaching, punctuated with periods of studying abroad in Berlin and Prague. He was one of those destined to participate in the eruption of knowledge in the four decades following 1890, most vivid in bacteriology but evident in other areas of the biological and medical sciences as well. Huber's tremendous enthusiasm for his subject was transmitted to his students. He also had a gift for presenting his material in an understandable way, probably because he himself understood it so clearly. Finally, Huber was remembered for "the encouragement and inspiration he gave to each one to render the very best that was in him." In the years that followed, Huber remained a model in Tinsley's mind as he himself labored to be the best teacher of medicine possible.

Huber's research focused largely on the sympathetic nervous system, neuroglia, and nerve endings. He was also interested in comparative anatomy and comparative neurology. One of his main collaborators in this later work was Dr. Elizabeth C. Crosby, with whom he published the extensive volume, *Comparative Neurology*. (In the 1960s Dr. Crosby spent several winters in Birmingham as a Visiting Professor at the Alabama medical school and despite her age brought a new enthusiasm to the teaching of neuroanatomy there.)

Tinsley was happy. He was on the Michigan tennis team and was popular with his classmates. He had been elected to membership in the medical fraternity and boarding house Nu Sigma Nu and had been designated to lead the fraternity brothers of his class. He enjoyed his classes and felt that the choice of medicine and the prospect of continuing such pleasant study for four years was sound. The prestige of the profession of medicine was being progressively enhanced by the development of scientific medicine and the elevation of the standards of medical education and practice. All in all, there was no reason to do anything but pursue his medical education at Michigan.

His father had different ideas. Throughout the fall his letters to his son contained frequent references to the desirability of getting the best medical education possible to stand him in good stead for the rest of his life. Tinsley initially disregarded these comments, hoping they would dwindle with time. They did not.

When Tinsley returned home to Birmingham for the Christmas holiday, he had several long and serious conversations with his father. He was happy at Michigan; it was a good school. He was doing well, and it was certain that he would obtain an excellent medical education and career if he completed medical school there.

Michigan had been a leader in medical education for nearly half a century and was still a leading school. The medical school was part of the original plan of the legislature in its act of 1837 organizing the University, and it had been educating medical students since 1850. Initially an annual course of about seven months was offered, which the student took twice, then, with a year of apprenticeship with a practitioner, qualified for examination. "In 1877 the curriculum was extended to two years of nine months each, and in 1880 three years of study of nine months each became necessary before a candidate could present himself for final examination. In 1890 the compulsory term of study was extended to four years of nine months each."[8] The additional years also facilitated a rational sequencing and grading of the curriculum, so that students could proceed through their studies in a logical progressive fashion rather than just taking a course twice: first the normal gross structure, interrelations, and function of the body's organs, then the microscopic structure and function, then the chemistry of the body, then abnormal structure and function (pathology, the science of diseases), and finally clinical applications. Nearly 20 years before the medical school at Hopkins opened, Michigan was one of the pivotal medical schools that initiated reforms elevating the standards of medical education in the 1870s.[9] By 1893, the year the Johns Hopkins school opened, the president of the University of Michigan commented on the marked improvements in the medical students at his school.[10] Michigan was also a rich school, probably the fourth wealthiest in the nation according to the statistics gathered by Flexner for his report of 1910.[11] The president of the university, H. B. Hutchins, was in

8. "An Historical Sketch of the Department of Medicine and Surgery of the University of Michigan" (*The Medical News*, April 20, 1901).

9. K. Ludmerer, *Learning to Heal. The Development of American Medical Education* (New York, Basic Books, Inc., 1985), 47.

10. University of Michigan, President's Annual Report, (1893), 17.

11. Abraham Flexner, *Medical Education in the United States and Canada* (New York: Carnegie Foundation of the Advancement of Teaching, 1910) 185–319 and appendix; also Ludmerer, *Learning*, 143.

12. Ludmerer, *Learning*, 227.

13. Ibid., Table 4.4, 97. Ludmerer agrees with Groce Harrison. In his ranking of U.S. medical schools in six tiers for the year 1910, Harvard, Michigan, Minnesota and Columbia are placed in the second tier. Hopkins alone is in the top tier; and the difference rests in "quality of clinical instruction."

the process of obtaining state funds to expand the university's hospital, an expansion which was to reach 450 beds by 1920 with an additional 800 soon thereafter. Each would be a teaching bed.[12] James Angell, the previous president, had pushed successfully for higher academic entrance requirements, so the other medical students would continue to be an excellent influence. The school had a long standing reputation for excellence in medical research. Ludmerer considered Michigan, along with Pennsylvania and Harvard and later Hopkins, one of four "pioneering medical schools of the nation."

So, Michigan was a superb school. Tinsley was happily ensconced there, making good progress. Why should he change?

For Groce, who had experience with formal medical education in three schools, including Hopkins, there was only one medical school in the nation that was really the best: Hopkins. He had been deeply impressed by what he saw firsthand in the differences between the teaching there and his own experiences at the Baltimore Medical College and in Nashville. He knew that Michigan was far better than either of the schools he had attended, but Groce was, in addition to being emotionally attached to Hopkins, extraordinarily well-informed about medicine and medical education for a physician of his time and place. He remained convinced that the clinical teaching methods introduced by Osler at Hopkins, on the foundation established by W. H. "Popsy" Welch, President Daniel Coit Gilman, and their colleagues, were not yet matched anywhere else, even though Osler was now at Oxford. To obtain the best medical education, Tinsley would have to leave Michigan and move to Hopkins to finish his M.D. degree.[13]

In later years Tinsley vacillated between saying that he had "transferred to Hopkins against my will" and that his father "never ordered or directed me to do anything but allowed me to make my own decisions." On his application for admission to advanced standing at Hopkins there was an item, "State why you desire to enter this School." To this Tinsley answered in his own handwriting, "My father believes Hopkins is the best place in the entire world to get a real medical education—a spirit of work." Although he made the decision to transfer for himself, that decision was made nearly completely on the basis of data supplied with evangelistic conviction by his father. He had little choice.

Tinsley later recalled that not only his classmates and colleagues in the Nu Sigma Nu fraternity, but also some of his professors, tried to dissuade him from making the change of medical schools. But the die was cast—to Hopkins he would go.

On May 5, 1919, Tinsley completed and dated his application form for admission to the Johns Hopkins University School of Medicine at the second-year level. It was complete with a note from his father.

There were in later years no intimations that the transfer had been an achievement of any difficulty. But there is one letter in Tinsley's file dated October 1, 1919, from Dr. Warren P. Lombard of the physiological laboratory at Ann Arbor. "He took the course in lectures in physiology provided for the medical freshmen [secretion, digestion, absorption, ductless glands internal secretion, nutrition, animal heat] and did first-class work—mark A," Lombard said. "He is all right."

THERE WERE SEVERAL PROBLEMS. Although Hopkins required a reading knowledge of both French and German, Tinsley had taken only a single course in scientific French and one in scientific German. He had received personal tutoring in German for seven years from Fraulein Schepke and felt at home in that language. Further, he had done very well in his four years of Latin as taught by Miss Thornton while in high school and had spent one year each reading Caesar, Cicero, and Virgil. With this background, he later found reading any of the romance languages (with the help of a dictionary) fairly easy. So he obtained French and German dictionaries and immediately began translating articles from medical journals into English, which he continued during the three months before being tested in Baltimore. He was allowed to use his dictionaries during the examinations, and he passed his language requirements with no difficulty.

The other problem was that Michigan offered biochemistry during the second year of school, but Hopkins offered it in the first year. If he simply transferred, he would miss the course. So in the summer of 1919 he studied biochemistry at the University of Michigan, eight hours a day for eight weeks straight. On September 24, A. G. Scott, assistant secretary of the University of Michigan Medical School, wrote to the Johns Hopkins Medical School, informing the secretary that Tinsley had received a final grade of B+. The tradeoff was not bad, though. At Michigan during his first year of medicine he had taken the course in bacteriology, and one of his teachers had been Paul Dekruif, who later moved to the Rockefeller Institute and gained popular fame with his book *The Microbe Hunters*.

The rest of the summer, Tinsley worked in the Birmingham Health Laboratory. In late September he moved to Baltimore and took up residence in rooms near the medical school. The weather was warm and mild, so he took his tennis racquet and

14. A. M. Harvey, Victor McKusick, and John Stubo, *Osler's Legacy: The Department of Medicine at Johns Hopkins 1889–1989* (Baltimore: The Johns Hopkins University Press, 1990), 128.

headed for the courts. As he walked onto the nearest unoccupied court, another young man about Tinsley's age came along with a racquet and a couple of tennis balls. They agreed to a game or two, and after two games the young man approached Tinsley and spoke in a slow drawl and "with an accent so thick you could cut it with a knife."

"Mah name is Alfred Blalock, and Ah'm from Jonesboro, Georgia." He extended his hand. Tinsley shook it.

"My name is Tinsley Harrison, and I'm from Birmingham, Alabama."

The two both loved tennis, so nearly every day after classes they played singles against each other—fairly evenly matched—for the rest of the fall until the daylight ran out. Al turned out to be in the same medical school class as Tinsley, and they enjoyed each other's company. Within a week they decided to room together, which they did for the remainder of medical school. Later they teamed up in tennis for doubles "and crucified everybody else around Hopkins." Years later, tennis for Tinsley remained synonymous with Blalock.

There were 90 students in the class, many of whom became lifelong friends of Tinsley. This was particularly true of Blalock, who became closer to him than anyone except his own family, and perhaps in some ways even closer. There were others. Chester S. Keefer, who became a good friend and later the Wade Professor and chairman of medicine at the Boston University School of Medicine, was one of the first clinicians to obtain and use penicillin at the end of World War II.[14]

One of the marks of a great school, and one of the attributes that keeps it great, is its ability to attract the most outstanding students. Good students stimulate other students and the faculty to maximum efforts and achievements then go on to their own achievements, helped by the network developed during their studies with others of similar character. Johns Hopkins was by this standard a great school. "School" here is used to include the Hopkins hospital and its house staff, integral parts of the system of medical education. In the middle part of the century, a large number of departmental chairmen, deans, officers of biomedical research and other professional societies, hospital and governmental officials, and contributors to the medical literature were alumni of the Johns Hopkins medical school and hospital. In joining Hopkins, Tinsley was becoming one of the elite of academic medicine for the coming generation.

His father was happy to pay the tuition of $250 per year, particularly since it could be paid in three installments.

Since by 1919 the medical curricula were becoming fairly standardized in the United States, at least among the more prominent schools, Tinsley had studied the same subjects during the previous year as his classmates, except for the physiologic chemistry which he had made up.[15] Physiology worried Tinsley. At Michigan the course consisted entirely of lectures, and apparently most of the second-year course at Hopkins was also lectures. He worried about his inadequate exposure, as he saw it, to the laboratory aspects of physiology, and he tried to compensate by memorizing as much as possible from the physiology text by William H. Howell.

Howell had been the first chairman of the Department of Physiology at Hopkins, having previously been head of physiology at Michigan then associate professor of physiology at Harvard, from which he was lured away by Gilman.[16] His work was largely on blood clotting, though his memory is more widely perpetuated by the Howell-Jolly bodies of abnormal red cells. His text was a classic and went through 14 editions. Memorizing this text must have given Tinsley a very solid base from which to launch his later physiological research. Howell, who had retired from the position then and was devoting much of his time to the School of Hygiene, gave some of the lectures on blood clotting, which Tinsley remembered well. He thought that the new chairman, Donald R. Hooker, who handled most of the teaching, "was an average teacher," but that Howell was outstanding. In the end, Tinsley's grade of 8.7 was the highest in the class.

Although "Popsy" Welch was still at Hopkins, and in fact remained there essentially all of his professional life, he had retired from the chairmanship of the Department of Pathology, which had been taken over by William G. MacCallum, a young and dynamic man known for his elucidation of the nature of post-thyroidectomy tetany (painful muscle cramps, spasms, and tremors) and its cause (loss of parathyroid hormone) and relief; the sexual reproduction of malarial parasites; and other work. He was also the author of a well-known text on pathology. MacCallum handled most of the teaching, but Welch gave several hours of lectures and served largely as an inspiration to Tinsley because of his stature in the advancement of medicine.

Welch was a towering figure in medicine and a major factor in bringing to the United States the creative energies for research systematized along the lines of 19th century German laboratories, where he obtained considerable experience before returning to New York in 1878.[17] In fact, it was in the Leipzig laboratory of Carl Ludwig that Welch was introduced to John Shaw Billings of Hopkins in 1876.

15. Alan M. Chesney, *The Johns Hopkins Hospital and the Johns Hopkins University School of Medicine: A Chronicle. Vol. III. 1905–1914* (Baltimore: The Johns Hopkins Press, 1963), 42–49. The details of the Hopkins curriculum of 1907–08 is given by Chesney for all four years in some detail. It had probably not changed greatly in outline and general arrangements when Harrison was there in 1919–22.

16. A. M. Harvey, G. H. Brieger, S. L. Abrams, and Victor McKusick, *A Model of Its Kind: A Centennial History of Medicine at Johns Hopkins, Volume I* (Baltimore & London: Johns Hopkins Press, 1989), 29.

17. Donald Fleming, *William H. Welch and the Rise of Modern Medicine* (Boston: Little, Brown and Company, 1954), 55.

Welch was later recruited to the new Johns Hopkins in 1884 as President Gilman's first appointment to the medical faculty and chairman of the pathology department.

Before starting work in Baltimore, Welch returned to Europe to learn more about the newly developing science of bacteriology. He returned to his old friend and mentor in Leipzig, Carl Ludwig, but left in the spring to study briefly in Goettingen under the bacteriologist Karl Fluegge. He missed Pasteur in Paris, but in July 1885 he took a month's laboratory course in Berlin with Robert Koch, to whom he had been introduced in 1877 at Cohnheim's laboratory at Breslau. Koch had discovered the tubercle bacillus just three years earlier, and it was an exciting and affable laboratory. Welch also missed studying with Virchow, but this was the result of direct advice from Ludwig to go with Cohnheim in preference to the Master, who was considered on the wane and then more interested in anthropology, politics, and Kulturkampf than the forefront of pathology. Cohnheim had a broader concept of pathology as including both the dynamic physiologic and chemical aspects of disease as well as the static anatomical side, and Ludwig correctly guessed that this would be the future science of diseases so absolutely fundamental to medicine and healthcare. This was also the thinking in Welch's choice of the name for his new department at Hopkins, the Department of Pathology, rather than the Department of Pathological Anatomy, "to stake out the claim that the chair really should cover, even if it did not actually cultivate, the whole broad field of the origin and nature of diseases," as Welch wrote later in his life. In the fall of 1885, at the age of 35, Welch moved to Hopkins, which would be his base for the rest of his long and amazingly productive life.

Fleming has called Welch's the most influential life in American science since Benjamin Franklin and the elder Benjamin Silliman. In an age when it was becoming increasingly difficult to be the Renaissance man, the list of his works is astonishing. In part it consists of being president of the board of scientific directors of the Rockefeller Institute, president of the American Association for the Advancement of Science, chairman of the executive committee of the Carnegie Institution of Washington, president of the American Medical Association, president of the Association of American Physicians, president of the National Academy of Sciences, chairman of the advisory council of the Milbank Memorial Fund, and an inspiring teacher who launched on their careers a host of the nation's and world's leading biomedical scientists and teachers—called "Welch rabbits." With the British physiologist H. Newell Martin, Hopkins President Daniel Coit Gilman, and planner and librarian

John Shaw Billings, Welch was "one of the four principal founders of the medical tradition at Johns Hopkins."

One of Welch's first pupils, Franklin P. Mall in 1886, became the first chairman of the anatomy department in the new medical school, and another, William S. Halsted, became the first professor of surgery. Welch was also instrumental in bringing Osler from Philadelphia, who led the search resulting in the appointment of Howard A. Kelly as the first chief of gynecology. And so the academic medical family at Hopkins multiplied and prospered, and Welch appropriately became its first dean. By this time, his research productivity had dropped off.

During Tinsley's course in pathology, Welch was still head of the new Hopkins School of Hygeine and Public Health, an institution which had been regarded as a turning point in public health education. Tinsley considered MacCallum a good teacher, but he regretted that Welch could give only a few lectures; Welch was an excellent speaker. Years later, Tinsley remembered these lectures as inspirational.

Tinsley made an 8.5 in pathology that year, near the top of the class.

PHARMACOLOGY WAS TINSLEY'S FAVORITE course. He made his highest second-year grade in this class: 9.5. In this case the leading star was John Jacob Abel, known for his isolation of epinephrine, crystalization of insulin, method of renal dialysis, and studies of pituitary physiology. Abel is considered America's first full-time pharmacologist and was appointed in 1893 to the first chair of pharmacology at Johns Hopkins. He had studied with H. Newell Martin and other academic ancestors of the Hopkins faculty. Like others on the medical faculty, he had returned from Germany to be a professor at Michigan, but he moved to Hopkins after only a year at Michigan. Tinsley considered Abel a superb teacher, one of the best.

Abel was prominent in pharmacology throughout the world and provided considerable stimulus to Tinsley's learning, but he was not the main pharmacology teacher remembered years later. That person was David Macht, an immigrant from Europe who spoke with an accent and was a local general practitioner among the less affluent members of the Baltimore Jewish community. "He was the best teacher I had in my second year of medical school," Tinsley recalled later. He loved his subject and could make everything crystal clear. Macht was an extraordinary man, a possessor of a keen mind. Even in 1919 he seemed rather old to Tinsley. But in 1950 Macht wrote and published a book on medicine in the Torah. "He must have been 90 years old or more then," Tinsley said.

18. An autopsy helper who fetches and transports bodies, opens skulls and chest and abdomens, bottles organs, and prepares remains for the undertaker.

19. Harrison, like many of his colleagues, believed that a thorough understanding of the pathology of individual diseases and their clinical manifestations is necessary to be a good clinician.

During 1919 as the troops returning from Europe were being demobilized, Tinsley had a striking experience in the autopsy room which illustrates the vulnerability of physicians, particularly pathologists, in those days. Edmond Clarke, who while working with MacCallum "almost got insulin before Banting and Best but didn't quite get it," was performing autopsies one Friday afternoon on six young soldiers from Fort Meade, and he showed Tinsley the six pairs of lungs. The soldiers had died from streptococcal pneumonia complicating influenza. On the following Monday after the weekend, Tinsley was shown the lungs of Dr. Edmond Clarke, dead of the same disease! One medical student in each class usually came down with tuberculosis during the four-year medical course. These were often detected early and satisfactorily treated, although with considerable loss of time. But there was no specific therapy for TB, and some of such students died. In this case it was streptococcal pneumonia complicating influenza. Tinsley was lucky he did not catch it.

The following summer between his second and third years of medical school, Tinsley obtained a job in MacCallum's department and helped with the autopsies, something of a diener[18] for the summer. It was a time of dead bodies; he was surrounded by corpses for the hot summer months. He attended all the autopsies and helped with some. He was assigned the stillborns on which he did the autopsies himself. In doing this he not only learned a number of facts about human diseases, but he also developed a feeling of kinship for Osler's path into internal medicine years before.[19]

After a brief few weeks vacation back in Birmingham, he returned to what became his real first love throughout his life: clinical medicine, with its learning and its teaching. He enjoyed his third year of medical school immensely—"really a great year, because now I was in clinical medicine. The main word was Osler. He'd been gone 15 years." Yet Tinsley was well aware that his father Groce had known Osler and had virtually worshipped him as the supreme physician and the embodiment of all he wanted his son Tinsley to become. Just how explicit he was with Tinsley in this is not clear. Osler stood as Tinsley's lifelong model as the perfect internist; this image had been transmitted to him through his father. Tinsley worked in Osler's shadow and under his indirect guidance, not only this year but throughout the rest of his life.

Tinsley's enthusiasm was reflected in his grades during his third and fourth years, generally 9's or 9.5's, even in operative surgery. He received an 8.5 in psychiatry and, ironically, in ENT. During his third year he took an elective in surgical pathology on Wednesday and Friday afternoons from 2 to 4:30, a pass/fail course which he passed.

In his third year he also took "clinical microscopy," taught three afternoons a week. This was really clinical pathology. He was taught various laboratory procedures, how to recognize various parasites such as worms and worm eggs in stool specimens, and how to run simple laboratory tests. There were several other parts to the course, but it was the parasitology that Tinsley best remembered later. He felt it was superbly taught and later said of it, "I learned a tremendous amount about [clinical] laboratory work."

The high point in his third year was the once-a-week clinic given by another town practitioner. Years later Tinsley recalled this experience: "We had a tremendous teacher with whom we spent one hour a week, Louis Hamman, who described Hamman's sign, the "Pop!" of mediastinal emphysema and pneumothorax [as well as the Hamman-Rich syndrome[20]]. And he was just a common ordinary practitioner. He was the greatest teacher I had in my third year. I've always learned more from the men in practice than from the ivory tower boys—full-timers. This is one of the great objections I've got to our medical school. We've forced out the Russakoffs."[21]

William Halsted, the professor of surgery, was senile and probably wasted by drug abuse. "He was the worst teacher I ever had in my life," Tinsley later said. Yet there was still a residual of inspiration even then, because Halsted was a towering figure in surgery. He had introduced the use of rubber gloves in the operating room and had been among the first to insist on asepsis [bacteria-free surgery], as opposed to Lister's antisepsis [use of antiseptics to control infection from surgery]. He held three absolutes in surgery: "No loss of blood; no trauma of tissue; no infection." For example, he prohibited the use of silk sutures as foreign material if there was a high probability of bacterial contamination.

Despite his enthusiasm for clinical medicine, Tinsley later thought the third and fourth years at Hopkins were poorly arranged for optimal teaching of medical students. Third-year internal medicine was entirely an outpatient experience, and only during the fourth year did the students have the opportunity to observe and begin practicing bedside medicine, to work up and follow hospitalized patients. Tinsley felt this third-year outpatient work was a tremendous waste of time, a backwards arrangement, because the students at this point had no bedside experience. The inpatient experience should come first, he thought, and the outpatient work only later. Medical students needed experience with patients. This required lots of time,

20. An acute interstitial pneumonia of unknown cause with diffuse alveolar wall damage (probably a subgroup of ARDS of unknown etiology). It is often rapidly progressive to death despite supportive care. Mortality is around 50 percent now and was much higher when described in 1935.

21. An excellent doctor, Abraham Russakoff was Tinsley's colleague, personal physician and close friend. He came to Birmingham from Baltimore to assist with lung disease in local coal and iron ore miners and was the only ABIM-certified chest physician in Alabama before 1968. Tinsley understood the push for full-time faculty, yet he still regretted the loss from part-time teaching of these talented practitioners like Russakoff.

22. From the material in Harrison's file at the Alan M. Chesney Archives at JHMI it appears this clinic was from noon till 1 P.M. on Saturdays as well as Wednesday and Friday.

23. Harvey, *Osler's Legacy,* 33–42.

24. Ibid., 40.

time for medical students and house officers to observe and examine hospitalized patients, listen repeatedly to cardiac murmurs or friction rubs, repeatedly palpate a nodular liver or an enlarged spleen, and observe changes in fever curves over the course of days or weeks. Medical students had large blocks of time available, and they needed the experience as early as possible. The students still needed to understand the clinical manifestations of the disease entities learned so diligently in pathology. Patients in outpatient settings were more hurried, though far less so than later in the century, and the opportunities to check details in the history, to demonstrate interesting or unusual physical findings, or to follow a patient for a prolonged period were more limited.

The system worked for Tinsley, despite his later reservations about it. During his fourth year, in addition to the inpatient rotations on medicine, surgery, pediatrics, and psychiatry, plus electives and one selective, he also took clinics three days a week.[22] He did very well on these and received a grade of 9.5.

The selective was a choice between pediatrics and obstetrics in the fourth year. Somehow Tinsley had missed or avoided taking third-year obstetrics, and now in the fourth year he chose pediatrics instead. The schedule was arranged in a way that did not permit him to take both. Thus, Tinsley never delivered a single baby in his life! This lack of experience was probably instrumental in bringing about his view in later years that physicians were not needed for normal obstetrics. He felt normal deliveries could be handled by a good nurse, provided she had back-up from a competent physician obstetrician in case of complications.

During Tinsley's final year at the Hopkins medical school, he was surrounded by other physicians who would play crucial roles in his own career. The head of internal medicine was G. Canby Robinson, on leave from his post as dean and professor of medicine at the new Vanderbilt medical school. Hopkins had borrowed him to serve as acting director of the department of medicine during the 1921–22 academic year following the resignation of William S. Thayer from that post and the departure of his designated successor, Walter W. Palmer, for New York's College of Physicians and Surgeons.[23]

Canby Robinson had graduated from the medical school at Hopkins in 1903, worked in a pathology laboratory at the Pennsylvania Hospital with Warfield T. Longcope, studied in Switzerland and Germany (especially with Friedrich Mueller in Munich), and had been the first resident physician at the new hospital of the Rockefeller Institute for Medical Research.[24] The interlockings of fate and personalities in

American academic medicine of the times were at work here. Canby Robinson had been "deeply disappointed" to find himself "in the middle of the class, just one place below the last student who wanted an internship at Hopkins."[25] His friend Longcope had graduated two years earlier and had replaced Simon Flexner, also a former Hopkins resident, as director of the Ayer Pathological Laboratory at the Pennsylvania Hospital. Flexner had left Ayer to become the director of the new Rockefeller Institute for Medical Research in New York.

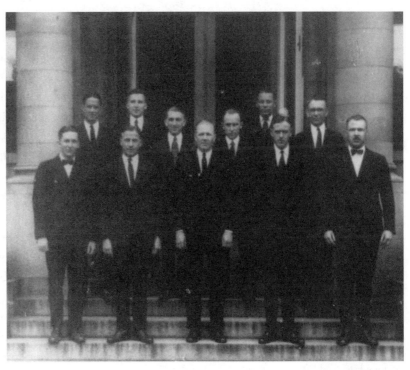

Tinsley Harrison (back row, far right) with a group at Johns Hopkins, circa 1921.

Through these personalities and their appointments, ties were formed that facilitated or led to later appointments and associations, as well as continued funding at Vanderbilt from the Rockefeller money. The people knew and respected each other, and they trusted each other to make the best possible job of anything they undertook and to be men of their word.

From the Rockefeller Institute, Robinson moved to Washington University in St. Louis in 1913 as an associate professor of medicine. In 1920 he resigned from that position to become the first professor of medicine (chairman of the department) and dean of the newly renovated and transformed Vanderbilt University School of Medicine.

The new medical school at Vanderbilt was embodied in new structures—at the university campus, and these new medical buildings would not be ready for occupancy until 1925. This was apparent to Robinson. A year as chief of medicine at Hopkins would give him additional valuable experience for Vanderbilt. So he took the job at Hopkins on an interim basis for a year, the post previously held by Osler, Barker, Janeway, and Thayer.

The chief resident in medicine during Tinsley's senior year at Hopkins was C.

25. Ibid., 40.

26. Ibid., 41.

27. T. R. Harrison, audiotape interview, Birmingham, 1974. (UAB Archives).

28. Proverbs 20:1— "Wine is a mocker, strong drink is raging: and whosoever is deceived thereby is not wise." Proverbs 31:4–7—"It is not for kings, O Lemuel, it is not for kings to drink wine; nor for princes strong drink: Lest they drink, and forget the law, and pervert the judgment of any of the afflicted. Give strong drink unto him that is ready to perish, and wine unto those that be of heavy hearts. Let him drink, and forget his poverty, and remember misery no more."

Sidney Burwell, with a house staff of five assistant residents and four interns from the class of 1921. This was the first year Hopkins began supplying standard white uniforms for the house staff,[26] and Burwell was the first medical chief resident at Hopkins brought in from the outside. On the recommendations of Drs. Paul Dudley White and Roger I. Lee of Harvard and the Massachusetts General Hospital, Robinson broke tradition and hired him, there being no satisfactory candidate in Baltimore at the time.

Robinson inherited from Thayer another staff member, Hugh J. Morgan, who seemed an unusually bright and effective young man.

These were Tinsley's friends and associates at Hopkins, who would play important roles in his later life. Alfred Blalock was Tinsley's best friend throughout their careers together at Hopkins and later at Vanderbilt. They remained close. Blalock obtained the job of running the medical bookstore where the students bought their books. According to Tinsley's later reminiscences, Blalock "bought the privilege to run the students' bookstore, and he earned his living all the way through by running the bookstore for the students. He was a good, but not an outstanding, student. He was a country boy from Jonesboro right outside Atlanta, and I was a country boy from Talladega, Alabama. Al wasn't a brilliant guy, really. I've known many more brilliant people. But Al was ambitious; he had the willingness to work a hundred hours a week. What he had was character and drive. He was not in the class with Bill Dock or Bill Resnick or Sam Levine or Sidney Burwell, among the really first-class minds I've known. But he was willing to work longer than anybody. Al would stay in the lab till midnight and go out and have a date. And the gals all would go 'Oooh' over him. He really had the touch with the ladies."[27]

GRADUATION CEREMONIES WERE ON a Tuesday, June 13, 1922. There is no record of Tinsley's family coming to Baltimore for the occasion, but whether they did or not, the entire Harrison family was delighted with their new physician. That evening some of the graduates had a party to celebrate. Until this time Tinsley never had taken a single drink of an alcoholic beverage, and he had never smoked. That evening he had his first drink and his first cigarette. He enjoyed both. During the declining years of his life he made up in these two respects for his early years of abstinence. He remembered not only Proverbs 20:1, especially in his youthful years, but later also Proverbs 31:4–7.[28]

After graduating, untested doctors moved through a chaotic transition to full-time

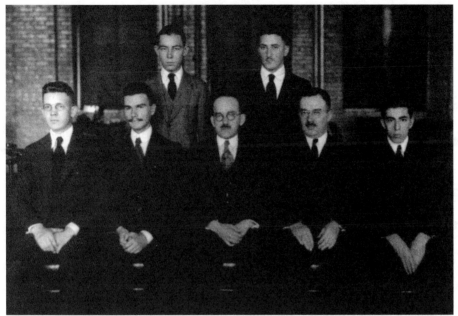

*Seven of the 1922
graduates of the
Johns Hopkins
Medical School.
Tinsley is at the
upper left in the
lighter suit.*

work. It was an informal process. New doctors could be recommended by staff. Then a series of phone interviews was offered. Finally a simple letter of notification from the chief of service to the appointee was sent. Tinsley obtained his appointment as an intern at Harvard's new Peter Bent Brigham Hospital in Boston. It is likely that his chief of medicine at Hopkins, Dr. G. Canby Robinson, telephoned or wrote to the chief of medicine at the Brigham, Dr. Henry A. Christian, to recommend Tinsley as a bright and promising young physician who would do an excellent job on the house staff. (Senior medical students slept in telephone booths for two days or more, awaiting word from an outstanding hospital so they could accept that in preference to an offer from another less desirable hospital which had given a solid offer but had also placed a deadline for its acceptance. The process became somewhat more organized in 1952. Such unformalized personal commitments and lack of coordination ceased with the institution of the National Internship Matching Plan, later the NIRMP, and still later the NRMP, for "Residency."[29]) At the time of Tinsley's graduation from medical school things were very much in the loose, informal, personal mode. He got the Brigham internship.

Young Doctor Harrison packed his belongings, took his new diploma crediting him with having earned an M.D. degree from America's best medical school, and boarded the train for Boston. He was 22 years old.

29. "Is the Match Legal?" Correspondence Section of the *New England Journal of Medicine* 348; 2259–62, May 29, 2003, especially 2260 with letters by James A. Pittman Jr. and especially W. Hardy Hendren. The account of Hendren states that the details of the Match were devised by him and his Harvard class of 1952. A letter from Leslie J. DeGroot, president of the medical school class at Columbia P&S in New York, disputes that the system originated at Harvard and states that it came from a meeting at Columbia. (Email from DeGroot to Pittman and Hendren, dated Friday, June 13, 2003). Regardless of how it started, it did get started in 1952.

30. H. K. Beecher and M. D. Altschule, *Medicine at Harvard: The First 300 Years* (Hanover, NH: The University Press of New England, 1977), 569 pp. plus index. There is an ironic sarcasm in this title and date of publication, since the year before "the best medical school in America" had published its history: James Bordley III and A. McGehee Harvey, *Two Centuries of American Medicine: 1876–1976* (Philadelphia, London, etc., 1976), 826 pp. plus index. Both books are well done, broad in scope, and interestingly written. They contain interesting items, like the fact that Harvard's David Edsall believed strongly that the famous *Flexner Report*, generally believed today to have led the reformation of American medicine, was inadequate for Harvard and could not help the school. In addition, Beecher and Altschule claim that *Flexner* was not at all the first serious effort, but the third. (176–). There were letters exchanged between Flexner and the Harvard administration, and Harvard appears to have won

UPON ARRIVING AT BOSTON's South Station a week after graduation, Tinsley took a taxi to rooms he had obtained through the assistance of the hospital. These were on Huntington Avenue some six blocks from the hospital and new quadrangle of the Harvard Medical School.

For many years Harvard's medical school, the third oldest in the nation, had resembled those elsewhere in this country.[30] It was operated by physicians and surgeons in practice as a commercial enterprise. However, when Charles Eliot became president of Harvard in 1869, one of his first priorities was the upgrading of the medical school.[31]

There are few records in the Brigham archives to document Tinsley's activities in Boston, other than to prove that he was indeed an intern there in 1922–23 and an assistant resident (called "JAR," for junior assistant resident) in 1923–24. We know several things from Tinsley's own reminiscences.

He started as a pup—he was responsible for the laboratory work on the patients in the ward to which he was assigned. As such he did the blood hemoglobin determinations, red and white cell counts using a micrscope and a hemacytometer, urinalyses, blood urea nitrogens, red cell sedimentation rates, and similar simple tests. He also had as one of his first attending physicians Samuel A. Levine, who was to become one of his closest friends and advisers.

The usual routine on the ward was for the house staff and students to make work rounds, draw blood for special tests, and carry out procedures from about 7 until they finished, usually around 9:30 A.M. The higher level residents would leave the group at 9 for morning report with the Chief until 10. At 10 they would present the patients admitted during the previous 24 hours or weekend and give follow-ups on especially interesting patients admitted earlier. This "morning report" was not universal; it was prominent at the Brigham but was omitted at the Massachusetts General Hospital, where it was regarded as a juvenile waste of time. Many hospitals copied this practice. It provided an excellent place for the exchange of medical information and the continuing education of not only the house officers but also the senior physicians who attended it. The teacher learns by doing.

After work rounds, staff spent 10 or 15 minutes in the cafeteria for coffee, a doughnut, and medical gossip for the younger house officers, completion of morning report by the others. After the cafeteria they would check special X-rays on their patients in the radiology department. At 10 A.M. the attending or "visit" (for visiting physician) would appear for attending rounds. The attending physician was a clinician who might be on the full-time regular faculty but was often a physician in private practice who used the Brigham exclusively. These private practice attendings held unpaid medical school appointments designated in the title: "clinical" as a code for voluntary or unpaid. This way the hospital acquired a physician staff of high quality and an assured flow of their patients, and the attending physicians or "visits" obtained appointments and staff privileges in an intellectually exclusive hospital and a famous medical school. Usually there was a quid pro quo, and the physician had to provide two months of service as an attending physician at no pay, or serve regularly in the outpatient department at no pay, in return for these appointments. In many places these or similar arrangements later grew into a group of geographic full-time physician staff supported entirely by their own practices. More recently some of these have developed into group practices and legal corporations of physicians. Hospitals were always complex.

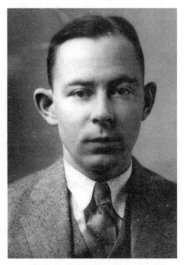

Tinsley Harrison, about 1923.

THE BRIGHAM HOSPITAL, JUST across Shattuck Street from the new basic science quadrangle of the Harvard Medical School, was a perfect starting place for Tinsley to launch a career in academic medicine. In addition to the chief, Henry A. Christian, and Samuel A. Levine, he had as colleagues Bill Dock, Emile Holman, and Samuel Grant. Grant "pointed Harrison toward clinical science. When Grant left the Brigham, Harrison moved into the laboratory that Grant had developed for studying blood flow by the Fick method."[32] All his colleagues were bright energetic young men, and most were enthusiastic about joining him in the laboratory to pursue questions of clinical interest.

TINSLEY WAS BUSY WITH his clinical duties and research activities. But he found time for other things at the Brigham.

During the latter part of his internship, Tinsley was walking through the corridors of the new Brigham Hospital when he passed some young nurses having a group photograph made for some publication. Always curious, he stopped to watch. His eye caught that of a tall handsome young woman in the group, strikingly beautiful. He stared without realizing it, and she stuck her tongue out at him! He stayed until the photo session ended and spoke to her. Her name was Elizabeth Woodward, and she was from Grafton, Massachusetts, outside Worcester near the middle of

at least a few points. Harvard also required that students admitted to its medical school possess a college degree before admission in 1893, the same year Hopkins did.

31. George E. Burch, and N. P. DePasquale, *A History of Electrocardiography* (1964; repr., San Francisco: Norman Publishing, 1990).

32. E. Braunwald, "The Pathogenesis of Congestive Failure: Then and Now" *Medicine* 70 (1991), 67–81.

the state. She had just completed her nursing training at the Boston Children's Hospital, but she was spending time at the Brigham to obtain additional experience in adult nursing. Tinsley asked her out on a date, then another. On February 21, 1924, they were married by a justice of the peace in a civil ceremony. This was on a Thursday, and they spent Friday, Saturday, and Sunday on a brief local honeymoon. To retain their respective statuses at the Brigham, they had to hide their marriage; it was strictly against regulations for either of them to get married. Neither wore a wedding ring or gave any other outward indication of change in marital status. They just kept working.

Thus it was that Tinsley and Betty continued to maintain separate quarters, and only a very few of their closest friends and their families knew they were married. At the end of June, Betty fainted in the operating room while assisting at Children's Hospital. During the medical workup she learned that she was pregnant.

They left for Baltimore shortly afterwards. The move was accomplished without difficulty, especially since neither yet had any great accumulation of belongings. Tinsley began his senior assistant residency (SAR) year. They no longer had to hide.

SAR WAS A YEAR for polishing clinical skills, doing research, and deciding on the course for later years. The two main options: pursue a primarily private practice of medicine or attempt a career in academic medicine of teaching and research with practice in a medical school setting. Tinsley had always enjoyed teaching and had obtained some experience in it as a resident at the Brigham, where he had junior and senior medical students from Harvard associated with him in his ward work. His father also seemed to hold a good teacher in very high esteem and had taken every opportunity to emphasize the importance of teaching to other individuals and to society as a whole. Teaching was a way of repaying a debt to society for the advantages society brought to the individual.

Academic medicine also involved research, perhaps even more than teaching, and certainly Hopkins, stimulated primarily by Welch and his followers, imbued the faculty and staff with the necessity of carrying on research to advance medical knowledge and practice. The staff was highly receptive and able, especially the bright young house officers chosen from the top graduates of Hopkins and a few other schools each year. These elite standards were winnowed by a pyramid system of appointment in successive years down to the very few who were most intelligent, alert, aggressive, and had the most initiative and ability to accomplish. Harrison had such colleagues, especially Drs. Emile Holman, later chief of medicine at Stanford University Medical School, and William Dock, later prominent in a variety of academic positions and son of George Dock, who had been a professor of medicine in Texas, then at Michigan, and was later chief of medicine at Washington University in St. Louis. Both remained Harrison's friends throughout their lives, especially Bill Dock.[33]

Tinsley was happy to be back in Baltimore, where he could again play tennis regularly with Al Blalock and enjoy his companionship. Pregnant, Betty worked for about three months as a nurse. They were happy with the prospect of their first child, but the living arrangements were terrible. Tinsley, who was on call full-time, every day, 24 hours a day, had a room in the hospital and was expected to be there all the time. Betty lived in a boarding house in a nearby neighborhood. The house staff were paid "in kind"—the experience and instruction they received from the senior staff was their payment; they earned no money). Betty and Tinsley's funds were extremely tight. At Betty's boarding house she was not comfortable. She had to share the bathroom facilities with numerous other roomers. She was developing in her pregnancy and she was often alone. In October she took the train for Massachusetts, where she joined her family for the last weeks of the pregnancy. Her brother in Grafton was a surgeon with a friend who was an excellent obstetrician. On November 10, 1924, the baby was delivered in Worcester Memorial Hospital. It was a boy. They named him Lemuel Woodward Harrison, choosing the first two names from Betty's family. She returned to Baltimore before Christmas, where her friends helped with the baby.

During this time Tinsley remained largely in the hospital, but the house staff were able to slip out for a few hours here and there, such as a few hours with Betty and the baby Woody, or a quick game of tennis with Al.

In Baltimore he teamed up with Blalock and another associate, C. P. Wilson, to study the effects of changes in hydrogen ion concentration on the blood flow of morphinized dogs.[34] With another colleague, W. A. Perlzweig, he published observations on patients with alkalosis in uremia, an unusual condition.[35]

Tinsley's chief of medicine during his senior assistant residency in 1924–25 was Warfield T. Longcope, who had replaced Robinson in 1922 as Tinsley was moving from Baltimore to Boston.[36] In what was becoming something of a Hopkins tradition of mixing up pathology and internal medicine, Longcope's training after his graduation from the Hopkins medical school in 1901 was in pathology.[37] After

33. Horace W. Davenport, *Doctor Dock: Teaching and Learning Medicine at the Turn of the Century* (New Brunswick and London: Rutgers University Press, 1987).

34. T. R. Harrison, C. P. Wilson, and A. Blalock, "The Effect of Changes in Hydrogen Ion Concentration on the Blood Flow of Morphinized Dogs." *J. Clinical Investig*, 1 (1925) 547–648.

35. T. R. Harrison and W. A. Perlzweig, "Alkolosis Not Due to Administration of Alkali, Associated With Uremia." *JAMA* 84 (1925) 671–673.

36. Harvey, *Osler's Legacy*, 43.

37. Osler was known for his expertise in pathology, even though he had been chief of medicine at Pennsylvania before moving to Hopkins. Longcope was trained in pathology. And years later an internist, Ivan Bennett, was named chief of pathology at Hopkins, much to the consternation of "real pathologists."

38. Harvey, *Osler's Legacy*, 44.

39. T. R. Harrison, to Dr. Rudolph Kampmeirer, May 6, 1976, 8–9.

Hopkins, Longcope had gone to the Ayer Laboratory to work with Simon Flexner, with a later appointment as assistant professor of applied clinical medicine at the University of Pennsylvania. He had then moved to New York as an associate professor of medicine and became the Bard Professor and head of the department before returning to Baltimore in 1922 as the new chief and third full-time professor of medicine. Longcope was "a bridge between the distinguished clinicians of the previous generation and the modern clinical investigator,"[38] and he was well trained in several related scientific disciplines.

As an assistant resident senior to those who had just completed their internships, Tinsley was less bound to the work of caring for patients in the wards and was given time to pursue research projects, which Longcope encouraged in every way possible. Since Longcope expected performance and proof of solid accomplishments for this measure of freedom from the clinical duties, the pressures on Tinsley to produce something substantial in the way of research were considerable.

In the meantime Robinson was busy planning the new Vanderbilt Medical School and overseeing the construction of the impressive new facilities. Robinson, who held Vanderbilt appointments as both chief of medicine and dean of the faculty of medicine, had the Hopkins arrangements in mind and wanted to create three divisions in his department of medicine: laboratories of physiology, bacteriology, and chemistry, each to be headed by an associate professor. But he only had funds for two positions.

In the fall of 1924, as he was shuttling back and forth between Nashville, Baltimore, New York, and probably other cities, Robinson had just observed dual coverages at Hopkins. Bill Resnik was running the emergency ward but also covering the electrocardiographic laboratory. Chester Keefer covered the bacteriology laboratory at night and on weekends. Tinsley had a similar responsibility for the clinical chemistry laboratory. Robinson was impressed by Tinsley's energy and abilities, as well as his knowledge of the technical procedures for the clinical chemistries of the day, and he offered him the chief residency in medicine at the new Vanderbilt Hospital along with the responsibility of running the chemical laboratory of the department of medicine. "He added that if I did well in both jobs there would in all probability be a place for me on the staff should I desire it, to climb upward on the academic ladder beginning as Instructor," Tinsley said. "I would be getting in on the ground floor during the development of a great medical school."[39]

It was an opportunity he could not refuse. Vanderbilt it was.

Nine Generations of Harrison Medical Doctors

Although little concrete information is available about the first two generations, Tinsley Harrison claimed to be a seventh-generation physician. That medical lineage has now extended to nine generations.

1st Tinsley's Great-Great-Great-Great-Grandfather

2nd Tinsley's Great-Great-Great-Grandfather

3rd Lt. Battaile Harrison (1771–?)

4th John Tinsley Harrison Sr. (1799–1875)
University of Virginia (?)

5th John Tinsley Harrison Jr. (1834–1915)
University of Nashville (ca. 1856)

6th William Groce Harrison Sr. (1871–1955)
University of Nashville (1892) and Baltimore Medical College (1893)

7th Tinsley Randolph Harrison (1900–1978)
Johns Hopkins (1922)

7th William Groce Harrison Jr. (1902–1988)
Johns Hopkins (1925)

8th John Bondurant Harrison (1938–)
University of Alabama Dental (1966) and Medical Schools (1971)

9th John Randolph Hutchinson "Hutch" Harrison (1961–)
UAB Medical School (1991)

6

THE VANDERBILT YEARS

1925–1941

1. Alfred Blalock, "A Clinical Study of Biliary Tract Disease," *JAMA* 83 (1924): 2057; "A statistical Study of 888 Cases of Biliary Tract Disease," *Johns Hopkins Hosp. Bull.* 35 (1924): 391.

2. The details of which are explained in W. P. Longmire Jr.'s *Alfred Blalock: His Life and Times* (Los Angeles: W. P. Longmire, 1991), 37–39.

3. Longmire, *Alfred,* 39; "Treatment of Chronic Middle Ear Suppuration," with S. J. Crowe. *Archives of Otolaryngology* 1 (1925): 267; Alfred Blalock, "The Incidence of Mastoid Disease in the United States." *South. Med. J.* 18 (1925): 621; Blalock, "The Recurrent Laryngeal Nerves

Tinsley's years at Vanderbilt were probably the happiest of his adult life. His childhood had been pleasant and instructive, but those years always seemed unreal, a romantic idyll. His Vanderbilt period was marked by study and intellectual rigor and friendship and success. During that decade and a half, Tinsley expanded his family, established himself as a clinician and a widely published academic researcher, became active as a member and leader of major medical associations, and nurtured existing friendships that would be important to him personally and professionally for the rest of his career.

Among his most meaningful relationships continued to be that with Al Blalock. When they graduated from medical school in 1922, Tinsley was selected for one of the best medical internships in the nation at Boston's Peter Bent Brigham Hospital, but Blalock failed in his attempt to win appointment as a Johns Hopkins surgical intern, probably due to his less than stellar academic performance in medical school. Blalock did win his second choice, a urology internship at Hopkins. This would permit three months rotation each on general surgery and gynecology, with the other six months in urology, which was, after all, a surgical specialty. During this year in urology, Blalock performed outstandingly and compiled an extensive study of "888 cases of biliary tract disease," which resulted in two publications.[1] He had chosen the topic because he knew of Hopkins surgery professor William Halsted's interest in it. Halsted died during the year, but Acting Chief of Surgery J. M. T. Finney was impressed and appointed Blalock to a residency in general surgery. Blalock was finally where he wanted to be.

Blalock's year of general surgery went well. He completed it in June 1924, however, because of political problems in the residency program,[2] he failed to gain another appointment in general surgery for the following year. This time he was saved by a senior faculty friend, Dr. Samuel J. Crowe, chief of otorhinolaryngology at Hopkins. Blalock spent 1924–25, his third postdoctoral year at Hopkins in the anomalous position of extern in ENT. Again he recognized the value Hopkins placed on research publications, and he produced five papers during 1924–25, three more or less on his own related primarily to otolaryngology,[3] and two from laboratory work done with his friend and supporter Tinsley, now back from Boston.[4] Longmire calls these last two papers Blalock's first serious effort in research.[5] By this time, the residency program in general surgery was filled, and he had no job as July 1925 approached.

As Tinsley, Betty, and the new baby were preparing for the move from Baltimore to Nashville, Blalock was distraught at the prospect of unemployment for the coming year, and Tinsley knew it. Blalock's friend and mentor Samuel Crowe telephoned neurosurgeon Harvey Cushing, his former Hopkins colleague and friend at the Brigham, who told him with some reluctance, "Send him along and I will see if I can't find something for him."[6]

Tinsley sought out his new and former chief, G. Canby Robinson, and discussed the problem with him.[7] It turned out that Vanderbilt's new chief of surgery, Barney Brooks, had been distracted by a terrible family tragedy. His only son had just died in St. Louis after a prolonged illness.[8] As a result, the new hospital was missing a chief of surgery. Tinsley was able to prevail upon Robinson, who was familiar with Blalock from his year at Hopkins and his connections there, to convince Brooks to appoint Blalock chief resident in surgery for 1925–26.[9]

Al had already arrived in Boston when he received Tinsley's call to tell him of the job and to insist that he take it: Blalock would be Vanderbilt's first chief resident in surgery; Harrison would be the first chief resident in medicine. Without even unpacking his bags, Blalock returned to the railroad station and left Boston for Nashville.

WHEN TINSLEY TOLD AL they would be "the first chief residents" in the school, what he meant was the newly constituted

in Dogs," with S. J. Crowe. *Arch. Surgery* 12 (1926): 95.

4. Alfred Blalock, "The Effects of Changes in Hydrogen Ion Concentration on the Blood Flow of Morphinized Dogs." *J. Clinical Investig.* 1 (925): 547; Alfred Blalock, Tinsley Harrison, and C. P. Wilson: "Partial Tracheal Obstruction: An Experimental Study in the Effects on the Circulation and Respiration of Morphinized Dogs." *Arch. Surg.* 13 (1925): 81.

5. Longmire, *Alfred*, 43.

6. Ibid., 41.

7. Rudolph H.

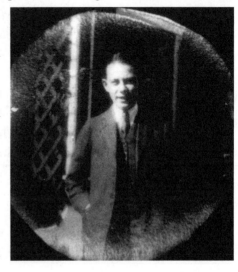

Tinsley Harrison, about 1924.

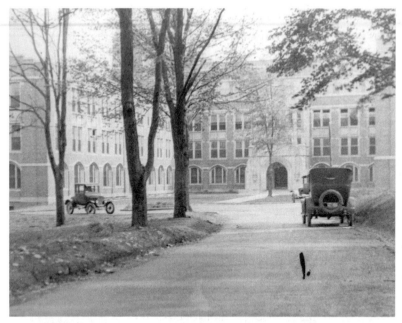

Vanderbilt medical school, around the time Tinsley Harrison and Al Blalock arrived in 1925.

Kampmeier, *Recollections, The Department of Medicine, Vanderbilt University School of Medicine 1925–1959* (Nashville: Vanderbilt University Press, 1980). Also Harrison, to Dr. Rudy Kampmeier, May 6, 1976. Vanderbilt University Medical Center Library, Special Collections, 2; S. R. Kaufmann, *The Healer's Tale: Transforming Medicine and Culture.*

Vanderbilt medical school. Medical schools had operated in Nashville for more than a century,[10] and this new school could trace its roots to two former schools. It is necessary to understand the background of the development of the Vanderbilt medical school in order to understand Tinsley's later career at the three other medical schools where he worked in North Carolina, Texas, and Alabama.

The vigorous and idealistic local management of James H. Kirkland, who became chancellor of Vanderbilt University in 1893 at the age of 34, and Cornelius P. Vanderbilt's gift of $1 million in the late 19th century were important factors in the rapid development of the new medical school in the first third of the 20th century.[11] Major financial help from the Carnegie Foundation and especially the General Education Board (Rockefeller Foundation), combined with several interesting personal associations formed through Hopkins and the Rockefeller Institute, helped with the new school's development.

Vanderbilt medical school's roots trace back to the Shelby Medical College of 1858–61, through Shelby's origins from the Central University of the Methodist Episcopal Church South. Bishops Holland McTyeire and Robert Paine urged the creation of this "Central University" for the church and its placement at the heart of their territory, Nashville.

McTyeire was a first cousin of Vanderbilt's wife. Mrs. Vanderbilt recognized that the university offered her husband the opportunity to leave a memorial. John Tigert IV, a biographer of McTyeire, wrote of Mrs. Vanderbilt, "Her task was somehow to help the Commodore, who loved her dearly, to decide that the Bishop's university was the enterprise he would like to endow."[12]

Philip Lindsley, the president of the University of Nashville, initiated the medical school. In 1824 he served as acting president of Princeton and was apparently a leading candidate to become permanent president, when he resigned to accept what appeared to be an excellent opportunity to build a new university in a developing part of the new nation, Nashville—the position of president of Cumberland College, forerunner of the University of Nashville.[13] The attitude of a South not yet humbled by the Civil War and Reconstruction is evident in comments made by President Lindsley in an address in 1837:

> How soon it may be practical to add the faculties of law and medicine, and what should be their character are questions more easily asked than answered. Such faculties might be organized immediately were we content to be on a par with Harvard, Yale and Virginia. But one or two professors of law and three or four of medicine would not meet our views—or equal to the ones of the profession.[14]

In April 1874, the merger between the medical faculties of the University of Nashville and the new Vanderbilt University arguably created the most prestigious medical school in the South:

> The effect of this agreement was that Vanderbilt without any expenditure whatsoever, secured, even before it opened its academic department, a medical school a quarter of a century old, famous in its day, and at that time well and favorably known. The alliance, however, at the same time brought to the medical school of the University of Nashville the prestige of an institution under the patronage of a great church and supported by an endowment far greater than that of any other school south of the Ohio River.[15]

It was Vanderbilt Chancellor James Kirkland, however, who played the role of Charles Eliot of the South in his management of the new Vanderbilt University and his interest in creating a leading medical school. A modest teacher who came to Vanderbilt in 1886 to be the chair of Latin, Kirkland was visionary—imaginative, vigorous, upward looking, and tenacious in pursuit of his clearly articulated goals. He was pragmatic and opportunistic, yet he never lapsed into the cynicism so apt to trap such an approach. He was consistently idealistic and charitable. He should serve as an inspiration for academic and medical administrators. In the accounts of his time as president,[16] he and he alone seems responsible for putting together the money, selecting and hiring Canby Robinson, then showing the flexibility to

(Madison: University of Wisconsin Press, 1993).

8. Kampmeier, *Recollections*, 1980.

9. Kampmeier states (20), "Canby spent the last half of 1922 visiting medical schools in Denmark, Germany, Holland, and England." Since Harrison and Blalock graduated in June of 1922, Robinson would have been with them during their last year of medical school, and since he was clinically active making rounds and the like with the medical students, it was likely that he knew both Tinsley and Blalock fairly well before Vanderbilt.

10. R. H. Kampmeier, Mary Teloh, Robert M. Vantrease, and William J. Darby, *Vanderbilt University School of Medicine. The Story in Pictures from Its Beginning to 1963.* (Nashville: Vanderbilt University Medical Center, 1990). However, Conkin in an excellent and detailed account of the old school, the transition, and the new school states, "Only in a very limited way did the old Medical School grow into a new one. The continuities were few." And, "The

changes wrought in less than a decade [in the new school] were revolutionary. In no other Vanderbilt school, in no other period, did change come so rapidly. Very few people on the campus, in any of the older schools, quite comprehended what was going on, at times least of all the professors in the old Medical School. Even Kirkland, at times, was less a guiding architect than an astonished observer." P. K. Conkin, H. L. Swint and P. S. Miletich: *Gone With the Ivy: A Biography of Vanderbilt University* (Knoxville: The University of Tennessee Press, 1985), 266–67.

11. Kampmeier, *Vanderbilt*.

12. Kampmeier, *Recollections*, 23.

13. Kampmeier, *Vanderbilt*, 2.

14. Kampmeier, *Recollections*, 12.

15. Philip M. Hamer, ed., *Centennial History of the Tennessee Medical Association, 1830–1930* (Nashville: Tennessee State Medical Association, 1930), quoted in Kampmeier, *Vanderbilt*, 13.

16. Kampmeier, *Vanderbilt*; Kampmeier, *Recollections*.

abandon his original plans and accept the more grandiose and expensive plans of Robinson for the new medical school.

Kirkland's efforts to raise the standards at Vanderbilt anticipated Flexner's coming review of medical schools.[17] Upon completing in Memphis his review of Tennessee's nine medical schools in November 1909, Flexner concluded:

> The state of Tennessee protects at this date more low-grade medical schools than any other Southern state. It would be unfair and futile to criticize this situation without full recognition of local conditions. A standpoint that is entirely in order in dealing with Cincinnati, Chicago, or St. Louis is here irrelevant. The ideals held up must indeed be the same; but their attainment is much further in the future. The amount of money available for medical education is small; the preliminary requirement must be relatively low. Practically all that can be asked of Tennessee is that it should do the best possible under the circumstances.
>
> This it does not do. The six white schools value their separate survival beyond all other considerations. A single school could furnish all the doctors the state needs and do something to supply the needs of adjoining states as well. Low as the entrance standard must be, it has been made lower in order to gather in students for six schools where one would suffice. The medical schools solicit and accept students who have not yet made the best of the limited educational opportunities their homes provide; and to this extent, not only injure the public health, but depress and demoralize the general educational situation.

After commenting on the waste involved in attempting to maintain duplicative resources at multiple medical schools and the senseless complexities illustrated by the management of a medical school in Knoxville by Lincoln Memorial University at Cumberland Gap simultaneous with Knoxville's University of Tennessee sheltering "an entirely superfluous school at Nashville," Flexner concludes,

> If our analysis is correct, the institution to which the responsibility for medical education in Tennessee should just now be left is Vanderbilt University; for it is the only institution in position at this juncture to deal with the subject effectively. . . . Improved teaching should compensate student defects. To this end, every effort should be made to secure endowment specifically applicable to the medical department; in the interval, fees must be employed not to wipe

out old obligations, however incurred, but to improve the school.[18]

The school might well have been called Flexner's medical school, or perhaps "the Rockefeller School of Medicine."[19] Kirkland apparently met Flexner for the first time during Flexner's famous tour of American and Canadian medical schools in 1909. The two got on very well together; Flexner was impressed with the vigorous efforts Kirkland was making to upgrade the medical school. As Kirkland attempted to implement the reforms suggested by Flexner, they became good friends. The two men soon had neighboring summer cabins in Ontario, Canada, and spent many a day fishing together on their lake. Flexner found no quality medical schools in Tennessee; Vanderbilt was the best of a sorry lot, the only one with real promise. In his book, and in even more detailed discussions with Kirkland, Flexner pointed out all its deficiencies. Subsequently, Flexner, who later would become intimately involved in the distribution of the Rockefeller money, recommended increased endowment for Vanderbilt in 1910.

In the wake of the Flexner evaluation, Kirkland made several decisions about the handling of the real estate and the approach to private individuals and foundations for money, essentially the only sources. The argument with the church over control of the university had already begun when Carnegie withheld $800,000 of his $1 million because of "his objection to the denominational status of Vanderbilt," and the issue was soon resolved in favor of a non-denominational status. Flexner intended for Vanderbilt to take the lead in developing medical education not only for the State of Tennessee, but for the entire South.

At the end of World War I, as Tinsley was entering medical school at Michigan, Vanderbilt's medical school was in chaos. The school had been running an operating deficit, which it was covering by withdrawing money from the Carnegie funds intended for other purposes. In order to upgrade to the minimum requirements set forth by the AMA to attain the status of a Class A school, "it had to require two years of college work for admission, which was sure further to depress enrollments" and to lower income from student fees.

At this point Kirkland "turned to his old friends, Wallace Buttrick and Abraham Flexner, both with the Rockefeller-funded General Education Board. In 1919 they committed $4 million to the building of a new medical school, the largest gift they had ever made to any university."[20] The financial support from the various Rockefeller charities over the years made John D. Rockefeller Sr. Vanderbilt's most generous

17. Flexner, *Medical.*

18. Ibid., 307–308.

19. Conkin, *Gone,* 202–208, 266–286, 374–377, 492–499.

20. Apparently the University of Chicago is excluded from this assessment on the basis that the $10 million given it by Rockefeller was a "starter grant" to begin that university.

21. Ibid., 267.

22. Ibid. One wonders, however, whether this would be so if the dollars were corrected for inflation to "constant dollars."

23. George W. Corner, *A History of the Rockefeller Institute 1901–1953, Origins and Growth* (New York: The Rockefeller Institute Press, 1964); Raymond B. Fosdick, *The Story of the Rockefeller Foundation* (New York: Harper and Brothers, 1952).

24. Gates and Buttrick probably quoted Romans 8:28 to Rockefeller in this connection, and especially Matthew 19:21-24.

25. John Ettling, *The Germ of Laziness: Rockefeller Philanthropy and Public Health in the New South* (Cambridge: Harvard Univ. Press, 1981), 73.

benefactor.[21] William K. Vanderbilt had also been generous with the university, and "after World War II, Harold S. Vanderbilt contributed much larger sums of money than ever provided by the GEB."[22]

How did these large sums of money become available to Kirkland? The story reveals a network of interconnections.

AROUND THE TURN OF the century John D. Rockefeller Sr. was the richest man in America, perhaps the country's first billionaire. His charities "grew in the new century into the largest such in the world." In many ways, Rockefeller was a simple, devout Baptist. With his success, he turned to the ordained Baptist minister Frederick T. Gates, to organize and manage all his philanthropies and charities. Gates was well-educated and had attended the Rochester Theological School, where he had come under the influence of Walter Rauschenbusch, who emphasized "a social gospel rather than . . . the doctrinal controversies that followed in the wake of Darwin." To Rockefeller, this must have seemed a good answer to the earlier attempts by Andrew Carnegie "to launch a new, carefully organized and administered philanthropy (a 'gospel of wealth')." Gates not only managed Rockefeller's investments with an effectiveness that substantially increased their yields and value, but he also organized the charities with brilliant originality. He picked Wallace Buttrick, another fellow-thinking graduate of the Rochester Theological Seminary and ordained Baptist minister, to head the new General Education Board (GEB).[23]

In another important connection of fate,[24] in July 1897 a New York medical student, who as a child had been in Gates's church in Minneapolis, gave him a copy of Osler's textbook *Principles and Practice of Medicine*, first published in 1892.[25] At this crucial time Gates was beginning his efforts to guide the Rockefeller charities toward science, education, and medicine, and he was astounded at the vastness of human ignorance about diseases and their management, a reaction which helped impel him towards his work in medicine and medical education. Conkin said:

> Inspired by the new work at the Johns Hopkins Medical School, incensed
> by the incompetence of so many American physicians, Gates helped set up the
> Rockefeller Institute for Medical Research in 1901. Significantly for Vanderbilt,
> he hired as its first director Simon Flexner, a pathologist, a brother of Kirkland's
> later close friend, Abraham, and a University of Louisville M.D. who had taken
> postdoctoral work at the Hopkins. In 1903 Gates formed the GEB, with Buttrick

as its secretary. Although the title did not suggest it, this board placed almost all of its early emphasis upon the South.[26]

In his book, *The Story of the Rockefeller Foundation*, Raymond Fosdick, its president from 1936 to 1948, recounts that, "More than satisfied with the promise of this initial venture at Johns Hopkins,[27] the Board over a period of six years voted funds for similar reorganizations on a full-time basis of the medical schools at Washington University in St. Louis, at Yale, and at Chicago. All its contributions in this field were invariably conditioned on specific funds being raised from other sources for the same purpose. This was the approach at Nashville, Tennessee, where with Chancellor Kirkland's statesmanlike co-operation, the Board developed at Vanderbilt an outstanding medical school to serve the South. As Flexner later stated, the first appropriation to Vanderbilt of $4 million (later increased to $17.5 million) acted like a 'depth bomb,' hastening the mortality of inferior schools, while those that were determined to survive made rapid plans to enlarge their resources and elevate their aims."[28]

In 1909 Gates created another agency, the Sanitary Commission (often called the Hookworm Commission), to work toward eradication of hookworm disease from the South. A 1911 estimate put the frequency of hookworm infection around 42 percent of the population, and much higher in some rural areas where they did not have outdoor privies.[29] To head this new commission he selected Wickliffe Rose of Peabody College, associated with Vanderbilt and a friend and strong ally of Kirkland's.[30] Rose later served as president of the GEB. Because of the peculiarly Southern problems, "in 1915 Gates and Rockefeller decided to disband the Sanitary Commission . . . [and] Under the auspices of a new, blanket agency—the Rockefeller Foundation—they turned to an international hookworm program but left the medical problems of the South primarily to the rapidly expanding GEB." The Rockefeller money was to provide annual funding for Walter Leathers's department of preventive medicine and public health at Vanderbilt for many years.

Gates's efforts were another example of Osler's presence, a large shadow over the development of medicine in this country.[31]

Abraham Flexner, his famous report having been published and Carnegie's $1 million having been allocated to Vanderbilt, left the Carnegie Foundation and joined the GEB as secretary with President Buttrick. Conkin's account is vivid:

26. Conkin, *Gone*, 269.

27. Fosdick, *Story*, 97. While Hopkins had full-time faculty in its basic science departments from the outset, those in the clinical departments remained part-time; i.e., they supported themselves largely with earnings from practice. In late 1913 Welch applied successfully to the board of the Rockefeller Foundation for funds to create an endowment to produce $65,000 annually to be used for full-time faculty in the departments of medicine, surgery, and pediatrics. Later obstetrics, psychiatry, ophthalmology, preventive medicine, the history of medicine, and radiology were added.

28. Ibid., 97.

29. Ettling, *Germ*.

30. Conkin, *Gone*, 269; Ettling, *Germ*.

31. Fosdick, *Story*, 80–. Osler and Hopkins, through Gates and Rockefeller, also influenced medicine elsewhere in the world. For example, Chapter VII of Fosdick's book is titled "The Johns Hopkins of China"

and recounts Rockefeller work at the Peking Union Medical College, still in operation in 1993. In 1972 a group of about 13 Chinese physicians came to America as the first such medical delegation since the communist government was established in 1949. Seven of the 13 were PUMC graduates.

32. Flexner was Jewish. However, this would not preclude his dedication to "Christian service." Indeed, he may have been more effective at it than some nominal Christians.

33. Conkin, *Gone*, 270–71.

34. G. Canby Robinson, *Adventures in Medical Education: A Personal Narrative of the Great Advance of American Medicine* (Cambridge, MA: Harvard University Press, 1957), 143.

As soon as the war ended Kirkland resumed his correspondence and his personal discussions with Buttrick and Flexner. Letters document only the surface of the story. By February, 1919, the members of the GEB gave a blank check to Buttrick and Flexner, and indirectly to Kirkland; they were to prepare a detailed proposal for a reorganized Vanderbilt Medical School. Buttrick and Flexner also visited Kirkland in Nashville. From this point on, the relationship was not one of a petitioner to benefactors. Flexner and Buttrick took a personal responsibility for the new school, and Flexner was as much or more involved in its planning than Kirkland. A dedication to Christian service guided all three men.[32] At critical junctures Kirkland seemed more cautious, less willing to think in terms of huge sums of money, than his two friends. From these discussions came plans for a reorganization that promised to cost at least $4 million. This the GEB granted in July 1919, but Kirkland postponed any announcement until November. The new plan was quite ambitious and entailed a new, full-time, research-oriented faculty, or a faculty modeled as closely as possible to the one at the Johns Hopkins and on Flexner's standards for a modern medical school. In its original grant the GEB emphasized medical training, research, and organized hygiene, particularly relating to venereal diseases, typhoid, malaria, pellagra, and hookworm disease. No medical school in the South (Hopkins they did not count as Southern) had the personnel or faculty to train physicians for these tasks or to carry out the needed research. The GEB selected Nashville as a strategic location, noted Vanderbilt's reputation for scholarly standards, and complimented the vision, energy, and leadership of Kirkland.

To get the work started in 1920, "the GEB encouraged Kirkland to make an early appointment of a dean for the new school. The dean needed to help plan the new buildings and to begin recruiting a new faculty. In a sense, Flexner picked the dean. He asked Kirkland to go to the medical school of Washington University in St. Louis to interview Dean G. Canby Robinson. This was a fateful trip, one that opened up problems and opportunities undreamed of by Kirkland."[33] Though Robinson did not resign from Washington University Medical School until July, the planning for the new school in Nashville began in earnest in the spring of 1920.[34]

ABRAHAM FLEXNER KNEW WHAT he was talking about. Canby Robinson was the ideal person for the task ahead at Vanderbilt. His career wove together strands from four institutions later important in recruiting money and people for Vanderbilt: Hopkins, University of Pennsylvania, Rockefeller Institute, and Washington University. Born in Baltimore in 1878, Robinson had attended college at the new Johns Hopkins then had studied medicine at Hopkins. He was a mediocre medical student, and when he graduated in 1903 he was disappointed and frustrated to learn that he ranked just one place below the last member of the class who wanted a Hopkins internship. He applied to the old New York Hospital and St. Lukes, also in New York City. When he took the two-day competitive examination at the former, he again failed by narrow margin.[35] At St. Luke's he was first on the alternate list, but no accepted candidate withdrew. Depressed and frustrated, Robinson consulted his good friend and fellow student at Hopkins, Warfield T. Longcope, who had graduated from Hopkins two years earlier and had just replaced Simon Flexner as head of the Ayer Pathological Laboratory at the Pennsylvania Hospital. Longcope, later to take Osler's old position as chief of medicine at Hopkins, found a position for Robinson in pathology for that year. The Simon Flexner just departed for New York was the brother of Abraham and the first director of the new Rockefeller Institute for Medical Research.[36] Matrices of families and friends formed the elite of the medical world. The same names continue to pop up.

The process of obtaining an internship in those days was still quite particular to the place. At Philadelphia, before he could be appointed, Robinson was required to be interviewed by each of the 12 hospital managers. The fact that he was a Quaker helped, as did his name "Canby," which convinced one of the managers that they were related. He was accepted as a qualified candidate, but, as the hospital started a new appointee every three months, he would have at least several months free before beginning. He spent this time helping Hopkins surgeon Martin Tinker start a service at the Clifton Springs Sanitarium in upper New York state. There he assisted Dr. Tinker with his surgical operations and acted as his anesthetist, worked in the clinical laboratory, and had charge of a few medical patients. He later obtained a position teaching anatomy at the Ithaca branch of the Cornell University Medical College, where he worked for Abram Kerr, who had been his instructor four years earlier at Hopkins. He was teaching anatomy when the call came from Longcope with news of the assistantship in the Ayer Clinical Laboratory.

After thirty months with Longcope, Robinson started his residency. It was what would later be called a rotating program and took Robinson through the various services of the hospital—medicine, surgery, on district obstetrics (such as home

35. Ibid., 63.

36. Harvey, *Osler's Legacy*, 40.

37. Robinson, G. Canby, and George Draper, "A Study of the Presphygmic Period of the Heart," *Arch. Intern. Med.* 2, (1910): 168-216.

deliveries)—experiences which were to serve him well in later years.

Robinson spent 1908–09 in Munich in the department of Professor Friedrich Mueller, where he worked with another American, George Draper, on "the presphygmic period of the heart"—the period between the time when the heart starts to contract and the beginning of the arterial pulse.[37]

Lacking the academic opportunity he sought, Robinson returned to Philadelphia in June of 1908 and entered private practice. Word of his experiences, capabilities, and desires spread (probably largely through Longcope, with whom he roomed during that period), and after 16 months he was called by Simon Flexner to become the first senior resident physician at the Rockefeller Institute Hospital. Though his period of private practice in Philadelphia was short, it was an experience which he later felt gave him a good perspective on what new medical graduates would face as they entered practice themselves.

In 1913 he moved to Washington University in St. Louis as an associate professor, where George Dock (father of Bill Dock, one of Tinsley's close friends) placed him in charge of the outpatient department, along with both laboratory and clinical teaching and a host of other duties. Robinson was to become acting dean during the war, then dean for the year immediately preceding his recruitment to Vanderbilt by Kirkland.

Even in these early years of the century, Robinson was familiar with the problems caused by the topsy-turvy growth and ad hoc arrangements of medical school-hospital complexes with buildings scattered to available land as various organizations were able to fund construction but wanted to preserve autonomy, or as new monies for construction became available to the university. The resulting lack of physical connections made coordination of patient care, education, and research difficult. Robinson was a hands-on manager and administrator. He personally prepared detailed sketches of plans for a large structure which would include all functions under one roof—a hospital with its wards and outpatient department, medical school teaching areas, research laboratories for clinical and basic science disciplines, offices for faculty and administration, a centrally located library convenient to all the rest, and even living quarters for the house staff. It was the first such large medical school/ teaching hospital combination under one roof in the United States.

A. McGehee Harvey, former chair of the Department of Medicine at Johns Hopkins, described the facilities for research by faculty of the clinical departments in 1925:

A new feature was the provision of facilities for research in the clinical departments, so that investigation related to patients could be closely correlated with the preclinical departments. In order to foster research that would not be confined to a single department, thought was given to correlating the teaching and research of the laboratory and clinical departments. Thus, in the department of medicine, a laboratory of clinical bacteriology adjoined the department of bacteriology; laboratories of medical chemistry and physiology led into the departments of biochemistry, pharmacology, and physiology; and the surgery laboratory was next to the departments of anatomy and pathology. These special arrangements were intended to break down barriers between departments, so that the influence of the medical sciences would be felt constantly by the clinical staff and students and that the knowledge and training gained in the laboratories would be carried into medical practice. This arrangement also served to keep laboratory teachers aware that the ultimate aim of medical education was the application of their sciences to the practice of medicine.[38]

When the new Vanderbilt opened in 1925 it was the only medical school in the South with any claim to prestige, unless the then still racially segregated Hopkins itself was considered a Southern medical school. Tinsley and Al were going to an excellent school clearly on the rise.

WHEN HARRISON AND BLALOCK arrived in Nashville to assume their duties on July 1, 1925, the new hospital/medical school was not yet finished. Groundbreaking began October 22, 1923, and construction had proceeded expeditiously. But the new school and hospital were still incomplete, and the only hospital for the school was still the old hospital across town at the south campus.[39]

The new dean, Canby Robinson, "had been there for some months, after two years of commuting back and forth from Baltimore to Vanderbilt."[40] The new associate professors Sidney Burwell and Hugh Morgan "were still in Europe spending a year as traveling fellows financed by the Rockefeller Foundation," as was Horton Casparis, who was to head pediatrics, then a part of the department of medicine. They, like Chief of Surgery Barney Brooks, would arrive some weeks later.

38. A. M. Harvey, *Science at the Bedside, Clinical Research in American Medicine 1905–1945* (New York: The Johns Hopkins University Press, 1981), 302.

39. Announcements, "Special Collections," VUMC Library.

40. Harrison to Kampmeier.

Tinsley Harrison, Vanderbilt, 1925.

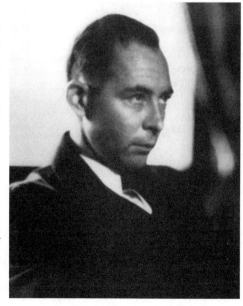

41. Ibid., 2.

42. Ibid., 2.

43. Harrison, interview.

Tinsley and Al therefore set to work in the old Vanderbilt Hospital, a pest house which had never had a full-time physician. "The men in practice did the best they could to help," Tinsley wrote in a letter to a friend, "but an almost complete lack of adequate facilities and janitorial and housekeeping help and deficiencies in Radiology made their job practically impossible."[41] The place was infested with rats, one of which bit Blalock. The deprivations were oppressive, aggravated by the sweltering humidity and heat. It was one of the hottest summers in memory in Nashville. Al and Tinsley threw open all the windows they could find, but the sweat-soaked heat aggravated the malodorous fumes drifting up and down the corridors.

"The only good thing about it was that the nursing was fair and probably better than we later had at the new hospital which had become University-oriented and had its own dean," Tinsley explained. "The dean was directly responsible to Dr. Robinson, the dean of the medical school. Robinson was too busy doing everything under the sun to insist that a patient-oriented rather than a lecture-oriented nursing course be instituted."[42]

Tinsley was opposed to the idea that nurses should, in order to enhance their professional standing, emphasize classroom studies in their educations and work more independently from physicians than they had in previous years. He felt free to comment on the work of nurses since his wife was one.

During his two and a half months at the crumbling old hospital, Tinsley spent much of his time working. Betty lived with the baby separately in another boarding house. Because of Tinsley's duties in the hospital and the lack of income, they essentially lived apart the following year. His salary for the year was several hundred dollars, "way under a thousand."[43] Money for the young couple was tight.

The original Vanderbilt house staff in 1925. Tinsley is in the center front, with the long tie. Al Blalock is to his immediate left.

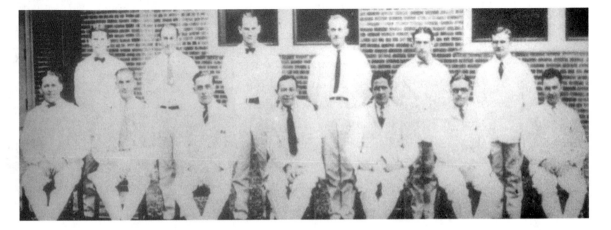

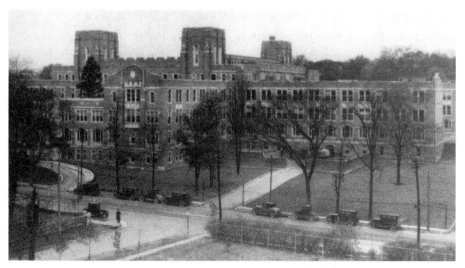

The new Vanderbilt University hospital and medical school shortly after completion in 1927. It was reportedly the first purpose-built medical school with facilities for research, outpatients, dining, and all other departments under one roof.

On September 16, 1925, the new Vanderbilt Hospital and Medical School opened. It was a great structure, by far the most grandiose yet and the most practical anywhere in the South. The only competitors would have been Tulane and the UTMB (University of Texas Medical Branch at Galveston), followed by the Medical University of South Carolina in Charleston, the University of Virginia at Charlottesville, the University of Georgia at Augusta, and Emory. In 1920 none of these others had access to $8 million for construction of a new plant and starting substantial endowments for operations and support of faculty research.

Clarence Connel was director of the hospital, an effective young administrator on good terms with Tinsley. Tinsley was appreciative of the excellent food, prepared under the supervision of Mrs. Robinson, the director of dietetics. The food was nutritious, attractively served, and always hot. This lasted until 1930, when the economic depression forced cutbacks.

Tinsley always felt that the hospital's size was a major advantage. "The great virtue of the place was its smallness," he later wrote. "Interns, residents, and faculty members all ate in the single hospital dining room. There were no fixed places. One day I might have lunch at the same table with the chairman of a preclinical department, or a junior full time teacher and one or more interns or assistant residents. The next day there would be a different group."[44]

Glenn Cullen, the chief of biochemistry, bubbled with enthusiasm and had worked at the Rockefeller Institute with Donald D. Van Slyke, probably the leading developer and promoter of new methodologies for clinical chemistries during

44. Harrison to Kampmeier.

45. Kampmeier, *Recollections*, 23.

46. Harrison to Kampmeier, 4.

47. Ibid., 5.

the first part of the 20th century, whose work was partly captured in his classic book on the subject with John Peters of Yale, often known simply as "Peters and Van Slyke." Interestingly, Peters had initially signed on in 1920 to join the medical faculty at Vanderbilt, but when he learned of the delay necessary before opening the new facilities in Nashville, he took a position at Yale.[45]

Though not a physician, Cullen took great interest in clinical matters and learned to relate his teaching of biochemistry to clinical problems so as to increase the interest of the medical students. Tinsley related an amusing experience with Cullen:

> Practical methods of chemical analysis of human blood had only come into being a few years before. The two pioneers were Wu of Harvard, who introduced practical techniques for obtaining multiple chemical studies on only a few cc of blood; and Donald Van Slyke, of the Rockefeller Institute, of whom Glen Cullen was an outstanding pupil. Glen was desirous that his first-year students should learn techniques by analysis of their own blood. He therefore taught them how to draw blood from their own veins. However he had one unique peculiarity. Whenever he himself was stuck he would faint. Not from the slight pain of the stick, but from the sight of his own blood. This angered him so that at his request I spent an entire Saturday morning repeatedly puncturing his own arm veins while he was sitting. Each time he proceeded to faint. With the aid of one of his own appointees I would simply lift him, who weighed probably 50 pounds more than me, to the floor, and he would immediately recover consciousness when recumbent. He would then insist that I stick him again. This went on for something like a couple of hours and not he, but I, finally refused to continue despite his desire that I do so.[46]

In 1930, Cullen moved to Cincinnati.

For Tinsley, Walter Garrey, the chairman of the department of physiology, was the elder statesman of the faculty. "He was a wee bit pompous," Tinsley said, "but he was a delightful person." Garrey's specialty was the heart. He had discovered the circus movement in atrial and ventricular fibrillation.[47] Because of his interest in the heart, he must have been a favorite conversation companion for Tinsley.

Paul Lamson, chairman of pharmacology, had come from Hopkins, where he had worked with John Jacob Abel and had taught Tinsley in the second year of medical school.

The giant of the pre-clinical faculty and for that matter of the entire school was

Ernest Goodpasture, a native Tennessean, and also from Hopkins. He was an excellent teacher and master of ceremonies at CPCs (clinical-pathologic conferences),[48] but his fame rested on his originating the use of the allantoic membranes (the membranes involved in the formation of umbilical cords and placentas) of chicken eggs for the culture of viruses—in his first case, the mumps virus. This discovery greatly facilitated later work in virology. Goodpasture's Syndrome was named after him.

The chief of surgery was Barney Brooks, a tough but highly respected chairman and later a patient of Tinsley's. Brooks was brought by Robinson from Washington University. Lucius Burch, head of gynecology and obstetrics, was the other clinical chairman. Burch was dean of the old school before the reorganization, and he soon resigned his job as chief of OB/GYN and became the chief mediator between the town and gown physicians.

Sidney Burwell and Hugh Morgan had returned before the new facilities opened in September. Burwell was chosen to head the physiology lab for the department, and Morgan headed the bacteriology lab. Syphilis became a major interest of Morgan's, and he later made a number of contributions to understanding and treating that disease.

IN THE WINTER OF 1925–26 Betty was pregnant again. Because of the local situation, with Tinsley on call most of the time, and because of the availability and willingness of her Massachusetts family to help, she returned there in the spring of 1926 to have her second child. On May 21, in the Worcester Memorial Hospital, Betty had a girl. They named her Emily Louisa from his mother and grandmother, but she was always known as Mimi. Betty returned to Nashville during the summer, as Tinsley's schedule became a little looser.

In 1926 when Tinsley completed his year as chief resident, Robinson continued his appointment as an instructor in the department of medicine. During his year as chief resident, Tinsley had managed to accomplish some laboratory research on top of all his other duties, particularly during the time of Betty's absence in Massachusetts. With the chief residency behind him, Tinsley hit his stride. His productivity increased, as evidenced by his publications, which are discussed separately in the next chapter.

48. Saul Benison, A. Clifford Barger, and Elin L. Wolfe, *Walter B. Cannon, the Life and Times of a Young Scientist* (Cambridge: Harvard University Press, 1987), 65. The CPCs and perhaps some early forms of "grand rounds" were developed from the case method of teaching, whereby real cases of patients' illnesses were presented for discussion by the group of assembled physicians. This method of teaching, though it seems so natural to us late in the 20th century, apparently was introduced into medicine in America by the famous physiologist Walter B. Cannon, who got the idea from Harvard law professor C. C. Langdell. Frustrated by the passivity of the clinical courses, Cannon almost exactly at the turn of the century (December 1899) "persuaded G. L. Walton, his instructor, to present one of the cases from his private practice as an experiment. Walton printed a sheet with the patient's history and allowed the students a week to study it. The discussion that ensued made Walton an immediate convert." Cannon published an article on this in the *Boston*

Medical and Surgical Journal (now the *New England J. Med.*) and sent reprints to Osler at Hopkins, George Dock at Michigan, and others, who responded enthusiastically. James Jackson Putnam immediately adopted the system, and in later years Richard C. Cabot popularized it to such an extent that his name became indelibly associated with it, particularly in regards to CPCs. Thomas D. Cabot, personal communication, July 7, 1993.

49. Tinsley thought Katy suffered from hypoglycemic spells, particularly late in the afternoons. Sometimes Betty would ask her to come by the house to check a minor complaint in Woody or later other children, and she would seem gruff and irritable, though not to the little patient. If they asked her to come in the early evening after dinner, on the other hand, she was "charming, witty, and a joy to have around."

50. Robinson, *Adventures.*

51. Longmire, *Alfred,* 45.

52. Ibid., 45.

All this was accomplished despite his administrative responsibilities overseeing the clinical chemistry laboratory as well as the outpatient unit, his seeing some private patients as a consultant, and his teaching duties as an attending on both inpatient and outpatient services. As Robinson later wrote, after commenting on the excellence of Burwell and Morgan, "we had a human dynamo in Tinsley Harrison to head the house staff and to show much vigor in teaching and in research."[50]

TINSLEY STILL MANAGED TO find time to play tennis with Blalock. In 1925, their first year in Nashville, they won the city doubles and played the final singles against each other. Blalock was powerful and tall, and possessed better service and net strokes. "But I had the ground strokes," said the victorious Tinsley.

Then catastrophe struck. In early 1927, Blalock developed tuberculosis.[51] A lesion in his left apex was detectable on physical examination and visible on X-rays. He also had acid fast organisms in his sputum. Longmire wrote:

> [Blalock] said that he always felt he had a lot of resistance to tuberculosis. That at the time he developed a pulmonary lesion he had really "asked for it," as he was working in the laboratory every night up until midnight and then carousing and raising hell until three or four o'clock in the morning until he got so run down he lost his resistance and developed the lung lesion.[52]

Blalock had to stop work and rest. On the best medical advice, he went to the place then considered to offer the best treatment of tuberculosis in the eastern U.S., the Trudeau Sanatorium at Saranac Lake, New York. Tinsley accompanied his friend to give what support he could. On the way Blalock worried about what this would do to his career. What would happen to all that beautiful research in dogs demonstrating that the shock of extensive soft tissue trauma was the result of fluid loss into the traumatized tissues? It was contrary to some published papers and a good find well done. Would someone else scoop him? And suppose he did not recover? Would the work be scooped, or would the field go elsewhere and all his hard work simply be forgotten? He fretted, and Tinsley knew that such agitation would not help Blalock's treatment at Trudeau.

"Where are the data?" Tinsley asked.

"Right here in my briefcase," Blalock answered.

"Well, then, that solves the problem. I'll just write the paper." And he did.

At Trudeau, Blalock chafed at the conservatism of his physicians, who would prescribe nothing but absolute bed rest, a healthy diet, and lots of fresh air. He wanted more aggressive therapy, at least pneumothorax treatments. But they would not listen to him. His roommate for a time was the Canadian Norman Bethune, who drew murals on the walls gloomily depicting their future tombstones with the dates of death; the one with Blalock's name on it had the date 1929.[53]

After a year of this forced inactivity in the hands of what he considered excessively conservative physicians, impatient, bored and probably depressed, Blalock checked out of the sanatorium and returned to Nashville. The outcome was far from assured, and the close view of his own mortality seemed to have a wildly invigorating if fatalistic effect on Blalock—he cashed in his insurance policy, took the money to buy "a sporty new Chrysler convertible coupe, and began to work harder and live faster than he had ever done before."[54]

He also used part of the money to travel to Europe.[55] After visiting several laboratories, he spent three or four months in Adrian's laboratory in Cambridge, and while there managed to generate enough data for two publications.[56]

From Cambridge, Blalock traveled to Berlin to visit Sauerbruch and his famous clinic. In Berlin, he suffered a serious pulmonary hemorrhage, which his hosts did nothing to help, a source of lasting bitterness later in Blalock's life. The hemorrhage stopped spontaneously, without treatment, and Blalock returned to the Trudeau.[57] He finally obtained the pneumothorax treatments he had been clamoring for. After several treatments, he returned to Nashville late in 1928, where the treatments were continued for about 30 months. During that time, with one lung collapsed, Blalock reactivated his lab and resumed work and publishing. Such was the spirit of the place and time.

During this period Tinsley and Betty introduced Blalock to Mary Chambers O'Bryan, a young lady "with soft dark hair, sparkling brown eyes, enticing dimples in her cheeks, and a generally pleasing personality, enlivened at times by her willingness to defend with an incisive tongue any challenge to Al's position."[58] She and Blalock were married on October 25, 1930, and the two couples were very close, working and playing together. However, tennis was no longer possible for Blalock and Harrison also gave it up: "When Al got TB, I hung up my racquet and never really played tennis again. I took up golf but have never been very good at it."[59]

CANBY ROBINSON, TINSLEY'S MENTOR and friend, left Vanderbilt in 1928 to

53. Ibid., 45. Bethune himself went on to ally with anti-fascists in the Spanish Civil War, then joined Chairman Mao in China, where he is still revered.

54. Ibid., 46

55. It is not known whether Blalock and Harrison met in Europe in 1928. Probably not, since colleagues do not remember either having mentioned such a meeting and nothing to suggest a meeting has been found in the records. They were probably too busy pursuing their own programs of medical (or surgical) research and clinical learning.

56. G. V. Anrep, A. Blalock, and M. Hammouda, "The Distribution of Blood in the Coronary Vessels," *Am. J. Physiol.* 95 (1930): 554.

57. Barney Brooks to Canby Robinson, April 23, 1928, Vanderbilt University Medical Center. "Dr. Blalock seems to be on the road to recovery. He is at present studying in Bern, Switzerland, on a fellowship granted by the GEB."

58. Longmire, *Alfred*, 48.

59. Harrison, interview.

60. Tinsley Harrison, memorandum, Vanderbilt University Medical Center. In this discussion, Harrison was contacted while in Europe. He favored Burwell at that time.

61. W. G. Harrison Sr., "Memoirs" (UAB Archives, University of Alabama at Birmingham), 201. Groce Harrison wrote some reminiscences, some of which apparently dated around 1947. In one titled only "Chapter LXIV" he recalls this trip to Europe: "Some 20 years ago, my older son was given a year's traveling fellowship by the Rockefeller Foundation to pursue post-graduate medical studies. He insisted that his mother and I accompany him and his wife on this Wanderjahr. We thought and talked about it for days, and it was finally decided to go and take the entire family, a total of nine. Our oldest daughter [Emily] had sailed in the early summer with a congenial group of teachers to visit Greece, Italy, and the Aegean Isles, but came by air from Athens to Venice to join the family on our arrival

become dean at Cornell and to undertake the building of the Cornell medical center. After much discussion and debate on whether Sidney Burwell or Hugh Morgan would be better for the job,[60] Burwell was named chairman of the department of medicine.

Before leaving for New York, Robinson had arranged for Tinsley to obtain a Rockefeller fellowship to spend a year in Europe, especially Germany. This was great news for Tinsley and for Groce. All those hours of tutoring with Fraulein Schepke were going to pay off. Betty and Tinsley made arrangements to leave the children, Woody and Mimi, with Betty's family in Massachusetts. In late spring of 1927, Tinsley and Betty took the train to New York, where they met Tinsley's parents, Groce and Lula, together with five other members of the family.[61] In New York, the group caught a steamship to Europe.

They first visited London and then Paris. In France they rented an old Cadillac with a chauffeur, who drove them from Paris to Vienna. Everywhere they stopped—for lunch, gasoline, or lodging—the males (Tinsley, Groce, and Groce Jr.) would seek opportunities to converse with local people.

After the initial touring was done, Tinsley began his fellowship work at Vienna's Allgemeines Krankenhaus, then after a few months transferred to Freiburg im Breisgau. The rest of the family went home after Vienna, but Betty, who was pregnant again, moved with Tinsley to Frieburg in the fall. Betty departed around Christmas time, sorry to leave the picturesque town. She went back to Grafton, Massachusetts, where she waited, and on February 8, 1928, her third child was born in the hospital at Worcester.[62] They named him Tinsley Randolph Harrison Jr., but they always called him Randy. Tinsley then joined her there before returning to Nashville. More about his fellowship year is told in the next chapter.

In July 1928 he reported back to Vanderbilt, where he was appointed assistant professor at a salary of $4,500 a year,[63] a nice salary for the times, and more money than the family had enjoyed before. Tinsley now had an excellent, well-equipped laboratory at his disposal, and a superb assistant from Texas—Miss Minnie Mae Tims, quiet and shy, but an excellent technician—all paid for by the departmental allocation from the chairman's office and, in turn, from the dean's office (and ultimately from Mr. Rockefeller).[64] Tims became Tinsley's secretary and lifelong friend. She earned $1,200 that year. There was also a black "diener/janitor," Tom Brooks ($910 annual salary), who helped with the dog experiments and was a friend and mentor of Vivien Thomas, the talented assistant who helped Blalock perfect his cardiovascular techniques.[65]

During 1927–28, a physician a few years younger than Tinsley joined the faculty to handle general internal medicine, with an emphasis on neurology and psychiatry—Seale Harris Jr. This young doctor from Birmingham also came from a storied medical family; his father was famous for having described "spontaneous hyperinsulism" shortly after the discovery of insulin.[66] Later Harris Jr. also taught physical diagnosis and clinical microscopy, a course in laboratory methods for third-year students named after the similar Hopkins course, but covering much laboratory work in addition to microscopy; still later he took over the supervision of the routine clinical laboratories in the hospital.

The Vandy faculty was always in flux. Two of Tinsley's colleagues left the department of medicine in 1928. C. P. Wilson moved to Portland, Oregon, where he entered practice and joined the clinical faculty of the University of Oregon medical school. Cobb Pilcher moved to the department of surgery at Vanderbilt to start an assistant residency under Barney Brooks. In November 1929 Harris Jr. left to join his father in private practice. (He returned in July 1930 to work full-time on the faculty, this time largely with Hugh Morgan in syphilology.) Another young doctor, Frank Luton—whom Burwell and Robinson had spotted as a medical student and sent to Hopkins for training—returned to take over psychiatry and neurology, working on a part-time basis. The administration wanted Luton well trained, so they also sent him to spend a year at the famous neurology hospital in London at Queen's Square. Years later Luton remained a fast friend and golfing partner of Tinsley's.

In 1928–29 Tinsley continued his research, teaching, and consultations with private physicians. John Youmans, several years older than Tinsley, had arrived from Michigan and had been given responsibility for the medical dispensary (also known as the outpatient department) during Tinsley's year in Europe, a job which Tinsley never again held at Vanderbilt. "Upon my return I was most grateful for this because then as now, I disliked administrative jobs," Tinsley said. "It was a real joy to work under John Youmans in the outpatient department. He told me that he hoped I would do as much or as little work there as I wished and urged me as Sidney Burwell had to devote much of my time to research and the remainder to teaching either on the wards or outpatient department."[67]

The loosening of Tinsley's schedule gave him and Betty time to become more socially active and for the first time money was not a major problem for them. They

in Vienna about the first of July. After 10 days sightseeing in England and a week in Paris, we rented the services of a chauffeur and his old Cadillac and drove across the country from Paris to Vienna. It was a most delightful experience. One of my boys, interested always in agriculture, remarked, 'Well, I'm going to talk to farmers on the way and shall try to find out something about these peasants—these people who feed Europe—how they feel toward things since the war.' The other son announced that he would be more interested in talking politics, economics, and about matters concerning the general life of the natives. Wherever we stopped for gas, for lunch, or to spend a night, he would engage as many people as possible in the questions that had to do with these special matters. My particular duties were to look after travel comforts, and, insofar as I could, when occasion allowed, I would inquire into the medical matters, the superstitions, the faiths and the beliefs and the practices of the people we met along the way."

62. The first child, Woody, was born November 2, 1924, when Tinsley was an assistant resident at Hopkins; the second, Mimi, was born May 21, 1926 as Tinsley was finishing a strenuous year as resident (i.e., "chief resident") at Vanderbilt. Randy was born while Tinsley was in Germany.

63. According to records in the Vanderbilt University Medical Center archives, in 1927 the salaries were as follows: Instructor = $800; Assistant Professor = $3,500; Professor = $7,500. Either these were changed substantially in 1928, or Tinsley obtained a special dispensation (as was his habit). The other possibility is that one or the other of the records is inaccurate.

64. C. Sidney Burwell to W. S. Leathers, May 14th, 1929, VUMC. Departmental salaries for 1928-29 and recommendations for 1929–30 are attached to the letters. Burwell had at that time replaced Robinson as chief of medicine. Miss Tims's salary was recommended for an increase by Dr. Burwell that year, from

hired a faithful live-in black nanny to help with the children and some of the household chores. Tinsley and Betty began hosting medical students and other faculty to the Harrison home for dinner and after-dinner discussion on various medical topics. Osler, as the chief of medicine at Hopkins, had devoted his Saturday evenings to similar gatherings with medical students at his home at 1 West Franklin Street, the same home where he had entertained Tinsley's father for dinner.[68]

Teaching required considerable time and effort on the part of the faculty, and the faculty took pride in doing the teaching well. Inspired by the example of Osler and the German professors, the chief of medicine or his designated attending physician would make teaching ward rounds from 8 to 9 A.M. with 16 or 17 medical students. This occurred daily (including Sundays in the later years) except Thursday, when medical grand rounds were held from 8 to 9 A.M. The chief or attending physician made rounds with the house staff later in the day several days a week, including Saturdays; in later years, this schedule often included Sundays. On these rounds a medical student would present the history and usually the physical findings of each patient in succession. After hearing the student's presentation of the history and physical examination, the attending would check these by his own discussion with and examination of the patient. Next the likely diagnosis and differential diagnosis would be discussed. After the attending had committed himself the laboratory and X-ray findings were presented. Often the attending would predict specific quantitative or visual findings before seeing the results. There would then be a discussion of the best course of management for the problem and of the prognosis. At the end of this exercise the attending would write a note in the patient's file. This sequence would be repeated at the bedside of the next patient and the next, until the end of the teaching ward rounds. A similar routine, at a faster pace and with fewer students, was followed in the outpatient department.

These rounds afforded opportunities for the attending physicians to teach not only "accuracy of diagnosis and effectiveness of treatment" but also "thoroughness of examination, accuracy of records, and recognition of the social and emotional factors concerned . . . [as well as] the best type of professional relationship to the patient and to other physicians."[69]

There was a belief that not only was the example of the teacher of essential importance in all this, but also that there needed to be a bond of personal relationship between the teacher and the student for the teaching to be effective. The personal characteristics of the teaching physician were therefore of prime importance: integrity, compassion for the patients, a serious sense of responsibility, and high standards of professional and personal conduct.[70]

Robinson and later Burwell and Morgan also provided examples for Tinsley in their manner and philosophy of teaching. They were all experts. Another format used by departmental chairmen at Vanderbilt was a weekly hour with medical students at which any topic could be discussed, often bringing up ethics, history of medicine, or even art as related to medicine. There was also the weekly CPC (clinical-pathologic conference) in the amphitheater, probably 11:30 to 12:30 on Thursdays as was the case at the Massachusetts General Hospital where Burwell had trained.[71] From 11:30 to 12:30 on Wednesdays, third- and fourth-year students and some house staff attended demonstrations of problems exemplified by ward patients. A third-year student would present the patient to the group, then the professor would query the patient and check important physical findings, after which there would be a wide-ranging discussion of the problems, diagnoses, management, prognosis, social and emotional problems, and relations with public health and prevention. There were didactic lectures on Saturdays from 11:30 to 12:30 for the review of special clinical topics, such as tuberculosis, syphilis, or various hematologic or other diseases. At these Saturday meetings patients from the wards as well as lantern slides would be used for demonstrations.

Tinsley handled many of these functions, especially in the late 1930s as he became more senior and experienced. And he was good. The students were impressed that he could come into a room, ask the students to suggest a topic they would like to hear about or review—any topic at all—and he would proceed with the topic and deliver a highly informative, well-organized, complete review of the subject as if reading from carefully prepared notes. His theatrical style captivated listeners. He would walk back and forth across in front of the audience with his eyes nearly closed as he spoke. Then he would stop, face the audience, and give some striking example or illustration, such as the heart sounds in a patient with a valve seriously damaged by rheumatic fever sequelae: "Lub-dub, swishshshshshsh, Lub-dub, swishshshshsh"; or a gallop, "Lub-dup-da, lub-dup-da, lub-dup-da"; and a seemingly endless variety of other sounds, complete with explanations of the underlying pathophysiology, polygraph tracings on the blackboard showing the relations of EKG, pressure curves, points of valve openings and closings, the heart sounds and pulse waves, and so on. He could give the same high-quality performance for the lymphomas, anemias, helminthiases (worms), arsenic poisoning, tularemia, malaria, or any other topic

$1,200 to $1,320. Department of Medicine Annual Report 1928, Vanderbilt University Medical Center, budget page.

65. Vivien T. Thomas, *Pioneering Research in Surgical Shock and Cardiovascular Surgery. Vivien Thomas and His Work with Alfred Blalock* (Philadelphia: University of Pennsylvania Press), 1985. Tom Brooks apparently served as a senior advisor and mentor to Vivien Thomas, as Thomas mentions on page 14 of his book. Brooks died in 1934, while Thomas lived to continue with Blalock through the Hopkins years in the 1960s. In 1928 Brooks was paid an annual salary of $910, and was recommended for an increase to $1,040 the following year (which would be $0.50 per hour for a 40-hour week, which they probably exceeded very consistently).

66. The elder Seale Harris was to play a crucial part in decisions regarding Tinsley many years later. J. A. Pittman, *Seale Harris*, eds. J. A. Garraty and M. C. Carnes (New York: Oxford Univ. Press, 1999). E. B. Carmichael, "Seale

Harris—Physician-Scientist-Author," *J. Med. Assn. State of Alabama* 33 (1954): 189–195.

67. Harrison to Kampmeier, 9.

68. Robinson, *Adventures*, 50; Harrison, "Memoirs."

69. Kampmier, *Recollections,* 88; C. S. Burwell, "Methods and objectives in the organization of the outpatient department of a teaching hospital," 1935, J. Amer. Med. Coll.

70. Kampmeier, *Recollections*, 105.

W. Groce Harrison Sr., circa 1930.

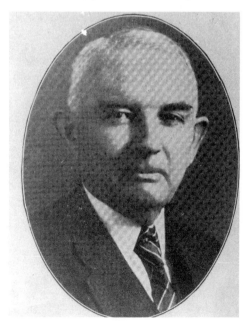

the students could think of. Many years later Sam Riven, a friend and colleague from the 1930s, wrote a book, *Worthy Lives,* about the Vanderbilt medical faculty. In it he caught the essence of each faculty member in a phrase of the chapter title: "The Professor of Medicine: Sidney Burwell," "Clinician and Southern Gentleman: Hugh Morgan," "Medical Humanist: John Youmans," "Virtuoso of the Scalpel: Alfred Blalock," "Physician to the Young: Katherine Dodd," and so on. He titled the chapter on Tinsley, "Teacher Without Peer."[72] It was true.

As BURWELL WAS PREPARING to leave Vanderbilt for Boston, where he was to become dean of the Harvard Medical School, he wrote a letter to Hugh Morgan in which he reviewed the department of medicine. "Dr. Harrison's lectures should supply a basis for the interpretation of symptoms, but can be used as an opportunity to inculcate some good habits," he wrote, thinking of the Oslerian idealism and dedication to medicine Tinsley often emphasized. Burwell continued: the teacher must seize the "chance to make an impression on students at a very impressionable time in their careers and in a way to set the pace and the standard for their whole course in medicine. I believe the imagination of the students could be captured and the drudgery of routine courses much lightened."[73]

During the first two trimesters of the third year Tinsley offered a series of one-hour weekly "lectures and demonstrations in therapeutics illustrating the general care of patients: the use of diets and drugs; their prescription and administration; and procedures such as venepuncture [obtaining a sample of venous blood for therapeutic purposes], pleural aspiration [using needle or tube to remove fluid from the space between the lung and chest wall], abdominal paracentesis [using needle to remove fluid from abdominal cavity], and lumbar puncture."[74]

Canby Robinson had from the outset given lectures on the history of medicine.[75] When Robinson resigned to take the job in New York, Tinsley suggested to new dean Walter Leathers that his father had a deep interest in this subject and could teach the course at little or no cost to the school other than expenses. This suggestion was accepted, and in 1929 Groce started an annual course in the history of medicine. Groce would take the train once a week from Birmingham to

Nashville, check in at Tinsley's house, lecture to the medical students, then return the next day by train to Birmingham. The course was well received and supported by the school's administration. Groce continued this weekly trek, through the 1940–41 academic year, when Tinsley left. At that time Groce was 70 years old.

As the 1930s progressed, Tinsley often substituted for the chief of service, Dr. Burwell or, after 1935, Dr. Hugh Morgan. During Dr. Morgan's tenure as chairman, Tinsley also regularly covered for Morgan during a three-month period.[76] Years later Tinsley wrote that the medical students were still the "single greatest feature of the school. That was the student body! I knew them well. Many were guests on repeated occasions in the home of Betty, my children, and myself." Some of these were from Alabama and continued close friendships with Tinsley throughout their lives. Among these were Robert Parker, who became a pediatrician in Montgomery for many years and served as director of the Alabama Board of Medical Examiners. Another was J. O. Finney Sr., later in the private practice of internal medicine in Gadsden, Alabama, president of the state medical association, and finally on the faculty of medicine in the medical school at Birmingham. His son, J. O. Finney Jr. later attended Vanderbilt, was twice a fellow with Harrison, and became a leading cardiologist in Birmingham.[77] John Chennault, a general practitioner in Decatur, served for years on the board of trustees of the American Medical Association (and, in a crucial vote during the time he was chairman of the State Committee of Public Health, cast the tie-breaking vote for "Tinsley's medical school" in Birmingham, thereby permitting major construction to continue).[78] These were just three of Tinsley's many students at Vanderbilt.

In Tinsley's enthusiastically positive statements about the students a Harrisonian tendency was becoming clear (which would be boon and bane in later years): he often emphasized his students above all else. He extolled them, sometimes uncritically or even intemperately. He cared about his students! In some ways, they were closer to him than his own family. They loved him in return as their great teacher, friend, and mentor. This was where he left his greatest mark in medicine.

In promoting these social activities, which he combined with excellent medical learning, Tinsley also contributed to the general atmosphere of friendliness and goodwill. Canby Robinson later wrote, "A fine spirit pervaded the medical school, and the members of the faculty were good friends, showing a remarkable cooperation in their work and in the school as a whole, and this spirit of comradeship extended to the members of the families of the faculty. Life was

Handwriting standards were, however, apparently not stressed. Kampmeier recounts an episode in which some medical students asked him to decipher a note in a patient's record many years later, which he identified as a note by Tinsley Harrison.

71. CPCs were still at 11:00 A.M. on Thursdays in 1993; but they were attended by only a half dozen people, and the discusser sometimes had his discussion written out in advance, with little discussion from the audience after his presentation, which seemed more to prepare for publication in the *New England J. Medicine*.

72. Samuel S. Riven, *Worthy Lives* (Nashville: Vanderbilt University Medical Center, 1993).

73. Kampmeier, *Recollections*, 100; Sidney Burwell to Hugh Morgan, May 17, 1935, VUMC Archives.

74. Kampmeier, *Recollections*. 86.

75. These lecture notes are on file in the Vanderbilt archives.

76. Kampmeier, *Recollections*, 84–85.

77. James O. Finney

Jr., personal communication, July 7, 1993. James O. Finney Jr. applied for admission to Vanderbilt medical school in 1960 and was referred to Tinsley Harrison for the evaluation interview. After they had talked, Harrison asked young Mr. Finney what he planned to do for the summer, and Finney replied that he intended to work in a local steel mill and earn $600 a month, or $1,800 for the summer. At this Harrison responded that if he would work as a special cardiology fellow with him for the summer, he (Harrison) would pay $200 per month "and get your father to make up the difference." Finney took the offer, had a great summer studying the kinetocardiogram and publishing a paper on the findings; but he never received the $400 per month difference.

78. The Alabama State Committee of Public Health at that time also served as the certifying board for hospitals and other organizations wishing to construct major healthcare facilities. There was considerable resentment

pleasant—happily industrious and stimulating, and everybody seemed to feel he was in the right place."[79]

EVEN IN THE SPRING of 1929, as Tinsley's first year as an assistant professor was drawing to a close, there were money problems at Vanderbilt. To establish a new assistantship in the department, Burwell wrote Dean Leathers[80] requesting that $3,500 be allotted for Tinsley for the coming year, rather than the $5,000 originally proposed. Tinsley knew this was not enough money. Hugh Morgan, besides Burwell the other senior person in the department, supported himself through private practice. Tinsley probably thought this would be desirable in furthering his academic career as well as enabling more money to be brought into the department and other personnel to be added.

On July 1, 1929, Tinsley joined his older colleague Lucius Burch, the obstetrician/gynecologist who had been dean at the old school, in practice at the nearby Eve-Burch Clinic. Tinsley practiced internal medicine and was the only internist in the group practice that was oriented primarily towards surgery and gynecology. He took a part-time faculty member salary of $3,500 from the school, thereby freeing up $1,500 to the department of medicine for an additional assistant or technician. Yet, if he worked hard enough at the private clinic, he would simultaneously allow himself to earn more than the $5,000 Vanderbilt had originally offered.

"When my rapidly growing family created pressing economic needs, I joined Dr. Lucius Burch and his son John, who remains one of my warm friends, in practice as their internist," Tinsley later wrote. "I learned more about the art of keeping sick people and their relatives happy from Lucius Burch than from any other man. He was more of a charmer than Hugh Morgan and that is saying a lot. My two years practice with the Burches were, even though they were not internists, perhaps the greatest educational experience of my entire life."[81]

TINSLEY WORKED ALL THE time. All this laboratory work, writing, reviewing drafts and galley proofs, and ancillary work required that he often return to the lab after dinner. He often came home after midnight. He would awaken at sunrise to depart for rounds. If an experiment got started in the afternoon, sometimes he did not return home for supper but took a break to eat with other Vanderbilt staff at the "Dog Wagon," a small all-night diner on 21st Street adjacent to the Vanderbilt Medical Center that was a convenient place for a quick bite and coffee among the late workers.[82]

During this time Tinsley's brother, Groce Jr., joined the Vanderbilt house staff as an assistant resident. Groce had completed medical school at Hopkins four years after Tinsley, and had then taken house staff training there. Now he was completing his house staff training at Vanderbilt, and as a research fellow he worked with Tinsley in the dog lab and at clinical research.

Groce did not have Tinsley's enthusiasm for academic life and in July 1932 moved to the Grady Hospital and Emory University Medical School in Atlanta to become chief medical resident with Dr. James Paullin. Though he kept open the possibility of remaining in some academic position, after some years Groce moved to Texas and spent the remainder of his life in clinical practice. Tinsley always maintained that his brother was an excellent clinician who simply was not interested in spending time in research.

In 1930, as the need for more good teachers grew in the face of the economic depression, John Youmans telephoned a friend at the University of Michigan, Sam Riven. Riven had taken house staff training at Michigan and had remained on the faculty. Youmans knew him to be an excellent internist and teacher and offered Riven a job. Riven accepted and moved to Nashville. Sidney Burwell introduced Riven to the local urologist Perry Bromberg. Bromberg, also on the clinical faculty at Vanderbilt, offered Riven the use of his office in the afternoons. Riven stayed in Nashville the rest of his life, adding yet another example of excellence in internal medicine for the Vanderbilt students, working every morning at patient care and teaching in the outpatient clinic on the first floor of the building.

Riven captures the spirit of the times and of Tinsley in his recollections and vignettes. He points out that Tinsley agreed with Youmans about "medical education's overemphasis on scientific technology. Over the course of a long, productive career in which he contributed to the scientific basis of cardiology, Harrison developed an interest in noninvasive methods of diagnosis and evaluation. But all along, his great gifts as teacher had depended upon his conviction that medicine was "much more a matter of the heart than of the mind." He did eminent work, was a superb clinician and scientist, and those who studied under him held him in something approaching idolatry."[83]

The new dean Walter Leathers was much less expansive and expensive—much better at controlling and balancing the medical school's budget—than Robinson had been. But the stock market crash of October 1929 and the subsequent economic depression of the 1930s aggravated financial problems. There is little discussion

among some of the "town physicians" in private practice against what they saw as the advance of "government medicine" (state government, aided by federal funds) to "build up the competition with my own hard earned tax dollars." This resulted in a 7-7 tie when a proposal for major construction at UAB came before the board which decided on the CON (certificate of need, without which the construction could not proceed). Chennault, as chairman of that board, cast the deciding vote in favor of UAB. This created a wave of resentment against him, which later resulted in a split in the state medical association of "pro-" and "anti-Chennault" delegates. This in turn resulted in Chennault's withdrawal from a race for presidency of the AMA and from the AMA board of trustees.

79. Robinson, *Adventures*, 185.

80. Annual reports of the Department of Preventive Medicine and Public Health, VUMC Archives. Walter Leathers, M.D., who had been dean of the medical

school of Mississippi and the state health officer there, had been recruited by Robinson to head the department of preventive medicine and public health. When Robinson left for Cornell, he followed as dean at Vanderbilt in 1928. His department became a recipient of Rockefeller funds and a vehicle through which the GEB pursued its goals for improving health in the South, especially the eradication of hookworm disease.

81. Harrison to Kampmeier, 7. Either Harrison's recollections of the time and dates are inaccurate, or the financial records of Vanderbilt are; or possibly there were arrangements not clear from existing records. In the Department of Medicine's Annual Report for 1929–30, prepared in May 1930 and reflecting both the record of the past year and plans for the coming year, Burwell comments that Tinsley Harrison wants to return to a full-time status. However, two years later (April 30, 1932) a letter from Burwell to Dean Leathers comments that Harrison's pay-

of this in the records of the department of medicine, other than the departmental chairman Burwell's continuing calls for more faculty and staff for the department and for more scholarship and loan money for students, who in his opinion were wasting time and talent by working for a living in local hospitals. Burwell was concerned that the large debts of some graduating students pushed them into more immediately lucrative jobs, but positions with far less potential for ultimate accomplishments in medicine than they were capable of. Burwell felt there was too much debt for the students' careers to bear. These problems were surely aggravated by the Great Depression, but Burwell had been voicing such complaints before, and he would later. The school continued along, relatively untroubled by the economic chaos around the land. In part, this relative freedom from economic verities was the result of the effective handling of these problems at the level of Chancellor Kirkland, who continued to obtain additional funding from the GEB. Until 1931 the GEB provided more than $14 million to the Vanderbilt Medical School and hospital, and, once its investments were secured, it again resumed its largesse to Vanderbilt.[84]

Tinsley did not like private practice, with its necessary schedules, routines, and structure. His style was much too unstructured to work well in such a regimented situation, with the great lack of freedom imposed by being on call most of the time—not at all a master of his own time or schedule. He soon came to long for the old days when his chief Sidney Burwell or John Youmans of the outpatient service would urge him to put research first."[85]

Burwell and other Vanderbilt administrators did indeed push Tinsley and others to research. In November 1930 the Southern Clinical Club met in Nashville for the presentation of papers, to show others what was being done there and to give young physicians another opportunity to make presentations of their work before groups. Younger colleagues were sent away for further research experience and training: J. L. Alloway, a resident and instructor in medicine, to become an assistant resident on the pneumonia service at the Rockefeller Institute, where he would work with Drs. Cole and Avery; Dr. Macdonald Dick, an assistant resident and assistant in medicine also to the Rockefeller to join a group doing physiological research; Dr. Albert Weinstein, an intern, to become an assistant resident on the metabolic division of the medical service of the Johns Hopkins Hospital; John Lawrence (later famous for cyclotron therapy of pituitary tumors at the Lawrence-Livermore Laboratory in California) to the Thorndike Laboratory of Harvard; and others.[86] Burwell's annual reports to Dean Leathers were filled with woeful complaints that the faculty were wasting away, consumed by "routine duties of patient care and teaching," as he put it, which prevented their achieving more in research.[87]

Burwell tried to promote research by arranging for his younger colleagues to have free time which they could devote to research. To this end Dr. Calhoun, after his assistant residency in medicine, became an assistant in medicine and worked at general medicine in the dispensary in the mornings, then devoted his afternoons to research in biochemistry under the direction of Cullen. He later worked with Tinsley. Dr. A. H. Bell also worked in the outpatient department half the day, then joined Goodpasture for research and teaching in pathology for the rest.[88] Everyone was expected to work at least half the day on Saturdays. Many, including Tinsley, worked most Sundays.

From February 14 to April 14, 1931, Sir William B. Hardy of Cambridge was visiting professor at Vanderbilt. He made rounds, met with student groups, gave other lectures on medical topics, and added greatly to the teaching and research atmosphere of the department and school. He also gave the annual Abraham Flexner Lecture. The lecture was on physiology in low temperature environments, but Hardy was widely accomplished and made contributions in other areas, such as endocrinology.[89]

In 1930 Dr. Alan Gregg succeeded Richard Pearce as head of the Division of Medical Education of the Rockefeller Foundation. The name of that division was changed to "the division of Medical Sciences, and the older interest in the training of competent practitioners was in large part superseded by a drive to widen the horizons of understanding in relation to unexplored or unsolved problems."[90] This division started a new form of assistance for research, the "fluid research fund," and made grants to Johns Hopkins, Oregon, Rochester, Stanford, Utah, Vanderbilt, and Yale. These were unrestricted funds except for the requirement that the recipient institutions use them for the support of research, lump sums which would support most of the work of Tinsley and others throughout the decade of the 1930s.

According to the book by Kampmeier and in the archives of the Vanderbilt Medical Center, Tinsley received the following amounts:

	TH	Technician
1932	$1,052	$3,770
1933	$902	$3,640
1934	$1,000	$3,290

ments from the Eve-Burch Clinic are being stopped because of the economic depression and recommends that he be taken back on the faculty at a salary of $5,000 with the option of increasing this to $6,500 by adding up to $1,000 from private consulting practice, which might or might not have been possible in 1932 Nashville.

82. The "Dog Wagon" operated from the mid-1920s through the mid-1930s. Identified on photo in VUMC Archives.

83. Rivens, *Worthy*, 29. Samuel S. Riven was born August 26, 1902, in Montreal. He died in Nashville in 1997.

84. Conkin, *Gone*, 282.

85. Harrison to Kampmeier.

86. C. S. Burwell, "Report of the Department of Medicine for the Year 1930–3," VUMC Archives, 1–3.

87. Department of Medicine Annual Reports, 1929–1935, VUMC Archives.

88. Burwell, "Report," 2–3.

89. Medicine Annual Report, 1931, VUMC Archives. Although Bayliss and Starling

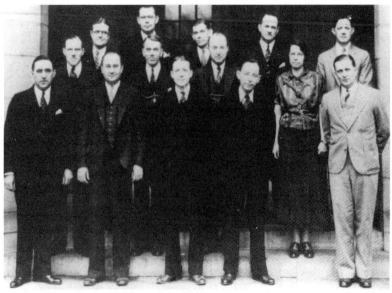

1935	$820	$2,940
1936	$1,000	$2,940
1937	$800	$2,940
1938	$600	$2,736
1939	-----	$2,763.50
1940	-----	$1,266[91]

Vanderbilt Medical School's assistant and associate professors, around 1932. Harrison is the front row, second from right, next to Katie Dodd, M.D.

are usually credited with coining the word "hormone" for the chemical messengers of the body in conjunction with their description of secretin, it was actually W. B. Hardy, a student in their laboratory at the time, who suggested

The item labeled "technician" would have supported several technicians at the then-prevalent salary levels, and it is likely that one of these was Minnie Mae Tims, who continued to work with Tinsley. The decrease in later years, even though some of the Vanderbilt faculty continued to receive support from the fluid research fund, probably reflects growing success by Tinsley in attracting funds from other sources. The fluid research fund distributed $39,029.90 over the years, supplemented with regular funds from the department of medicine, and increasingly by grants from other private entities. The first grants from the U.S. Public Health Service began in the early 1940s.[92] The Roosevelt administration was more than willing to support Tinsley and his laboratory, which was responsible for about half the publications coming from the department of medicine. The 1932 departmental annual report by Burwell states, "the nearer full-time he [Tinsley] is, the better."[93]

The Vanderbilt school earned a lot in grants. That same year, from the Rockefeller Foundation, Leathers received for the department of preventive medicine and public health $23,514 for work on hookworm disease and other helminthiases. Goodpasture received $2,500 from another foundation. Cunningham, chairman of anatomy, received $3,000 from the National TB Association, $2,000 from the Commonwealth Fund, and another $1,000 from the National Research Council. The NRC also awarded $250 to Goodpasture and $750 to Burwell and Cullen. The American Social Hygiene Association gave $1,000 to Morgan.

In the summer of 1932 Tinsley returned to the full-time faculty at a salary of $5,000 and the option of keeping another $1,000 from practice (if there were sufficient paying patients in 1932). His return was marked by an important academic advance; he was promoted from assistant professor of medicine to associate professor of medicine, a tenured position.[94]

Finances were tight in 1933. A proposed across-the-board salary reduction of 8 to 10 percent was avoided in most cases only by money shuffling and leaving vacancies empty. The general budget of the school was reduced by 8 percent. Most of the schools at Vanderbilt and elsewhere were suffering from the depression. Twelve percent of the Vanderbilt students were relief clients from the government, and 25 percent received some kind of external aid.[95] The fraternities curtailed formal dances; the students gave up their junior prom.

In *Gone With the Ivy*, Conkin wrote:

> The most threatening effect of the depression seemed to be an ever greater provincialism. Vanderbilt had practically ceased to be a Southern university, becoming in effect a local college. Only a sprinkling of College undergraduates now came from distant parts of the South, let alone from the North. Over three-fourths came from the Middle Tennessee-Southern Kentucky region, and in 1933 exactly two-thirds came from the Nashville area. The Graduate School and the School of Religion drew from a larger area, but only the Medical School had anything close to a national constituency.[96]

The fortunes of the hospital were waxing and waning. Negotiations were carried out with the city of Nashville for payments for indigent care and with Meharry Medical College for sharing in this. Attempts were made to increase the numbers of private patients in the hospital.[97] Forty percent of the patients in Vanderbilt Hospital were private patients, but many of these could not pay. A research grant of $300 was received from the American Medical Association. Youmans was studying nutritional edema then prevalent among the patients in the dispensary, helped by a young man from the department of physiology, Herbert Wells, later to be important in Tinsley's career.[98]

For years Burwell's annual reports complained about the lack of individual treatment rooms for the wards, lack of isolation arrangements for patients with acute infectious diseases, the need to use the general medical wards for psychiatric patients, and even (though he was chairman of medicine) the need to place ob/gyn patients on the general surgical wards. Now, the "only Vanderbilt school with a national constituency" was the only one which dared expand in the face of these dire financial

that word to them, as they credit him in a footnote to the physiology text published in 1915. However, it was not really Hardy who suggested the term. Rather it was his classics professor Veasey who suggested the term to Hardy. This Dr. Hardy of Cambridge, who visited Vanderbilt, was likely the same man.

90. Fosdick, *Story*, 124.

91. Kampmeier, *Recollections*, 300.

92. Medicine Annual Reports and Medical School Budgets.

93. Burwell, "Reports," 26.

94. Ibid.; Tinsley R. Harrison, curriculum vitae, UAB Archives.

95. Conkin, *Gone*, 377.

96. Ibid.

97. Medicine Annual Report, 14. The work of the hospital grew dramatically in some areas, such as the laboratory service. For example, Wasserman serological tests for syphilis were done in the following numbers: 1926-7, 5,341; 1927–8, 7,684; 1928–9, 9,500; 1929–30, 15,120; 1930–1, 17,804; 1931–2, 19,721. Similar in-

creases were occurring in other laboratories. One problem was the cost for these tests, which started as the responsibility of the department of medicine. This meant that the medical school was subsidizing the hospital. The counter argument would have been that it made no difference overall, since many hospital patients could not pay. As the financial situation grew tighter, sharing agreements were worked out, and the philosophy was developed that "the hospital should pay for itself." The free beds were therefore sharply reduced. This had a twofold effect. First, students became much more aware of their patients' finances than before, which some of the professors considered undesirable. Second, teaching became more difficult, since there was more reluctance to teach with paying patients, which again raised ethical questions for some of the faculty. These questions were to remain.

98. Even the applicants to the school of medicine diminished during these hard days: (Year—Number

straits. Kirkland tried to obtain funds from the new Public Works Administration for the school, but was unsuccessful. The GEB came to the rescue, awarding Vanderbilt $2.5 million in 1935, "with just over a third for hospital construction, the rest for endowment to operate the expanded facilities. This was its first large grant in six years, proving once again the esteem it had for Vanderbilt, although the gift came after a tough fight within the board. The days of GEB funding were about over."[99]

Thus the major construction to make a substantial addition to the Vanderbilt medical center began: another hallway parallel to 21st Street on the far side of the building parallel to "B" corridor, which housed Tinsley's office and laboratories on the second floor. The new "D" corridor completed in 1937 was huge: eight stories high with 155 new beds. The new space provided room for psychiatry and for patients with infectious diseases. In the financial climate of the times, however, the endowment produced too little money to pay the expenses of the new addition. The opening of some units was delayed. Dean Leathers juggled soft money, tuition income, and what "hard money" there was to keep things running.[100]

Tinsley continued his rapid pace of research and publications, working hard on his new book to be published in 1935. Ben Friedman left for New York, and Seale Harris was promoted to assistant professor, but without any salary increase. Morton F. Mason, Ph.D., a bright young biochemist, started collaboration with Tinsley which was to last for many years. The extramural research grants to the department of medicine totaled $27,320.[101]

LIFE CONTINUED FOR TINSLEY and his family. His and Betty's fourth child, Helen Elizabeth, was born July 17, 1934—the first born in the town in which they lived. She was called Betsy, but Tinsley called her "Sunshine."[102]

Then 1935 saw a tragedy in the Harrison family. Tinsley's younger sister Weeze (Louisa Dabney Harrison, 1907–65) began acting strangely. She had married a young medical student, Walter Davis. They had three children in rapid succession, and with her husband working hard at his internship and residency at Arkansas, she cared for the children alone. The stress of raising three young children, with her husband away all the time and very little money for a much-needed break, was too much for her to bear. She became preoccupied, lost in her own thoughts. She wandered around, distracted. She went home to stay with Groce and Lula, then came to visit Tinsley and Betty. She was out of money, so they loaned her $25. She took this and went shopping. She disappeared for a whole day. The family was very concerned. Weeze returned in the evening with no clear recollection of where she had been or what had happened—the $25 was gone. She returned to Birmingham by train. The family was unsure of what to do; she was clearly mentally disturbed.

Groce paid for the best psychiatrists available. She went to Atlanta, Hopkins, and other centers. She tried shock therapy. Nothing worked. She remained in a strange, disaffected funk. Two years later, Weeze was committed to Bryce Hospital, the state mental institution in Tuscaloosa, with a diagnosis of schizophrenia. She remained there the rest of her life.

Tinsley provided insight into his amazing work ethic when he later spoke of Weeze. "She was the only schizophrenic in the family," Tinsley later said. "The rest of us, especially me, were all manic-depressive."[103]

BETTY WAS PREGNANT MOST of 1938, and the day after Christmas she delivered in the Vanderbilt Hospital a husky boy. They named him John Bondurant Harrison, the first name from Tinsley's grandfather and the second from his mother's family. In 1938 Tinsley carried a full teaching load at Vanderbilt and often substituted for the department chairman, Hugh Morgan. He was in charge of the laboratory which did the clinical electrocardiograms on patients, both inpatient and outpatient.[104] He served on various committees of the medical school, graded students, and otherwise helped with the chores. He continued his vigorous pursuit of laboratory and clinical research and publishing.

For Tinsley and Betty, 1938 was a good year.

Blalock had a good year, as well. He was promoted to the rank of full professor at Vandy in 1938.[105] This was unusual. The rank of full professor was usually reserved for the single individual in a department who also held the administrative position of chairman of the department. Around this time Blalock was offered the position of chief of surgery at the Henry Ford Hospital in Detroit, an excellent teaching hospital and a tempting offer. A series of bargaining meetings must have gone on. Blalock was awarded the academic appointment without the administrative job. While Tinsley surely was happy for his friend, Blalock's appointment probably also provided additional motivation for greater achievement for himself.

In 1938–39, Robert H. Williams served as chief resident in medicine at Vanderbilt, having just returned from his year with Warfield Longcope

of Med. School Applicants) 1927—251; 1928—373; 1929—447; 1930—604; 1931—541; 1932—427; 1933—374; 1934—361; 1935—474. The number continued to increase thereafter.

99. Conkin, *Gone*, 375.

100. Ibid., 375–76.

101. Medicine Annual Reports.

102. "Variety Shade Landowners of Virginia Association" meeting, audio-tape, Lake Martin, Alabama, June 18–20, 1993. The VSLVA is

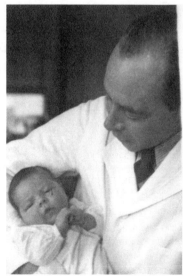

Tinsley with his youngest son, John, 1938.

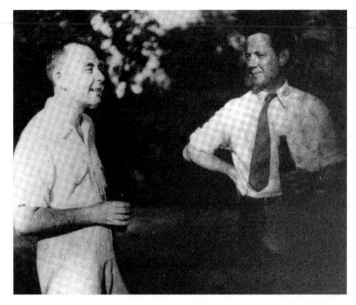

Tinsley with Al Blalock at the annual Vanderbilt medical student graduation party, about 1940.

a family corporation initiated by Tinsley Harrison which owns the remnants of the old Bondurant plantation in Virginia. The area of some 1,600 acres is used to grow trees, the proceeds of which finance a biennial meeting of the living Bondurant progeny.

103. Harrison, Audiotape. However, the manner in which this diagnosis was determined is of interest. A daughter of "Weeze" later related that she had obtained the medical record from the Bryce Hospital, and this showed that "the diagnosis was made by a vote of the 15 doctors there at the time. The vote was 8-7 in favor of schizophrenia, so that's what the diagnosis was." ("Variety"). In 1997 I obtained a copy of the hospital record, and Leon Eisenberg, M.D., of the Department of Social Medicine at Harvard Medical

at Hopkins. Williams had interned at Vanderbilt in 1935–36 and taken an assistant residency the following year, followed in turn by the year at Hopkins. Williams, a superb internist and excellent resident, was a fellow Southerner (a Tennessean), a Hopkins graduate,[106] and a coworker with Tinsley on renin and other aspects of hypertension.[107] He was a quieter presence, but his ambitions, ideas, energy, and enthusiasm matched Tinsley's, and their personalities went well together; they became fast friends. Williams went on to the Massachusetts General Hospital where he worked in the Thyroid Unit with J. H. Means, then to the Thorndike Memorial Laboratory in Boston where he proved himself an able clinician and investigator, studying endocrinology and the pharmacology of the new antithyroid drugs.[108] In 1949 he was chosen to become chief of medicine at the new University of Washington medical school in Seattle, where he remained active in endocrinology and academic medicine the rest of his career. He was important in Tinsley's life, and played a vital role later.

THE ACADEMIC WORLD OF medicine was not impervious to outside affairs. The world had slipped back into war as the 1940s began, and Tinsley was aware of the consequences. He gave an address in Ann Arbor in September 1940 at the opening of the medical school. Hitler's armies had invaded Poland just a year and a month earlier. It was a timely occasion for assessment of what makes human institutions good and great. His first sentence recognized the situation: "When sorrow, oppression and madness reign where Harvey, Pasteur and Virchow worked, one may well be fearful for the future of medicine." In his presidential address before the Young Turks, Tinsley expressed concern for the future of medicine and what was needed for continuing progress. The crux of the matter, to Tinsley, was the kind of *people* one recruits and comports his activities with.

He included a paragraph which inadvertently is key to some of his later problems:

> The distinction between administration and leadership should be clarified in the minds of our younger faculty members. The man who concerns himself too much with administration merits comparison with Penelope. "All the yarn she spun in Ulysses' absence did but fill Ithaca full of moths." If we can choose young men who possess both the urge to turn for themselves the pages of "Nature's book of infinite secrecy," and the capacity to stimulate still younger men to give their best efforts, the details of administration will—in the main—take care of themselves.[109]

Tinsley was at the pinnacle of academic success for a young physician, already often substituting for Hugh Morgan, his own chairman in Nashville. In 1940–41 he took Professor Morgan's place and fulfilled most of his functions for three months. Morgan at that time was writing chapters on syphilis, aortic diseases, and hypertension for new editions of the decade-old multi-authored textbook of internal medicine edited by Russell L. Cecil—*The Cecil Textbook of Medicine*.

The faculty, staff, and students had looked forward to a two-month visiting professorship that year by Sir Edward Mellanby, director of the Medical Research Council in Great Britain, but he was unable to come because of the war. The gastroenterologist Chester M. Jones of the Massachusetts General Hospital spent a whole year at Vanderbilt, which he later related to others as one of the happiest years of his life.[110] Morton F. Mason, the young Ph.D. from the biochemistry department who had worked and published with Tinsley, returned from England and the continent with 12 publications to his credit (including those at press), five with J. N. Barcroft.

In 1940–41, Mason and Glenn Cullen, chairman of the department of biochemistry, made rounds once a week with an attending physician in the department of medicine. They also attended the weekly journal club meeting of the department of medicine. This reflected not only the variety of their interests and recognition of the ultimate source of their support, but also the obvious increasing importance of chemistry and physiology in clinical medicine and investigation. Their participation was particularly helpful to Tinsley as he prepared extracts of kidneys. The fluid research fund would exhaust itself this year, but Tinsley had private support. John Williams, who had served as chief medical resident and instructor during

School, former chief of psychiatry at the Massachusetts General Hospital, and a highly respected leader in psychiatry, was kind enough to review it. Though the half-century old records were sparse and not in good condition, Dr. Eisenberg thought the diagnosis of "schizophrenia" was probably correct, certainly given the state of psychiatric knowledge in the 1930s. (L. Eisenberg, M.D., personal communication, UAB Archives, 1997).

104. Hugh J. Morgan, Department of Medicine Annual Report, 1939–40, 7. It is amusing today to read in Professor Hugh Morgan's annual report for the department of medicine, 1939–40, that there was then a great "increase in the number of requests for electrocardiograms and the necessity for taking multiple records. The latter is an outgrowth of the recent developments in electrocardiography. Instead of three standard leads, now as many as seven leads are employed, which more than doubles the work." In addition, the EKG technician

Harrison and Dr. Mort Mason in a laboratory at Vanderbilt University, 1935.

Miss Lowe also served simultaneously as secretary for Drs. Luton and Mahoney.

105. Longmire, *Alfred*, 62.

106. Like Harrison, Robert Williams had taken his first year at one medical school (Vanderbilt) then transferred to Hopkins for his last three years.

107. Maxwell Finland, *The Harvard Medical Unit at the Boston City Hospital* (Boston: Harvard Medical School, 1983), vol. 1, 456.

108. Ibid., vol. 1, 455–481; vol. 2, part 1, 433–434, 479–480.

109. T. R. Harrison, "Some Thoughts About Medical Education," address, opening of the Medical School, University of Michigan, September 30, 1940, VUMC Archives.

110. Walter Lincoln Palmer, "Chester Morse Jones," obituary, trans. Assn. Amer. Physicians, 1973, 19. "Some of the happiest experiences of Ches-

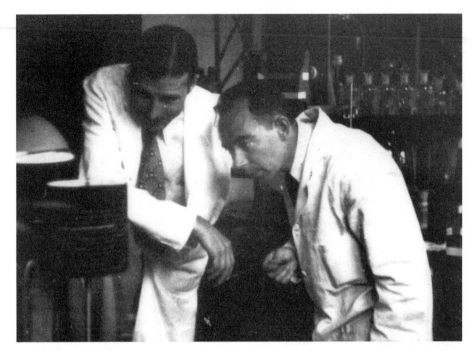

the previous year, joined the research group as an assistant in medicine.[111] Things were moving along. Hugh Morgan's salary as professor and chairman was raised to $10,000 annually, and technicians made $13 a week (up from $12). The largest grant that year was to Ernest Goodpasture, $30,000 for the study of chemotherapy of infections due to filtrable viruses. The Rockefeller Foundation gave money for work on nutrition, and the Commonwealth Fund supported Youmans's work in that area. Exchanges with other academic medical centers continued—"Josh" Billings to Hopkins to work with Longcope, and J. Allen Kennedy to the Brigham, thence to Barcroft in Cambridge, and back to Vanderbilt.

Tinsley was comfortable, ensconced in a staff that supported his work. The future seemed set and the next step in his life and career seemed inevitable.

IN OCTOBER 1940 TINSLEY received a letter from his friend Herbert S. Wells—the earnest young physician with wire-rimmed glasses who had started at Vanderbilt as an instructor in pharmacology in 1927 but had switched to physiology as assistant professor in 1932. A large endowment was coming to Wake Forest College from the late Bowman Gray, head of the Reynolds Tobacco Company, headquartered in Winston-Salem, North Carolina, and there might be an opportunity for Tinsley to

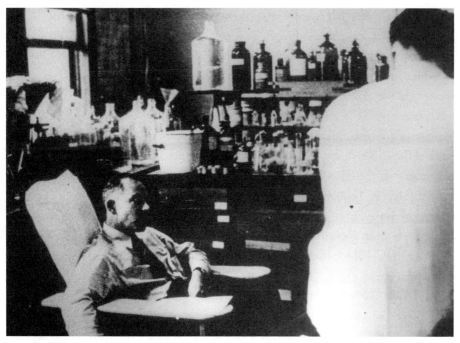

An exhausted Harrison in one of the Vanderbilt research labs.

ter's life, frequently recalled with joy and appreciation, occurred in the year 1940, spent as Acting Associate Professor of Medicine at Vanderbilt University in Nashville, Tennessee. Old friendships were renewed and new friendships formed, all cherished in later years."

111. Morgan, "Annual Reports."

112. Kampmeier, *Vanderbilt*, 73.

113. Tinsley Harrison to Herbert Wells, October 22, 1940, Dorothy Carpenter Medical Archives, BGSM.

114. Robert P. Morehead, "The contribution of a great man to Wake Forest University and its Bowman Gray School of Medicine—Tinsley R. Harrison, M.D." *North Carol. Med. J.* 44:809–811, 1983.

115. This trip almost surely occurred in late November 1940.

116. Meads, Manson, *The Miracle on Hawthorne Hill: A History*

build his own excellent department of medicine. Wells himself had already moved to Wake Forest to help with the move into new quarters the next year.[112]

Tinsley responded from Vanderbilt on October 22, 1940, thanking Wells for suggesting him and stating that while "there is no particular desire on my part to leave Vanderbilt, I am thoroughly open minded on the subject and the possible prospect of being able to start from the ground up and build a department is one which has considerable appeal to me. As you know, I would not be happy anywhere without the opportunity to keep on doing investigation. The whole thing would have to depend on what the immediate and future plans and prospects are at Wake Forest, and particularly on the question of whether there would be opportunity to build a department second to none. If there is to be such an opportunity I would very definitely be interested."[113]

Wells suggested Tinsley's name to Coy C. Carpenter, the dean of the Wake Forest medical school.[114] Dr. Carpenter contacted Tinsley and arranged for Tinsley and Betty to travel by train to Winston-Salem.[115] They stayed at the Carpenters' home and spent two full days looking at the city. Tinsley met with Carpenter and reviewed plans for the new school, and he could see the construction underway. The entire medical school and hospital would be under one roof just as it was at Vanderbilt, *of the Medical Center of The Bowman Gray School of Medicine of Wake Forest University and the North Carolina Baptist Hospital* (Winston-Salem: Wake Forest University, 1988), 19.

117. Morehead, "Contribution," 809.

118. Ibid.

119. W. C. Davison, *The Duke University Medical Center (1892–1960)* (Durham: Duke University Medical School, 1960), 1–4, 8. Duke medical school (together with the hospital and nursing school) received $4 million from the original bequest of $10 million. But even before that the ever-helpful GEB had given Dr. William P. Few, president of Trinity College, $3 million of Rockefeller money in 1920–23, with the collaboration of Abraham Flexner. This was used to help convince James B. Duke to provide the endowment. Few had been working to persuade Duke to support a medical school for a decade. On December 11, 1924, he created the Duke Endowment, and on December 29 Trinity College became a component of the new Duke

and Carpenter must have assured him there would ultimately be more construction for a larger physical plant—though Tinsley preferred a small, high-quality school.

Around this time Dean Carpenter was asked by Dr. Felda Hightower, then a part-time instructor in anatomy and later a faculty member in surgery, "How much money do we really have to develop a four-year medical school?" "Unlimited," Carpenter replied.[116] For him it was a matter of faith; he knew the resources were finite, and how much there was in fact in the bequest of Bowman Gray. Carpenter wanted the rising young talent at his school. He likely offered similarly optimistic estimates over the school's finances in the next few years.

On this trip, Tinsley also met with Wingate Johnson, chairman of the board of trustees of Wake Forest College and a leading internist in Winston-Salem. Johnson had already been picked by Carpenter to become chief of the private diagnostic clinic, or PDC—the faculty practice plan modeled after the successful operation of the same name at Duke. This might have sent a cautionary warning to Tinsley, but Johnson was such a gentleman and diplomat, as well as such an excellent internist and general practitioner, that no trouble was foreseen.

"The impression Johnson made on me had a great deal to do with my decision to accept the position," he said later.[117] He was also struck by his meeting with heirs of the tobacco magnate Bowman Gray. "I was impressed by the rather striking charm and obvious integrity the family showed," Tinsley said. After he had talked with them, he felt "completely satisfied with the financial status of the school. . . . They indicated to me they were behind the school and were going to stay behind it."[118]

The Harrisons returned to Nashville full of optimism for the future at the new medical school in North Carolina. James B. Duke, another giant of the tobacco and electrical power industries in the region, had left a bequest of more than $10 million for the establishment of Duke University medical center at his death in 1925. The new school (which opened in 1930) was doing very well.[119] Duke looked poised for greatness, as Vanderbilt had been two decades earlier. It was the right time in Tinsley's career, and he felt himself the right man for the job.

Tinsley was not the only member of the faculty of medicine at Vanderbilt receiving inquiries. Al Blalock had already declined an offer from Henry Ford Hospital; he had negotiated a full professorship and a higher salary at Vanderbilt in the process. Ernest Goodpasture had received an excellent offer from Harvard Medical School but had also opted to remain, after negotiating a substantial increase in his compensation. Now Blalock was involved in serious negotiations with Johns

Hopkins for the position of chief of surgery originally held by William Halsted. It looked as if he would take it.

Tinsley did not yet have an offer, just an inquiry. Carpenter was a careful dean, and before finalizing the offer he traveled to Nashville and talked with some of Tinsley's colleagues, then to Tinsley. Exactly when the offer was made by Carpenter is not known, but after the end of November the decision was made. Tinsley would leave Vanderbilt.

On February 10, 1941, Tinsley wrote his chief, Hugh Morgan, that he was resigning effective July 1, 1941. The following day Morgan wrote a similar letter to Dean Walter Leathers informing him of the forthcoming resignation.

THE SPRING ENDED BRINGING summer. The changing seasons seemed to represent Tinsley's changing situation. Friends had a series of parties for those departing, the biggest hosted by the entire department of medicine at a large private clubhouse on the banks of the Cumberland River. It was a grand party with much wine and beer; a good time was had by all. The party ran late into the night. Many imbibed into the late hours. As the guests departed, on the way down the steps Tinsley fell awkwardly into the mud. He righted himself, a little embarrassed but okay.

In 1925 Tinsley and Alfred Blalock had officially taken their positions on the Vanderbilt house staff the same day. Now they were to leave the same day for careers in their separate fields, surgery and medicine. In the years that followed, their careers differed in many respects. But they remained the closest of friends for the rest of their lives.

As July 1941 approached, the Harrisons departed. After 16 happy and productive years in Nashville, the Harrison family was moving on to greater responsibilities and great adventures in North Carolina.

University. Even this was far from the total received. When the first dean of Duke's medical school, W. C. Davison, in 1927 "asked Mr. George G. Allen, chairman of the trustees of the Duke Endowment, for a special appropriation for the Medical Library," Allen "inquired whether the Medical Library was a University library or a Hospital library. I promptly replied, 'Hospital library, of course.' He said, 'Thank you. You will get it [$100,000] and more when you want it.' (Both of us knew that Mr. Duke had designated in his Will that 90 percent of the income from his residual estate, which was larger than the original Duke Endowment, should be used for hospitals and left the remaining 10 percent 'to and for' Duke University.)"

7

Publications and Professional Activities

Given Tinsley's interests and his capacities, it was probably inevitable that he would become widely published in academic medicine and would be a member and leader of the major professional medical associations in his specialties.

During his two years at the Brigham, in addition to carrying out his clinical duties in an excellent fashion, Tinsley managed to publish four papers as senior author or co-author. The first, with Bill Dock and Emile Holman, was an experimental study of the effects of arteriovenous fistulae on the cardiac output in dogs.[1] The co-authors demonstrated an increase of cardiac output of approximately 100 percent in the presence of a sizeable fistula, as compared with the flow before it had been created and after it had been blocked or removed. They also showed the effects on the heart (myocardial hypertrophy and often dilatation) and demonstrated that the results were to some extent dependent on how long after creation of the fistulae measurements were taken. The publication in the British journal *Heart* revealed a certain ambition on the part of the authors—ambition for high quality, but also for academic achievement in the world of medical research. The editor at the time was Thomas Lewis, aided by A. R. Cushney of Edinburgh, Leonard Hill of London, Sir James MacKenzie of St. Andrews, Frank Wilson of Ann Arbor, Ludwig Aschoff of Freiburg, Willem Einthoven of Leiden, George Dock of Los Angeles, and Yandell Henderson, G. Canby Robinson, and William H. Howell of Baltimore, as well as many others prominent in clinical medicine and physiology of the day—especially cardiology.

Tinsley's second paper was "Notes on the Regional Distribution of Rheumatic Fever and Rheumatic Heart Disease in the United States" with Sam Levine as his co-author.[2] They called attention to the apparently greater frequency of rheumatic

1. T. R. Harrison, W. Dock, and E. Holman, "Experimental Studies in Arteriovenous Fistulae. Cardiac Output." *Heart* 11 (1924): 337.

2. T. R. Harrison, and Sam Levine, "Notes on the Regional Distribution of Rheumatic Fever and Rheumatic Heart Disease." *South. Med. J.* 17 (1924): 914.

fever and heart disease in the northeastern United States. "The disease is most common in cold, damp places," they argued. They speculated that it might be helpful to patients with a history of rheumatic fever or rheumatic heart disease to move to places with lower frequencies of those disorders. They also cautioned: "Further statistics are needed in order to ascertain the basic facts upon which a campaign for the sanitarium treatment of rheumatic fever may be established." The wave of optimism that followed identification of so many infectious causes of diseases during the previous 40 years is illustrated by a statement in their introductory paragraph: "While awaiting the discovery of the specific cause, any light that can be thrown upon the general etiological factors may possibly prove to be of benefit in combating this insidious and crippling disease."

Another paper, based solely on reviews of the work of others, was probably stimulated by his famously having missed the diagnosis of myocardial infarction in a patient during rounds with Levine, as well as the developing awareness of the disease by clinicians everywhere. "Obstruction of the Coronary Arteries" was published in the 1925 edition of *Transactions of the Medical Association of the State of Alabama*, primarily for the assistance of physicians in his home state in recognizing this newly understood clinical entity.[3]

The final paper from Harrison's 24 months at the Brigham again used the Fick principle to determine blood flow through the lungs of rabbits with and without a pneumothorax, then a standard method of collapsing a tuberculous lung as a means of therapy.[4] The results showed that flow through the collapsed lung remained high at first then diminished, suggesting that the therapeutic effect in tuberculosis must be associated with hypoxia.

These four papers, while not earthshaking, were sensible and worthy contributions which introduced Harrison both to the medical investigators of the world and to the laboratory and clinical studies, and most of all to the method of procedure used by world-class experts such as S. A. Levine and Samuel Grant.

By 1925, HARRISON was in Nashville, and he published four papers in 1925, four in 1926, and nine in 1927.[5] The papers were not disposable clinical reviews but reflected many hours of labor in the laboratory generating data with colleagues. He had three in the new *Journal of Clinical Investigation* before 1927, including one in the very first volume of the journal.[6] The nine which came into print in 1927 were all based on laboratory work—no reviews, book chapters, or clinical

3. T. R. Harrison, "Obstruction of the Coronary Arteries," *Tr. Ala. State Med. Ass'n.* (1925): 1.

4. W. Dock and T. R. Harrison: "The Blood Flow Through the Lungs in Experimental Pneumothorax." *American Rev. of Tuberculosis* 10 (1925): 534.

5. The lag in publication time accounts for the fact that, although his work at the Brigham ended in mid-1924 and he produced four publications while there, only two appeared in print that year.

6. Harrison, "Effect," 547.

7. C. P. Wilson, T. R. Harrison, and C. Pilcher, "The Action of Drugs on Cardiac Output. IV. The Effects of Camphor and Strychnine on the Cardiac Output of Intact Unnarcotized Dogs," *Arch. Int. Med.* 40 (1927): 605.

8. C. Sabiston Jr., "Alfred Blalock," *Annals of Surgery* 188 vol. 3 (1978): 255.

9. Harrison, interview, 1974.

10. Russell L. Cecil, ed. *Textbook of Internal Medicine* (Philadelphia: W. B. Saunders Co., 1927).

11. Vienna was historically the most prominent, and there was an "American Medical Association of Vienna" extant that year which published a guide (unsigned: The American Medical Association of Vienna. Cafe Edison, Alserstrasse 9, Vienna VIII. 1927–1928. Printed by E. Kainz Vorm. J. B. Wallis-Hausser, Viena.). However, this guide, known to visiting American physicians and medical students as "the Blue Book," was oriented more toward short-term visitors than serious faculty members such as Har-

commentaries, though some of the basic animal physiology work was published in clinically oriented journals such as the *Archives of Internal Medicine*.[7]

Tinsley also published a paper in 1927 that appeared without his name on it. As related in Chapter 6, when his friend Al Blalock had to be hospitalized for tuberculosis in 1927, Blalock fretted over what would happen to his research in dogs demonstrating that the shock of extensive soft tissue trauma was the result of fluid loss. Tinsley analyzed the data, arranged the references, wrote the paper, handled the submission and revisions, reviewed the galley proofs, and saw it published under Blalock's name.[8] Tinsley later said this was only right: "I didn't really do the work."[9]

During all this activity at Vanderbilt, another new enterprise was being launched in New York and Philadelphia: the *Textbook of Internal Medicine*, a large multi-authored text published by the W. B. Saunders Company of Philadelphia and edited by Russell Cecil, M.D., who was then professor of medicine at Cornell in New York, but who had been born in Kentucky and had lived as a child in Selma, Alabama. This text, which appeared for the first time in 1927,[10] replaced the fading *Principles and Practice* of Osler (who died in 1919) during the 1930s, '40s, and early '50s.

IN 1927, THANKS TO the Rockefeller fellowship midwifed by Canby Robinson, Tinsley headed to Vienna and the famous Allgemeines Krankenhaus to see first-hand how the great continental clinical and research enterprises operated.[11] He was disappointed. The Allgemeines Krankenhaus was an inspiring place, with its great history,[12] its statue of Billroth in the garden, the feeling that the ghosts of Skoda and Rokitansky were watching from the shadows, and the somewhat gruesome museum with the stuffed human skin. It was a very large physical structure, and it had large wards; each housed 40 patients in a single room. Privacy was minimal. Stands with curtains for screens were sometimes put up when a patient wanted to use a bedpan or bathe, though at times there were no screens if the staff was too busy or the screens were already in use. There were similar arrangements, or lack of arrangements, for a patient who died in the ward.

The place was too impersonal and the classes were enormous. For Tinsley, Vienna was too big. It seemed over-organized for commercial exploitation of visiting American physicians.[13] He enjoyed the town, but he was never very musical, and he longed for the sort of personal attention he had heard Carl Ludwig had bestowed on Welch years ago in Leipzig.

After several months he arranged for another place in Freiburg im Breisgau.

Tinsley and Betty moved there, probably around mid or late October. The rest of the family had returned home to America, and Betty was pregnant with a third child so would also have to return soon.

Freiburg was much more to Tinsley's liking, a lovely little town in the Black Forest. The school was small and the people friendly. The faculty seemed more interested in helping him accomplish some research. One study was published: "Ueber die Beziehungen des Nervus vagus zum Atmungs-mechansmus," with R. L. Moore.[14]

As nice as it was, Frieburg, like much of German-occupied Europe, would become a haunted place, a grotesque example of misguided science. The chief of medicine at the medical school was Hans Eppinger.[15] As World War II erupted, Eppinger became a prominent Nazi and chief of medicine at the Allgemeines Krankenhaus. After the war ended, Eppinger was implicated in experiments on Jews, Gypsies, and other "undesirables." He was to be tried at Nuremburg, but committed suicide. Tinsley must have seen Eppinger quite a bit, but he worked daily with more junior members of the faculty. Tinsley's single published paper from the time is not closely related to the work Eppinger was doing, which concentrated on metabolism, body composition, and the like.

Tinsley rejoined Betty in Grafton, Massachusetts, in the early spring of 1928 and worked for several months before returning to Nashville. He spent this time with Barcroft and working with others in an ongoing study of the measurement of the oxygen-carrying capacity of hemoglobin.[16] It was excellent experience in an area of growing clinical importance, and it introduced Tinsley to the biomedical science community and their mode of working.

BACK AT VANDERBILT IN the late 1920s and early 1930s, Tinsley continued to pursue laboratory and clinical research. He published six papers in 1929, 12 in 1930, 10 in 1931, and seven in 1932. Of these 35 papers, one was in the *American Heart Journal*, one was in the *American Journal of Medical Sciences*, three were in the *American Journal of Physiology*, five were in the *Archives of Internal Medicine*, and 12 were in the *Journal of Clinical Investigation*. Four others were published in surgical journals (*Archives of Surgery* or *Surgery, Gynecology and Obstetrics*) with his surgical private-practice colleague, John Burch, and involved cardiovascular changes during and after spinal or general anesthesia. The other eight were primarily clinical papers on cardiovascular problems, published in the *Southern Medical Journal* or the *Memphis Medical Journal*.

rison. It lists pensions for lodging, shops where one could purchase "electro-medical and X-ray instruments and apparatus, ENT equipment, diathermy apparatus, and a revolving chair by Prof. Dr. Barany," as well as theater tickets, jewelry, etc. The Blue Book also provides an extensive list of "courses" or lectures, which could be attended singly or in a series. Though these were named after famous physicians (Chvostek, Wenkebach, etc.), these well-known physicians do not appear to have participated personally in this instruction. There were strict rules for use of the Association's rooms. Similar guides existed for Berlin (in German, also unsigned: Das Medizinische Berlin. Ein Fuuehrer fuer Aerzte und Studierende. Berlin, S. Karger, 1905, 7th edition), France, and perhaps other countries and cities, though none has been found for Frieburg. The Countway Medical Library at Harvard Medical School contains one previously owned by C. Sidney Burwell and donated by him in 1943. J H. Honan,

Honan's Handbook to Medical Europe. A Ready Reference Book to the Universities, Hospitals, Clinics, Laboratories and General Medical Work of the Principal Cities of Europe (Philadelphia: P. Blakiston's Son and Co., 1912). Because of his Hopkins connections, Harrison was probably also aware of the then recently translated book by Billroth on German universities (Billroth, Theodor: *The Medical Sciences in the German Universities. A Study in the History of Civilization*. [translated and with an introduction by William H. Welch]. New York, Macmillan, 1924).

12. Erna Lesky, *Die Wiener Medizinische Schule im 19. Jahrhundert*. 1908. Trans. by L. Williams and I. S. Levij, *The Vienna Medical School of the 19th Century* (Baltimore: Johns Hopkins University Press, 1976).

13. Helmut Wyklicky to J. Pittman, February 26, 1997, UAB Archives. Professor Wyklicky, recently of the Institute for the History of Medicine at the University of Vienna, called this "the American Curse."

Miss Minnie Mae Tims, Harrison's technician and secretary, even received a then-unusual reward for her work during this period: her name is listed as a co-author with Harrison on two papers in 1931.

Vanderbilt colleague Seale Harris Jr. did some work with Tinsley and published one paper with him in 1931 on a test of respiratory function as an index of congestive heart failure. It was a clinical test they termed "the respiratory index."[17]

Tinsley's brother Groce joined the Vanderbilt house staff in the early 1930s, and as a research fellow he worked with Tinsley on clinical research. During the years 1932–36 they co-published seven papers relating to the shortness of breath experienced by patients with congestive heart failure.[18]

DURING THE MID-1930S PERIOD another significant professional event occurred, with typically little fanfare from Tinsley. As Tinsley went through his mail one day, his father was sitting beside him and noticed that Tinsley threw one letter and envelope into the trash with extra force and an epithet.

"What was that?" Groce asked.

"Some damn fool wants $10 to tell me I'm an internist," Tinsley replied.

"Let me see that, son, it might be worth sending them the money."

The letter was retrieved, the money submitted, and Tinsley became a board-certified internist, having been "grandfathered in" by the newly formed American Board of Internal Medicine.[20]

UNDERLYING TINSLEY'S NUMEROUS PUBLICATIONS during his Vanderbilt years was constant research, including methods others sometimes found odd, and collaboration with colleagues that often led to lasting friendships as well as substantial professional contributions to academic medicine.

One evening around midnight most of the house staff had gone to bed and were fast asleep in the quarters on the second floor in the "S" corridor. They were awakened by a loud clattering crash. They jumped out of bed and rushed down the corridor, as the clattering continued. It was coming from one of the laboratory rooms just around the corner on "B" corridor. When they opened the door, they were amazed to find their teacher Tinsley doing cardiac output determinations on a patient, while an assistant sat high on a stepladder with a large box filled with pots, pans, and various other noise-making articles which he would suddenly dump to the floor on a signal from Tinsley. The aim of the exercise, it turned out, was to study the effect of sudden change from tranquil sleep to an alarmed awakening on the cardiac output in the patient.[21] One of these young house officers was Ben Friedman, who had just completed medical school at Washington University and was doing his internship at Vanderbilt.

This was Ben Friedman's introduction to Tinsley Harrison. It was a bit unusual, but so had been much else in Friedman's odyssey. He was born in a small town near Odessa, Ukraine, near the Black Sea in 1904. His father, a merchant, heard about an upcoming pogrom in 1913 and moved the family by wagon across the land to Riga, then by boat to London, and finally to New York. There he worked as a cantor, while Mother made most of the money for the family as a seamstress. Ben was bright. He managed to gain entrance to City College of New York, where he was a classmate of Mark Altschule, himself to become a famous professor of medicine at Harvard. In 1927 Ben was admitted to the newly Flexnerized medical school in St. Louis, Washington University School of Medicine. Upon receiving his M.D. in 1931, he started his internship at Vanderbilt, where he met Tinsley in his cardiac output lab in the middle of the night.

The two became good friends, and after his assistant residency in 1932–33, Ben took what amounted to a research fellowship with Tinsley in 1933–34. The following year he spent as a research fellow continuing work begun the year before with Tinsley. During this year, 1934–35, Ben supported himself financially by working in Hugh Morgan's syphilis clinic (known as "Clinic L," L for lues—a serious infectious disease). He learned a great deal about that disease during the year, especially cardiovascular syphilis; but his real research was with Harrison. His first eight publications were based on work done in Harrison's lab, seven of them with Harrison as co-author, all on various aspects of congestive heart failure or improvements in the technology of studying congestive failure.[22]

In July 1934 Ben returned to New York for a research fellowship at the Cornell University School of Medicine. After two more years as a Sutro Research Fellow at Mount Sinai Hospital, during which he continued to publish chiefly with the well-known cardiologist Myron Prinzmetal[23] on studies of depressor substances from the kidney, he entered private practice in 1937 with E. T. Oppenheimer. With Oppenheimer he continued to practice, do research, and publish until he joined the U.S. Army Medical Corps in 1942. He and Tinsley kept track of each other during the war years; they would work together again.

14. "Ueber die Beziehungen des Nervus vagus zum Atmungsmechanismus," *Zeit. fur Die Gesellschaft Exper. Med.*, 31 (1928): 305.

15. See *Die Medizinische Facultät der Albert-Ludwigs-Universität Freiburg im Breisgau, Grundlagen und Entwicklungen* by Eduard Seidler. Berlin, Heidelberg, New York, Springer-Verlag, 1991–1993, 269.

16. J. Abeloos, N. Barcroft, T. R. Harrison, and J. Sendroy, "The Measurement of the Oxygen Capacity of Hemoglobin," *Am. J. Physiol.* 66 (1928): 252

17. T. R. Harrison, S. Harris Jr., and J. A. Calhoun, "Studies in Congestive Heart Failure. XVI. The Clinical Value of the Ventilation Test in the Estimation of Cardiac Function," *Am. Heart J.* 7 (1931): 157.

18. T. R. Harrison, J. A. Calhoun, and W. G. Harrison Jr., "Afferent Impulses as a Cause of Increased Ventilation during Muscular Exercise" *Am. J. Physiol.* 100 (1932): 68; T. R. Harrison, W. G. Harrison Jr., and J. P. Marsh,

"Reflex Stimulation of Respiration from Increase in Venous Pressure," *Am. J. Physiol.* 100 (1932): 417; T. R. Harrison, W. G. Harrison Jr., J. A. Calhoun, and J. P. Marsh, "Congestive Heart Failure. XVII. The Mechanism of Dyspnea on Exertion," *Arch. Int. Med.* 50 (1932): 690; W. G. Harrison Jr., J. A. Calhoun, and T. R. Harrison, "Studies in Congestive Heart Failure. XVIII. Clinical Types of Nocturnal Dyspnea," *Arch. Int. Med.* 53 (1934): 561; W. G. Harrison Jr., J. A. Calhoun, J. P. Marsh, and T. R. Harrison, "Studies in Congestive Heart Failure. XIX. Reflext Stimulation of Respiration as the Cause of Evening Dyspnea," *Arch. Int. Med.* 53 (1934): 724; T. R. Harrison, C. E. King, J. A. Calhoun, and W. G. Harrison Jr., "Studies in Congestive Heart Failure. XX. Cheyne-Stokes Respiration as the Cause of Paroxysmal Dyspnea at the Onset of Sleep," *Arch. Int. Med.* 53 (1934): 891. T. R. Harrison, J. A. Calhoun, and W. G. Harrison Jr. "Congestive Heart Failure.

IN 1938, FIVE FULL publications of Harrison's work appeared, three in the prestigious *American Journal of Medical Sciences*. Two more were submitted for publication the next year, (another in the *AJMS* and one in the *Journal of Clinical Investigation*). Several other publications had resulted that year from the work on the renal pressor substance, which appeared to be a very promising course of pursuit; though he was not one of the authors on these, it was recognized that the work came from his laboratory. Two were authored by his new young assistant and co-author on other papers, John R. Williams, a recent graduate of the University of Rochester medical school. These publications added to Harrison's academic standing. His research funding was solid, likely to continue in reasonable abundance. In addition to support directly from the medical school's budget, which could now be decreased in view of his increased extramural support, Tinsley had support from the fluid research fund of the Rockefeller Foundation, and support from other private sources was increasing. He had just received $3,500 from the Josiah Macy Foundation, a large grant for those days.[24] His revision of the manuscript for the second edition of *Failure of the Circulation* had gone well and was published in 1938.

In 1940 Tinsley authored or co-authored nine publications, nearly a third of the entire department of medicine's output of 28 that year, and far more than any other faculty member.

On January 6, 1941, Miss Minnie Mae Tims wrote an interesting letter in response to an inquiry from Carpenter to Tinsley about his most significant work, probably to prepare publicity. Miss Tims wrote Miss Nola Reed, secretary to Carpenter and what amounted to financial officer for the school, giving Tinsley's view of what "Dr. Harrison considers as his most important work." The first is in a separate category: his book, *Failure of the Circulation*. In addition he gave her four articles, or sets of articles, to list:

1. Pathogenesis of Congestive Heart Failure, a review published in *Medicine*, 1935, 14:225.

2. The Pathogenesis of the Uremic Syndrome, a review, published in *Medicine*, 1937, 16:1.

3. Arterial and Venous Pressure Factors in Circulatory Failure, a review in *Physiological Reviews*, 1938, 18:86.

4. Various publications in 1940 dealing with the problem of hypertension, as listed in the attached bibliography.

Unfortunately, the "attached bibliography" has been lost. However, since eight of the 10 papers Tinsley authored or co-authored that year concerned the work on antihypertensive substances derived from kidneys and other organs, it is clear that Tinsley thought this would be the next phase in research and perhaps his most important work. The only authors on these eight papers besides Tinsley were Williams and Arthur Grollman. Perhaps most interesting of all is that the first three references (or four, counting the book) are to *reviews*, rather than to single research papers describing specific discrete discoveries.

Tinsley authored or co-authored 10 papers in 1941, eight with Grollman and Williams on the renal depressor agent. This was the apex of Tinsley's output; he would never again publish so many papers in one year.

ONE REASON FOR THE slowdown in Tinsley's academic publishing was that medical school administration and increasing participation in professional associations were taking more and more of his time.

Academic travel to meetings, for conferences, to act as a visiting professor, and similar functions consumed appreciable time, energy, and resources. Tinsley's predecessor Burwell had served for a week as visiting professor at Emory several years earlier. But the real excursions of academic medicine in the 1930s centered on the annual clinical research meetings in Atlantic City, New Jersey.

These meetings were dominated by the Association of American Physicians (AAP), a clinical research organization started in 1886 by prominent professors in prestigious medical schools and hospitals in the northeastern United States. Although originally in Washington, D.C., in early June, and later in September in attempts to meet with other organizations (such as the American Surgical Association), these came to be regularly scheduled to include the first weekend in May and were the most important of the year for physicians engaged in clinical research. For many years there were comparable meetings for the basic science departments sponsored by the Federation of American Societies for Experimental Biology, or FASEB, held two weeks earlier, often at Atlantic City.

The AAP considered itself an exclusive group of medical leaders. The membership was limited to 100, then 125, then many years later to 500 (more recently the AAP includes larger numbers). Only members could present papers or sponsor colleagues to present at the Atlantic City meetings or enter into the discussion of papers. This exclusivity and the desire of others, especially younger investigators, to

XXI. Observations Concerning the Mechanism of Cardiac Asthma" *Arch. Int. Med.* 53 (1934): 911.

19. (Omitted)

20. Harrison audiotape, UAB Archives.

21. Ben Friedman, interview, 1992, UAB Archives. It appears this study never made it into print.

22. A. Grollman, B. Friedman, G. Clark, and T. R. Harrison, "Studies in Congestive Heart Failure. XXIII. A Critical Study of Methods for Determining the Cardiac Output in Patients with Cardiac Disease," *J. Clin. Invest.* 12 (1933): 751; B. Friedman, T. R. Harrison, G. Clark, and H. Resnik, "Studies in Congestive Heart Failure. XXII. A Method for Obtaining 'Mixed' Venous Blood by Arterial Puncture," *J. Clin. Invest.* 13 (1934): 533; B. Friedman, T. R. Harrison, G. Clark, and H. Resnik, "The Effect of Therapeutic Measures on the Cardiac Output of Patients with Congestive Failure." *Trans. Am. Assoc. Phys.* 69 (1934): 158; B. Friedman, H. Resnik, J.A. Calhoun, and T. R. Harrison. "Effect of Diuretics on the Cardiac Output of

Patients with Conges-
tive Failure." *Arch.
Int. Med.* 56 (1935):
341; B. Friedman,
G. Clark, H. Resnik,
and T. R. Harrison,
"Effect of Digitalis on
the Cardiac Output of
persons with conges-
tive Heart Failure,"
Arch. Int. Med. 56
(1935): 710; H.
Resnik, B. Friedman,
and T. R. Harrison,
"The Effect of Certain
Therapeutic Mea-
sures on the Cardiac
Output of Patients
with Congestive
Heart Failure," *Arch.
Int. Med.* 56 (1935):
903; H. Resnik and
B. Friedman, "Studies
on the Mechanism of
the Increased Oxygen
Consumption in
Patients with Cardiac
Disease," *J. Clin. In-
vest.* 14 (1935): 551;
T. R. Harrison, B.
Friedman, G. Clark,
and H. Resnik, "The
Cardiac Output in
Relation to Cardiac
Failure," *Arch. Int.
Med.* 54 (1934): 239;
T. R. Harrison, B.
Friedman, and H.
Resnik, "Mechanism
of Acute Experimental
Heart Failure," *Arch.
Int. Med.* 57 (1936):
927. All of these
papers were published
in excellent journals
with international
circulations.
23. Famous for

present and discuss papers led to the formation of the American Society for Clinical Investigation in 1908, sometimes called the Young Turks for their revolutionary approach to dignity.[25] Their annual meetings were scheduled also for Atlantic City at a time adjacent to the AAP meetings. In 1940, Henry A. Christian and some of his colleagues found both the Young Turks and the AAP to be so hopelessly hidebound and exclusive that he and some colleagues led in the formation of a third group, the American Federation for Clinical Research, or AFCR.[26] To encourage young people to join the AFCR, the only requirements for admission were sponsorship by a current member and publication of one research paper. For many years after World War II the three societies met together at Atlantic City, where there were few distractions and one could meet colleagues strolling up and down the boardwalk during breaks or in the late afternoons or evenings. The doctors and professors would dine together at Hackney's, the Brighton Punch Bowl, the Knife and Fork, or other congenial places. It was the perfect place for discussing work with colleagues around the world and for medical politics and academic advancement.[27]

Tinsley started attending these meetings in the early or mid-1920s, particularly as his first paper was published in the ASCI's new *Journal of Clinical Investigation*. The first issue appeared in October 1924 (unsynchronizing the years and volumes for later years, so volume 1 was 1924–25). The journal was introduced by an inspiring article on "Purposes of Medical Research" by the great New York cardiologist and electrocardiographer Alfred E. Cohn. In that same issue, two separate papers were published by C. Sidney Burwell and G. Canby Robinson, both on the relations of blood gases to cardiac output, exactly Tinsley's interests. The next two issues contained cardiology articles by Tinsley's classmate William Resnick. Finally, in the August 1925 issue, just as he was about to get started in the new Vanderbilt hospital, his article with Charles Wilson and Al Blalock on pH and circulation appeared.[28]

Tinsley was a prolific medical scholar during the 1920s and '30s, and by spring meeting time in 1928 he had 22 papers in respectable journals, including one from Germany, one from Barcroft's lab, and three in the *Journal of Clinical Investigation*. By the age of 28, he was a leader in understanding cardiac output and cardiovascular physiology and pathophysiology in general. That year he was elected to the Young Turks of ASCI. Now he had even more reason to attend the spring rites in Atlantic City.

By 1933 he had published a total of 54 papers, including a number in the *American Journal of Physiology*, the *Archives of Internal Medicine*, the *Journal of*

Biological Chemistry, and 15 in the *Journal of Clinical Investigation*. In May that year at Atlantic City the Council of the AAP elected Harrison an associate member, a five-year election. Full members of the Association were chosen from the associate members.[29] At the May 1934 AAP meeting, Tinsley presented a paper titled "The Effect of Therapeutic Measures on the Cardiac Output of Patients with Congestive Heart Failure." During 1934, working with Ben Friedman, his brother Groce Jr., and several other colleagues, he authored or co-authored another eight papers, including one in the *JCI* and one in the *Transactions of the AAP*. This was more than twice the number published by any other member of the department and more than a third of the department's total output for the year. Tinsley was a leading scholar.

The pressures on younger faculty members to research and discover and publish as much as possible were immense. These pressures for academic advancement undoubtedly played a large role in the competitive Tinsley's motivation to perform well in medical science. He seemed to have deeper wellsprings of motivation for scientific understanding. First, he was genuinely interested in trying to understand human physiology and pathophysiology, especially as related to the cardiovascular system. This stemmed from his own intellectual curiosity and energy, but also from his belief gradually developed over the years that only through such understanding could medical diagnosis, prognosis, and treatment be optimally pursued. Many years later, at a meeting of medical investigators honoring him, he said that he valued many things in academic medicine—the tear in the eye of a grateful patient, the sudden gleam of understanding in the eye of a student, and the dawning of understanding in his own consciousness. He also believed that a medical school, as an educational institution emphasizing the intellect, must vigorously pursue research and investigation of all sorts if it is to fulfill its functions in society.

The biggest splash, and Tinsley's greatest single contribution to understanding in cardiology, came in 1935 with publication of his first book, *Failure of the Circulation*. His lifelong friend Ben Friedman said years later, "It served as a clear beacon of light in a heretofore beclouded sea of obscurity."[30] This was accurate. For more than 10 years, Tinsley had been intensely studying congestive failure and cardiovascular pathophysiology, especially as related to congestive heart failure, and he was an astute observer, an imaginative and careful investigator, and a perceptive synthesizer of a wide array of facts. It is amazing that Burwell a few years earlier had to write an article titled "The Progressive Nature of Heart Failure" to call attention to the usual course of the disorder. *Failure of the Circulation* was written by someone who

his description of "Prinzmetal's angina."

24. Kampmeier, *Recollections*, 188.

25. J. A. Pittman and D. M. Miller, "The Southern Society for Clinical Investigation at 50: The End of the beginning," *Am. J. Med. Sciences* 311 (1996): 248–253. This article discusses the formation of the SSCI (Southern Society for Clinical Investigation) but also the "Old Turks" (Association of American Physicians started in 1886 by Osler, Pepper, and others) and the "Young Turks" (ASCI, American Society for Clinical Investigation, started in 1907).

26. The American Federation for Clinical Research (AFCR) was sometimes confused with the FASEB, presumably because the word "federation" is a part of both titles. AFCR is supposed to focus on clinical research, and FASEB on basic research, though obviously there is much overlap.

27. The last meeting at Atlantic City was in 1975.

28. Harrison, "Effects," 547.

29. One was elected an "associate member"

for five consecutive years. It was a sort of probationary period, and full members, of which there were only 125 total at the time, were chosen from among the associate members. Thus, associate membership served as a stimulus to keep producing research publications, or increase the effort and results.

30. 110, 113 Friedman, Ben to George E. Burch, Tulane, dated January 22, 1970 (attachment), UAB Archives; James Howard Means, "Birth of the Association," *The Association of American Physicians, Its First Seventy-five Years* (New York, Blakiston Div., McGraw-Hill Book Company, Inc., 1961). The Association of American Physicians formally originated with a meeting of "the original seven" physicians in the New York office of Francis A. Delafield (12 West 32nd Street) on October 10, 1885. "The original seven" were Robert T. Edes of Boston, Francis Delafield, William H. Draper, and George L. Peabody of New York, and William Pepper, William Osler, and

knew the field as well as anyone else at that time, far better than most, and it was still remembered as a landmark work by cardiovascular physiologists as the twenty-first century began.[31] This book, more than any single paper, marks Tinsley's most significant contribution to cardiology.

IN 1936, TINSLEY WAS elected to full membership in the AAP. He also worked out a method for cannulating the coronary sinus of dogs without opening the chest, thereby facilitating studies of cardiac metabolism. He worked with Blalock studying pericarditis and concretio cordis (an interest of Burwell's) and their effects on cardiac output.

He lost a friend and confidant, however, when his faithful assistant Tom Brooks died. Little is known now about Brooks, but he appears to have been a talented and skilled colleague and an important member of the research team. He helped and guided his younger colleague and pupil Vivien Thomas, the black technician who became famous for his work with Alfred Blalock.[32] Tinsley was fortunate to locate James E. Lewis, an able and energetic younger man. Lewis started at an annual salary of $840.[33]

Following publication of *Failure of the Circulation* in 1935, Tinsley changed the emphasis and direction of his research program to a pursuit of understanding hypertension. This consisted of attempts to extract from kidneys substances which would raise or lower the blood pressure, among other things. Interesting and tantalizing results were obtained at times, and the work brought Tinsley close to such advances as the discovery and the naming of "angiotonin" and "hypertensin" (later negotiated to the name "angiotensin") and familiarized him with the field. The work also brought his colleague and collaborator Grollman very close to a field in the early stages of its explosion into the clinical arena, that of adrenal cortical steroids. But their Vanderbilt lab made no major advances in the field of renal or adrenal agents responsible for control of blood pressure. This was perhaps in part because of Tinsley's departure from Vanderbilt just as the work was becoming most productive.

A second edition of *Failure of the Circulation* was published in 1938, and in the early 1940s Tinsley worked on a planned third edition with Franz Reichsman, a younger colleague from Vienna. Though he was Jewish and in Vienna, Reichsman was able to escape after the *Anschluss* in 1938 because he was a citizen of Yugoslavia. He came to the Jewish Hospital in Baltimore, then Hopkins, then followed Tinsley to Bowman Gray School of Medicine. There he worked as a clinical fellow (paid with a grant from the Dazian Foundation) and in his spare time searched the literature for articles concerning congestive failure and shock. Reviewing the literature was much more difficult then. There were fewer journals, but there were also fewer aids to finding articles. The *Index Medicus*, founded by Billings and Robert Fletcher, had existed since the 1890s.[34] But other print media, and of course computer searching systems, did not yet exist. The young Reichsman annotated the references he found in a copy of the second edition of *Failure of the Circulation*, then he and Harrison would review them together. Tinsley then began work on a revision of the material for a third edition. Tragically, the manuscript was among papers burned when a moving van caught fire during the Harrisons' relocation to Dallas, Texas, in March 1944 (see Chapter 9).[35] Burned in the truck fire, the manuscript for the projected new edition was irretrievable. Tinsley never again took up a revision of the book, his greatest success up to that time. Instead he asked a colleague at Dallas, Carleton B. Chapman, M.D., to undertake doing the third edition. Chapman demurred—a decision he later said he regretted—soon left, and later became dean of the Dartmouth Medical School and still later head of the Commonwealth Fund of New York.[36]

THE LATTER HALF OF the 1930s in Nashville continued the intense pace of activities. Tinsley served on the promotions committee of the medical school and on the library committee. He continued or increased his other activities. He enjoyed the library committee because of his lifelong love of books. He often brought armloads of books to rounds or journal club meetings to demonstrate a point appreciated by multiple authors on the subject at hand.[37] The meetings and travel continued.

In 1938 Tinsley served on the governing council of the Young Turks (American Society for Clinical Investigation), along with Isaac Starr. Starr later worked on the ballistocardiograph and encouraged Tinsley in his attempts to develop non-invasive methods of studying cardiovascular physiology and pathophysiology. John R. Paul was president of the ASCI that year; he later became chairman of medicine at Yale. Tinsley was also selected president-elect of the ASCI in 1938 and served during the 1939 meeting in Atlantic City.

The council that year included Eugene M. Landis of Virginia, later chairman of physiology at the Harvard Medical School, and William B. Castle, who had already done his famous work leading to the identification of the "intrinsic factor," critical in the pathophysiology of pernicious anemia. In his presidential address for the Young Turks, Tinsley discussed the reasons for stagnation and decline in established

James Tyson of Philadelphia. Osler had written Tyson in 1881 shortly after his first visit to Philadelphia to suggest forming such an organization, and James E. Graham of Toronto may have suggested it to Osler before that. The founders of the AAP were probably well aware of The Clinical Society of London, founded in late 1867 by leading clinicians of that city. It was founded for "the cultivation and promotion of practical Medicine and Surgery, by the collection of cases of interest, especially of such as bear upon undetermined questions in Pathology or Therapeutics." The organization appears to have been relatively open, and all qualified practitioners were welcome for nomination. The early reports were of individual cases or series of cases representing interesting clinical problems, thyroid problems being particularly prominent. One of the significant early accomplishments of this Clinical Society was the delineation of myxedema as a specific disease entity and the careful and remarkably complete description of its clinical semiology and pathophysiology. See "Statement of the Origin and Objects of the Society" Transactions of the Clinical Society of London," 1 (1868) and "Report of a Committee Nominated to Investigate the Subject of Myxedema," *Trans. Clin. Soc.* 26 (1888): 298. The Society also published a substantial book describing 109 cases of myxedema in detail. See also James A. Pittman and D. M. Miller, "The Southern Society for Clinical Investigation at 50: The End of the Beginning," *Am. J. Med. Sciences,* (1996).

31. Braunwald, "Pathogenesis," 67; Ralph S. Bates, *Scientific Societies in the United States* (Cambridge: M.I.T. Press, 1965). The Society for Clinical Investigation was formed in 1908, and apparently another group, the "American Association of Clinical Research" was formed in 1909. It should not be confused, however, with the much later AFCR (American Federation for Clinical Research).

32. Thomas, *Pioneering,* 14; Sherwin B. Nuland, *Doctors, the*

institutions, especially medical schools. There were always external causes difficult to control, he recognized, but the most important cause was failure to find and appoint the very best person for the job. This was a theme he was to repeat often in his life. He was particularly concerned with appointments at junior levels, those who would be available for senior leadership positions in future years. "Every instructor should carry in his knapsack the baton of a field marshal!" he said.[38] At the meetings in 1940 Tinsley presented a paper at the "Old Turks" meeting: "Pressor Properties of Extracts from Normal and Abnormal Kidneys." There was some discussion by Dr. George Harrop, the famous Hopkins specialist in metabolism and endocrinology who in 1936 had joined the pharmaceutical company E. R. Squibb and Son as director of research laboratories.[39]

Tinsley had attracted so much attention in academic medicine by this time that his alma mater, the University of Michigan, awarded him an honorary master of science degree in 1940.[40] Such honors and professional recognition would continue throughout the next two decades. For example, he was elected in 1956 to honorary membership in the Sociedad Medica de Santiago (Chile).[41]

IN 1943, WHILE AT Bowman Gray (Chapter 8), Tinsley was named to the advisory committee of the American Board of Internal Medicine, which set standards for certifying internists. In mid-November 1944, after Tinsley had moved to South-western Medical School (Chapter 9), the Southern Medical Association's annual meeting was held in Cincinnati. Tinsley was awarded the association's Research Medal, which had been established in 1912. Though the SMA had been founded in the Old Confederacy and was based in Alabama, many of its meetings were held outside the South. In the 1960s, after the AMA deserted both clinical medicine and scientific presentations at its annual meetings to address itself mainly to the improvement of medicine and defense of physicians by political means and scientific publications, the SMA meetings became the largest physician meetings in the country devoted mainly to the practice of medicine, with thousands of physicians strolling through acres of exhibits by pharmaceutical companies and device manufacturers. The SMA held its annual meetings in November to avoid conflict with the dates of the AMA, which held its big annual meeting in June and its smaller interim meetings in December. In numbers of physician members, the SMA was and remained throughout the 20th century second only to the AMA.

At the other end of the spectrum was the annual meeting of the Old Turks—the

Association of American Physicians (AAP) founded in 1886 by William Osler, William Pepper, and other leaders of academic medicine to promote clinical research.[42] Throughout the end of the 19th century and all of the 20th, the Old Turks represented the acme of achievement for faculties of internal medicine in schools around the country, finally becoming so exclusive that by the end of the 1900s it threatened to make itself extinct, a progression aggravated by the explosion of specialty societies, which became the preferred venues for presentations of hot research results. Tinsley had been elected a member of the AAP in 1933 while still at Vanderbilt. In May 1947, at the annual meeting of the Old Turks, Tinsley gave his famous "black crow-white crow" discussion about the nature of congestive heart failure.[43]

At that 1946 meeting groups of academic physicians strolled the Atlantic City boardwalk in the sun and brisk sea breeze of early May as they discussed the postwar future of American medicine. One group composed largely of chairmen of departments of medicine and other leading internists throughout the South, such as Rudolph Kampmeier of Vanderbilt, Tom Finley of the University of Georgia, Paul B. Beeson of Emory (later chair at Yale then at Oxford), and Tinsley discussed the need for a more local group, and a smaller less exclusive group, devoted to clinical research, but still senior to the American Federation for Clinical Research[44] to counteract the excessive exclusivity of the two most senior clinical research organizations in the country: the Association of American Physicians (founded 1886—the Old Turks) and the American Society for Clinical Research (founded 1909—the Young Turks). Since no one except members were even permitted to speak at the AAP meetings, unless invited by a member, and since the Young Turks were becoming almost as exclusive, these academic leaders felt they needed a less formal meeting where their younger colleagues could present and discuss their research. Thus, this group formed the Southern Society for Clinical Research (later Clinical Investigation, the SSCI) in 1946. Harrison was the first president, and the organization grew and thrived as a primarily regional organization devoted to clinical research. As the 21st century began, it continued to thrive, as did similar organizations in the western, central, and, to some extent, eastern parts of the country.[45]

In 1948 the American Heart Association (AHA) underwent a major change. It had been a rather small group of researchers and academics devoted to publishing research results and holding meetings for discussion and debate. But in 1948 it began accepting members who were neither physicians nor scientists but anybody interested in heart disease and physiology. At the same time it converted itself from

Biography of Medicine (New York: Vintage Books, 1989), 440–442.

33. Medicine Annual Report.

34. Carleton Chapman, *Order Out of Chaos. John Shaw Billings and America's Coming of Age* (Boston: The Boston Medical Library in the Countway Library, Harvard Medical School, 1994), 196.

35. F. Reichsman, personal communication, April 1993.

36. C. B. Chapman, personal communication, May 1993. Chapman had also been born in Talladega, Alabama, and he and Harrison had many mutual friends there as well as in medicine.

37. Riven, *Worthy.*

38. T. R. Harrison, presidential address, *J. Clin. Invest.* (1939).

39. Harvey, *Osler's Legacy,* 46. In view of Harrison's ties to Johns Hopkins and its staff and his need for money to support his research, it is surprising he did not try harder and obtain support from Squibb. Harrop had worked at Hopkins on adrenal steroids with George Thorn, and Squibb

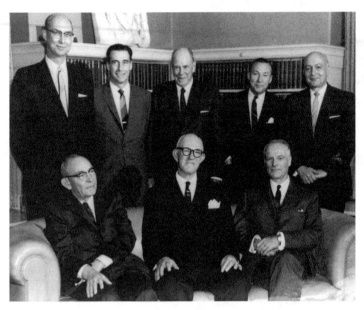

Tinsley, seated, left, with the first NHI council, 1948.

might have been expected to take an interest in a possible agent for lowering blood pressure. Probably Harrison, having already cast his lot with Lilly, was not free to pursue possibilities with other companies. But Harrop was clearly interested, as shown by his attendance and discussion here.

40. Harrison, curriculum vitae. A letter from Harrison to Mr. Frank E. Robbins regarding the robes & cap for this ceremony

a group interested primarily in doing and discussing research to one advocating such research, raising money to support it, and lobbying for public support. It was into the management of these transformations that Tinsley was propelled by his election as first president of the new and different AHA.

The same year, lobbying largely by lay people led to another event which elevated the status of cardiology: the creation of the National Heart Institute (NHI). Heart disease had become the number one killer of Americans and commanded increased attention from everyone. In this climate the early and indefatigable health lobbyist Mary Lasker said to her friend, U.S. Surgeon General Dr. Leonard Scheele, "Len, why shouldn't there be a Heart Institute?"[46] Scheele wrote the bill, modeling it on the earlier National Cancer Act of 1937, and though it was late in the congressional session and Truman was on the west coast, got it passed and signed on June 16, 1948. As one of the leading cardiologists in the world at the end of the war, and now as incoming president of the American Heart Association, Tinsley was appointed to the first "council" of the new National Heart Institute.

THE SINGLE NATIONAL INSTITUTE of Health had become plural, Institutes. The NIH was to play an increasingly important role in academic medical centers throughout the nation and in medicine and health throughout the world—and in Tinsley's life.

Even before World War II, momentum had been building for support of biomedical research, and the contributions of scientific research to the war effort greatly accelerated interest and faith in such research as an answer to problems, a sort of second-stage booster for the Enlightenment. The main impetus came through the OSRD (Office of Scientific Research and Development), headed by Vannevar Bush of "Endless Frontier" fame. "The laboratory, as much as the factory, proved to be the great arsenal of democracy. Radar. Missiles. Radio-controlled fuses. Mass-produced penicillin. The atomic bomb."[47] As the OSRD closed with the war's end, it devolved into two main groups: the expanded National Institutes of Health and the National Science Foundation.

The NIH was derived from the Hygienic Laboratory opened in 1887 by the U.S. Marine-Hospital Service as bacteriology and infectious diseases were coming to the fore. The Marine Hospital Service itself had been established in 1798. The NIH as such was begun in 1930 out of the Hygienic Laboratory under the aegis of Louisiana Senator Joseph Ransdell, who dreamed "of creating a great medical research institution in which hundreds of scholars would work on the underlying basis of all the diseases of humankind."[48] But the new name provided the new National Institute little additional funding because of the deepening economic depression.

One crucial advance did occur in the mid-1930s: the Luke Wilson family donated 95 acres of land to the federal government for "a worthy purpose."[49] This land, a rural farm in 1930, is 12 miles from downtown Washington and is now directly across the highway from the National Naval Medical Center and the federal Hébert School of Medicine. The original NIH first expanded with the creation of the National Cancer Institute in 1937. The NCI had legal authority to make grants to extramural institutions, such as universities and research institutions. The NCI was created with separate legislation and for a time considered itself co-equal with the NIH, but it soon became the ninth division of the NIH.

Next, buildings were constructed on the Wilson farm: Building 1, later to become the Administration Building with the NIH Director's office, was started in 1938 and dedicated by Franklin D. Roosevelt in 1941; Building 2 was for "Industrial Hygeine," Building 3 for "Public Health Methods," and Buildings 4 and 5 for "Infectious Diseases," all clustered around Building 1.[50]

As the OSRD itself completely disappeared, the last of its funds moved to the U.S. Public Health Service or were retained to be phased out. The funds appropriated to the NIH were then either used intramurally or, the majority, distributed to extramural institutions as research grants and contracts. The post-war amounts rose dramatically: $4 million in fiscal year 1947 (beginning in July 1946), $15.6 million in 1950, and $36.6 million in 1955. By the end of the 20th century the total NIH budget was more than $20 billion current dollars. Tinsley, along with his institutions, was by virtue of his training and experiences one of the relatively few physicians in the country poised to receive maximum benefit from these events.

STILL AHEAD, OF COURSE, was the 1950 publication of what has been described as

is in the University of Michigan Archives, Bentley Historical Library (copies in the UAB Archives), and gives the following physical data on Harrison: height: 5 feet 6.5 inches tall; hat size: 7–1/8; chest: 35 inches

41. Perhaps through the promotional efforts of his research fellow from Chile, Cecil Coughlan, M.D.

42. Pittman, "Southern Society."

43. During the discussion following presentation of a paper, Harrison remarked: "Some time ago, some philosopher said that if it can be shown on incontestable evidence that there is a white crow, then the statement that all crows are black can no longer be considered tenable. This well-studied patient would seem to represent a white crow." Tinsley Harrison, "Beri-Beri Heart Disease by C. Sidney Burwell and (By Invitation) Lewis Dexter," *Trans. Ass'n. Amer. Phy.* 60 (1947).

44. Later changed to the American Federation for Medical Research (AFMR).

45. Pittman, "Southern Society." The SSCI

continues into the
21st century and has
taken over publica-
tion of the old and
established *American
Journal of the Medical
Sciences*, where many
classics of medicine
first appeared—an-
other story in itself.

46. D. S. Fredrick-
son, "Science and
the Culture Warp" in
*Emerging Policies for
Biomedical Research*,
eds. W. N. Kelly, M.
Osterweis, and E. R.
Rubin (Washington,
DC: Association of
Academic Health
Centers, 1993), 33.

47. G. P. Zachary,
*Endless Frontier. Van-
nevar Bush, Engineer of
the American Century*
(New York: Free Press,
1997), 1.

48. Fredrickson, "Sci-
ence," 16.

49. This land was
directly across the
Rockville Pike (from
Washington to Rock-
ville, Maryland) from
the National Naval
Medical Center, which
owned a golf course
adjacent to the NIH
campus. Later this golf
course was absorbed
in by the NIH, so
that at the end of the
20th century the NIH
campus was well over
100 acres.

50. Fredrickson, "Sci-
ence," 22.

the most recognized book in all of medicine, *Principles of Internal Medicine*, which Tinsley began editing in 1945 and oversaw through the fifth edition in 1965. Now titled *Harrison's Principles of Internal Medicine*, the current 18th edition was published in 2011.

Modern mass-circulated textbooks of medicine came only after Gutenberg revolutionized printing in the 1450s, but medical texts had probably existed in some form since the times of Hippocrates or Imhotep in the west and Sheng Nung in China. Prior to the late 19th century, most of the medical textbooks used in America came from Britain, with exception of self-help and sectarian books (those of the Thomsonian "steam doctors," homeopaths, etc). A few general medical texts originated in America, which, though excellent for the times, did not long survive their original single authors.[51]

From 1892 through the first third of the 20th century Osler's *Principles and Practice of Medicine* dominated U.S. and Canadian texts.[52] Up through the seventh edition published in 1909, it was a one-man book. In April 1908, as that edition was nearing completion, Osler wrote to Lewellys F. Barker, his successor in the chair at Hopkins, and invited him and his associate W. S. Thayer to come in as joint authors.[53] They declined, probably in part because they had to earn most of their income from clinical practice. Former Osler resident Thomas McCrae, later a professor at Jefferson Medical College in Philadelphia, participated in the textbook for the 1912 eighth edition, and, after Osler died, for the ninth edition in 1919. The latter listed "the late Sir William Osler"—he died December 29, 1919—and McCrae as authors and included a portrait of Osler as the frontispiece. McCrae continued alone through the 12th edition in 1935. The 13th–15th editions (1938–45) were overseen by Henry A. Christian, chief of medicine at Harvard's new Brigham Hospital. Thereafter the book went out of print until revived in 1968 as a *Johns Hopkins Textbook of Medicine*, which had been Osler's desire when he wrote Barker 60 years earlier.[54]

Osler had many advantages in writing his book between 1890 and 1892. He had an excellent basic education and had been a general practitioner in a rural community. He was also an expert pathologist, the main foundation, with bacteriology, of medical science in those days. And he had experience in Europe and on the faculty of three medical schools where he gained valuable experience teaching both medical students and practicing physicians. Further, as the new chief of medicine at the not-yet-opened Johns Hopkins medical school, with young physicians to carry much of the clinical load, Osler could devote himself to writing. Thus, he worked an average of five hours a day, four or five days a week from October 1890 through June 1891. He sent the first five sections to the publisher on July 1. He took a two-week breather in Toronto in August, then returned to non-air conditioned Baltimore and the same routine, essentially finishing the manuscript by mid-October. Though he was a master of the English language, he had it checked by a Mr. Powell of the Hopkins English department. He later said, "Without the help of [H. A.] Lafleur and [W. S.] Thayer, who took the ward work off my hands, I never could have finished in so short a time. My other assistants also rendered much aid in looking up references and special points. During the writing of the work I lost only one afternoon through transient indisposition, and never a night's rest. Between September, 1890, and January, 1892, I gained nearly eight pounds in weight."[55]

An immediate success, the book was ultimately translated into French, German, Spanish, Portugese, Russian, and Chinese[56] and sold hundreds of thousands of copies.

In 1927, as McCrae was struggling to maintain Osler's great book alone, a new competitor appeared: *The Textbook of Medicine* edited by Russell L. Cecil, a practicing New York microbiologist and rheumatologist with an appointment at the Cornell University College of Medicine. Cecil (1881–1965) was born in Nicholasville, Kentucky, but moved to Selma, Alabama, in 1889, where his father became pastor of the First Presbyterian Church. He remained there until 1900. Thus, like Osler, Cecil spent a formative decade in a rural community. Young Cecil earned his A.B., cum laude, from Princeton, then he obtained an M.D. from the University College of Medicine (later Medical College of Virginia) in Richmond in 1906. His father became "the Presbyterian Pope," Moderator of the General Assembly in 1911.[57]

Like Osler, Cecil trained in pathology, taking a residency at Presbyterian Hospital of New York from 1907 to 1910, after which he served as an instructor in medicine at Columbia. In 1916 he moved across town to the Cornell Department of Internal Medicine, where he remained the rest of his life, doing much of his early clinical work at Bellevue Hospital.

Most of his early research concentrated on infectious diseases, especially pneumonia and its treatment with vaccines, on which he became a considerable authority. During his Army years (1917–19) he headed the surgeon general's commission for the study of pneumonia, resulting in a major 1918 report in the *Journal of Experimental Medicine* and 10 papers with Francis Black, later a professor of medicine at

51. These included those of Austin Flint Jr. with 6 editions between 1866 and 1886, Robert Bartholow of Philadelphia (1880), Alonzo B. Palmer of Michigan (1882), Nathan Davis Smith of Chicago (1884), and Alfred L. Loomis of New York (1884).

52. James A. Pittman Jr., "Prominent Textbooks of Internal Medicine in the 20th Century," (paper presentation, International Society for the History of Medicine, Galveston, Texas, 2000).

53. A. M. Harvey and V. A. McKusick, *Introduction to Osler's Textbook of Medicine Revisited* (Birmingham, Alabama: Gryphon Editions, Ltd., 1978).

54. The 1968 edition was produced by Hopkins internal medicine faculty, led by chair A. McGehee Harvey. Quoted in *The Principles and Practice of Medicine*, 17th edition, eds. A. M. Harvey, L. E. Cluff, R. J. Johns, A. H. Owens, D. Rabinowitz, and R. S. Ross (New York: Appleton-Century-Crofts, Educational Division, Meredith Corp., 1968), preface.

55. Harvey, *Introduction*.

56. Garraty, *Oxford's*, 804–807.

57. Ibid., 599–600; Interview with assistant, First Presbyterian Church of Selma, AL, 1999.

58. K. Francis, "A Textbook Case of Medical Innovation: Austin Flint's *Principles and Practice of Medicine* and the Germ Theory of Disease," in *American Association for the History of Medicine*, Abstracts of the 73rd Annual Meeting, Bethesda, MD, 2000, Session 16.

59. James A. Pittman, "The Most Prominent Internal Medicine Textbooks of the 20th Century" (paper presented at International Society for the History of Medicine, Galveston, Texas, 2000). By the late 1940s it was apparent to Cecil that most practicing physicians, who at that time were still general practitioners trained mostly with rotating internships or no internships at all before the war, could not hope to keep up with the ever-increasing specialization. He therefore initiated and edited a

Yale. He served from 1920 to 1928 as chairman of the U.S. Public Health Service Hygiene Laboratory's commission to study pneumonia.

As early as 1917, Cecil was focusing on rheumatoid arthritis, establishing an arthritis clinic at Cornell and a bacteriologic research laboratory at Bellevue. He pursued the idea that infection is the cause of RA, often then referred to as "chronic infectious arthritis." His work identified typical strains of streptococci as the causative agent. Although later disproved, the work led others years later to the discovery of the rheumatoid factor in the blood of such patients. In 1934, he became a charter member of the what is now known as the American Rheumatism Association; he served as its third president 1936–37. In 1948 Cecil formed the Arthritis and Rheumatism Foundation for support of research and education. He remained a major actor in that organization the rest of his life.

Cecil typified, participated in, and caused some of the march of medicine to the specialization and sub-specialization of his time—as biomedical knowledge and technologies multiplied and became too much for a single person to master. Recognizing this, and as a teacher of medicine in a major medical school, he initiated the multi-authored single-volume textbook of internal medicine, which by this time had also become quite distinct from specialties such as ophthalmology, surgery, obstetrics/gynecology, and to some extent pediatrics, psychiatry, and neurology. There had been earlier multi-authored works, such as *Tice's Practice of Medicine* in the U.S. and several in Europe, but these were multiple large volumes suitable mainly for libraries rather than for most practicing doctors. Others were single volumes but intended mainly as family guides rather than for practicing MDs. Textbooks of medicine not only summarize the knowledge of the day, but they also solidify it and establish a platform for later developments.[58] The American Board of Internal Medicine was established in 1936, less than a decade after the appearance of the first edition of Cecil's textbook.

Cecil's explanation was published in the preface of his book in 1927:

The rapid growth of medical science during the last few years has made it almost impossible for a single individual to master the entire field. In internal medicine, as in other branches of human knowledge, the age of specialism has of necessity arrived, and some of our ablest practitioners even devote themselves in great measure to one disease. In order that physicians and students of medicine might have the benefit of an authoritative and up-to--date treatise on every medical subject, it seemed desirable to prepare a text-book of medicine in which each disease, or group of diseases, would be discussed by a writer particularly interested in that subject. This book represents an effort to carry out such a plan. In all there are one hundred and thirty contributors, each of whom is a student or investigator of the subject upon which he has written. . . . Most of the contributors to this book are teachers of medicine in university medical colleges, and have, therefore, presented their material in a form especially acceptable to medical students. . . .

The result was a multi-authored single volume written by scholars most knowledgeable about their subjects. Cecil wrote the sections on arthritis and lobar pneumonia, and the long section on neurology was written by Foster Kennedy, who garnered a special place on the title page. The book quickly outpaced *Osler* and by mid-century dominated the market. By the end of the 20th century it was still one of the two main textbooks of medicine, probably second in sales only to *Harrison*.[59]

IN THE SUMMER OF 1945, as the war raged on in the Pacific theater, and as Tinsley struggled to make Southwestern, his new medical school in Dallas, "the best medical school in the world," he received a call from Morris Fishbein, M.D. Fishbein had recently retired as editor of the *Journal of the American Medical Association* and was working for Doubleday, which had just bought the Blakiston company of Philadelphia. "The new owners wished to produce a book on internal medicine to compete with *Cecil*, published by Saunders. *Cecil* had come to enjoy an almost complete monopoly in the United States. Tinsley was invited to come to New York and discuss with Fishbein and Ted Phillips, the chief executive of Blakiston, the question of becoming editor-in-chief of the projected book. All expenses would be paid, there would be a small honorarium, and tickets to the two most popular shows on Broadway would be provided."[60]

The invitation to prepare a new comprehensive textbook on internal medicine launched Tinsley on the aspect of his career which was to become the most successful and rewarding. It is the reason his name is probably the most familiar of any American physician, although most students, physicians, and even scholars know little about him even as they hold his book in their hands or read it on their computers. The only modern American competition to *Harrison* is *Cecil*.

In response to Fishbein's invitation, Harrison stated that he thought that *Cecil* was out-of-date and that there was no textbook that presented internal medicine

companion text, *The Specialties in General Practice* (Philadelphia-London: W. B. Saunders Co., 1951), which was published in three editions in 1951, 1957, and 1964. A new edition was due in 1970. But in 1969 the nation's general practitioners (GPs), unhappy with their decreasing numbers, esteem, and hospital privileges relative to the burgeoning numbers and prestige of the post-World War II specialists who had received residency training on the GI bill (unavailable to the GPs because there were few GP residencies), had reorganized to promote the specialty of "family practice" and formed the American Academy of Family Physicians, which then created the American Board of Family Practice and established residency training programs and board certification. Robert E. Rakel, an able and leading GP physician, now formally a specialist, wrote Saunders and suggested a new textbook (see R. E. Rakel to J. Pittman, December 4, 2001, UAB Archives). Saunders then decided to publish a textbook in family practice with Howard Conn, who had edited *Conn's Current Therapy* for them for many years, with Rakel as his co-editor. Saunders also wanted representation from the American Academy of Family Physicians, then called the American Academy of General Practice. Thomas Johnson was a physician employed by the AAGP and he agreed to be a third co-editor. Thus, they had a known and trusted editor in Conn, an academician in Rakel, and a representative of the national organization of family physicians in Johnson. I suggested the title be *Textbook of Family Practice* to match their other two famous textbooks, *Textbook of Medicine* and *Textbook of Pediatrics.*" They agreed and the first edition of the *Textbook of Family Practice* was published in 1973, nine years after the last edition of *The Specialties in General Practice.* Conn and Rakel edited the second edition published in 1978, and Conn died in 1982. Rakel was editor of the next four editions published in 1984,

the way it was taught in the better medical schools. He had certain definite ideas concerning a different arrangement and a more modern approach to the subject, but he had neither the desire nor the time to edit such a book.

Fishbein stated that the trip to New York would involve no obligations other than an open mind and the willingness to describe his ideas about a new book and to make suggestions concerning possible editors. After such discussions Harrison would be free to decline participation if he wished. The invitation was accepted. Harrison would arrive in the late afternoon, attend the theater and join Fishbein and Phillips for breakfast and lunch. After an afternoon matinee he would take an early evening flight back to Dallas.

The more Harrison thought of the matter the less was his desire to become editor. Therefore, to avoid embarrassment he devised a list of conditions that he thought no publisher would accept. Likewise, in order that the Blakiston Division might receive something in return for its expense, he clarified his ideas concerning the optimal arrangement of the book under discussion.

The evening show was excellent (unless memory, after 25 years, is playing tricks, it was *Oklahoma*). Upon being introduced to Phillips at breakfast, Harrison was favorably impressed. Here was personal charm, a rapid grasp of new ideas, and insight into features of a book that might facilitate its sales and enhance its intellectual value to the reader.

The discussions initially centered on arrangement. All agreed that the arrangement of current textbooks had changed little since the first edition of *Osler* when nothing was known about the physiology and biochemistry of disease. Hence, clinical medicine at that time was mainly empirical and related to morbid anatomy and, in lesser degree, to microbiology. Much was known concerning the "what" of disease and diagnosis but almost nothing about the "why" or about treatment.

During the ensuing 50 years a revolution had occurred. A major part of teaching was now devoted to pathophysiology and pathochemistry. Since these topics related to reversible alterations in function rather than irreversible changes in structure, a knowledge of pathophysiology was fundamental if treatment was to be based on reason rather than on rote. But against such heresies the textbooks of medicine had remained as firm as Gibraltar.

Patients do not usually come to physicians with known diseases but rather with complaints or symptoms. Likewise, many present with abnormal physical signs. These manifestations of disease, and especially the symptoms, provide the initial clues to diagnosis. Therefore, a textbook should begin with the major manifestations of internal disorders and then discuss specific diseases.

Both hosts expressed strong agreement with these ideas concerning arrangement. This was not surprising. Feeling that he had thus repaid his obligation and sung for his supper, Harrison proceeded to conditions he deemed would be unacceptable to the publishers.

There would need to be an editorial board which Harrison would select. This group would personally write much, perhaps most, of the book. They would have a free hand in selecting such additional authors as they deemed necessary. In choosing editors and authors there should be no consideration except the intellectual quality of the book. Thus, the tendency, then current in some textbooks and systems of medicine, to pay large attention to a wide geographic distribution with one or more writers from practically every medical school to augment sales, would not be followed.

At this point, Fishbein remarked that in his capacity as editor of the *JAMA* he knew those authors who would meet deadlines and those who would not. He also knew those writers who submitted polished manuscripts and those likely to submit "sloppy," poorly written versions that would put large burdens on the editors. Therefore, he believed that he could aid Harrison in the selection of editors and that he could help the editors select authors. However, after receiving such advice the editor-in-chief and subsequently the other editors would be free to accept or reject it.

Then came the surprising statement. Ted Phillips said, and Fishbein agreed, that they concurred completely with the idea of disregarding geographic distribution and other considerations of medical politics in choosing authors. They were in favor of one criterion only—the probable contribution of an individual to the quality of the book.

Harrison had now been partially disarmed. He had assumed there would develop irreconcilable differences that would justify his polite withdrawal from the venture. Although his disinclination to participate was weakened by the cooperative attitude of Fishbein and Phillips and by their insight into what the projected book should be, Harrison was not yet convinced that he wished to undertake the job. He still had certain weapons that might induce the publisher to prefer a different editor-in-chief.

There would need to be fairly frequent, brief meetings of the editors with the publisher and with each other. In addition, there should be occasional leisurely meetings of perhaps 10 days to two weeks, held in pleasant places, divided between work and recreation, and including the editors' families. Thus, friendships would be

1990, 1995, and 2002.

60. Wilson, *Harrison's*. The account and quotations here of the founding of *Principles of Internal Medicine* are taken from reminiscences compiled and edited by Jean D. Wilson, M.D., distinguished endocrinologist from Southwestern and former editor-in-chief of *Harrison* for three editions. Wilson's remembrance was published as the eleventh edition and the millionth copy of *Harrison* were coming out. The notes of Tinsley's own recollections are recorded in the first chapter of Wilson's book.

developed, and high morale could be established. In the long run, a strong *esprit de corps* would produce and sustain, through multiple editions, a first-class textbook.

Phillips promptly remarked that the publisher would be willing, at least for the first edition and possibly for later ones, to provide an expense account of $10,000 for such meetings. The editors could spend this as they deemed best in terms of facilitation the job. He then discussed royalties and agreed to provide, over and beyond the expense budget, royalties somewhat larger than was customary for textbooks.

At this stage in the discussion Harrison had only one remaining trump that might relieve him of the necessity of proceeding further. Even though he was for the first time beginning to question whether he wished such relief, he decided to play his card and rest his decision on the issue.

Harrison stated that while he was still reluctant to become editor-in-chief it might be fruitful to consider individuals to be selected as possible editors. He added that in his opinion at least one of them should be a person in the private practice of medicine. The proper type of person would provide a feet-on-the-ground point of view and keep the other editors, presumably academicians, from producing a volume far removed from the realities of day-to-day patient care. Harrison suggested Bill Resnick and, assuming that neither of the others had heard of him, started to explain the reasons for his choice.

Fishbein interrupted. He stated that although he did not know Resnik personally, he considered him one of the finest internists in the country. Furthermore Fishbein agreed with the idea of having one editor who was concerned, not with academic medicine, but with the realities of practice.

Other members of the editorial board were then discussed. Tinsley's next suggestion was Bill Dock. Fishbein said that he undoubtedly had one of the best minds in American medicine and was a broad scholar, a superb clinician, an excellent pathologist, and a charming raconteur. However, he was a chatterbox who monopolized all conversations and a prima donna who was not likely to function as a smooth team worker. Tinsley replied that Bill Dock had been a close, personal friend since they had been colleagues as interns more than two decades previously. He was well aware of Bill's defects which were small relative to his virtues. Both hosts then said this was a decision to be made, not by them, but by the editor-in-chief.

The next person suggested by Tinsley was Bill Castle. Fishbein said that the field of hematology was developing rapidly and that an editor who was an expert in this field was highly desirable. Bill Castle was certainly such an expert. However, experience had shown that he was a procrastinator on deadlines. Max Wintrobe was not as well known as Castle, but his book on clinical hematology was acclaimed. His reputation was growing rapidly. His style of writing was clear and concise, well adapted for a textbook. Further, he was reliable with deadlines. It was agreed that Wintrobe would be invited to become an editor.

The next question involved an editor with a strong background in infectious disease. Harrison stated that Chester Keefer was such a person and was also an extraordinarily able clinician. Fishbein agreed but said that Keefer was deeply involved in the penicillin program and would probably decline. However, there was nothing to lose by asking him.

The final understanding and conclusion of this initial meeting was that Harrison would consent to become editor-in-chief provided he could assemble a strong editorial group.

SOME MONTHS LATER A second meeting was held in New York. Those attending were Ted Phillips, his administrative assistant, Mrs. Eunice Stevens, who kept notes of the proceedings, Bill Resnik, Bill Dock, Max Wintrobe, and Harrison. As yet, no one had agreed to join the editorial board, but all were willing to discuss participation.

There was general agreement that the first part of the book should consider "Manifestations" and then "Mechanisms of Disease." There would be strong emphasis on pathophysiology and on pathochemistry. The consideration of specific diseases would follow and presumably would constitute the last two-thirds of the book.

All present considered it desirable to secure Chester Keefer, who had declined to attend the meeting. It was decided to phone him and ask him to meet Phillips and Harrison in the late afternoon at the Boston airport. Chester agreed.

During the flight, the two passengers discussed the meeting that had just ended. Wintrobe and Resnik had displayed considerable interest and some enthusiasm. However, little had been actually accomplished. Most of the time had been spent listening to Dock's delightful but mainly irrelevant comments. It seemed clear that future meetings would be fruitful only if some means could be found to prevent him from converting the discussion into a monologue.

The conversation with Keefer lasted only a half hour. He stated that he appreciated the invitation to become a member of the group and under other circumstances would probably have accepted it. However, his responsibilities concerning the distribution of the limited supplies of penicillin to the civilian population made it impractical to assume additional obligations. He agreed with the tentative decision made earlier to ask Paul Beeson to become an editor if Keefer should decline.

During the return flight from Boston it was agreed that Tinsley would communicate with Beeson and attempt to arrange for him to meet with the group at an early date. Beeson agreed to attend a meeting but would reserve judgment concerning his own final decision.

At the next meeting, also in New York, Wintrobe urged that an additional editor with a background in metabolism and endocrinology was needed. Some progress in arriving at a tentative chapter outline was made. However, once again Dock did most of the talking, much of which was unrelated to the matter at hand, but entertaining. Despite this serious but very enjoyable handicap, the morale of the group was high. It was now clear that not only Harrison but also Resnik, Wintrobe, and Beeson were emotionally committed to participation.

Shortly after this meeting Dock wrote that he had decided to withdraw. At no time had he agreed to become an editor. Despite the strong bonds of friendship between him and both Resnik and Harrison, the latter two were pleased with his decision. Fishbein had been correct—Dock was simply not a good team worker. His withdrawal did not stem from pique or any clash of personalities. His friendships with the other editors have remained as warm as before. He has contributed chapters whenever requested. In the absence of definite knowledge of his reasons for withdrawing, one suspects that he realized his digressions during the meetings were hindering progress and that he could best aid the book by declining to be an editor.

Harrison and some of the others had been loath to expand the size of the editorial group. Dock's withdrawal made it possible to add a metabolic editor without expansion. Wintrobe suggested George Thorn, but at the time Thorn was ill with hepatitis and was unwilling to accept new responsibilities. The decision was made to delay the appointment of a metabolism editor in the hope that Thorn might later participate.

THE NEXT MEETING WAS held at Phillips's home in Philadelphia (1946 or 1947). The spring flowers were at their peak. Ted was not only a superb host but an excellent chef who specialized in steaks. His white chef's hat, almost two feet tall, emphasized his culinary artistry. At this meeting the chapter outline was considered in detail.

During the discussions a general pattern emerged. Much of the talking was done by Harrison, Wintrobe, and Phillips who, despite the lack of technical knowledge, had sound ideas about arrangement. Beeson was relatively quiet, but such suggestions as he occasionally offered had great merit. Resnik often remained silent. So long as decisions met his approval he said nothing. Even when he disapproved he would withhold comment for a time. Eventually, no longer able to contain himself, he would explode. "Tinsley, you are crazy!" Since Resnik had been his intimate friend and arguing with him for more than two decades, Harrison knew that Resnik's anger was not personal, therefore, no offense was intended or felt. After a time, the others in the group took a similar attitude toward Resnik's explosions, which in most instances were based on valid reasoning. The net result of his outbursts, which recurred throughout the first five editions, was healthy. He and Wintrobe were effective in preventing complacency and acceptance that criticisms were only fair and that sections could be improved by rewriting. When the atmosphere became tense Beeson and, later, Thorn were good arbitrators and peacemakers.

In 1946, but also in '47 and '48, the first edition of the book consumed Tinsley's attention, time, and energy. As editor-in-chief, he felt obligated to set the pace. He not only prepared his own sections and rewrote them in response to criticisms, but he also carefully reviewed the work of other participants. It was necessary to recruit other authors to work on cardiovascular, renal and electrolyte, and other areas, then to recruit (unpaid) critics to criticize the work once it was done. His faithful secretary since Vanderbilt days, Miss Minnie Mae Tims, handled all the transcribing and typing (Tinsley "wrote" most of his work, including manuscripts, by dictating it then reviewing the typed material); she also handled much of the logistics. Tardy authors and reviewers had to be prodded. References and the specific numbers for doses, laboratory values, and so on, in the text had to be checked. There were also the negotiations with the publisher, but these were made easier by Ted Phillips. Much communication was required by frequent letters and telephone calls as well as the physical meetings of the editors to coordinate everything. Then there was the constant pressures of deadlines. The book exacted a large toll on Tinsley, perhaps consuming more attention, time, and energy than he could afford.

IN JANUARY 1947 OR 1948, the group gathered at New Orleans. This meeting undoubtedly occurred at or adjacent to the time of the annual meeting of the Southern Society for Clinical Investigation.[61] Probably most of these editorial meetings were held in connection with meetings of interest to internists.

Thorn indicated that he would be able to participate [at New Orleans] as an

61. Pittman, "Southern Society."

editor and planned to attend the long meeting to be held during the summer of 1948. This was good news indeed. The other major event of this meeting was the introduction by Wintrobe of what was immediately named the "wolf system." He had not only read personally the chapters that had been sent to him but had passed each of them along to whichever colleague on the Utah faculty that he deemed best qualified to criticize that particular subject. He had insisted that their criticisms be anonymous but frank, with no punches pulled. The rationale was that if criticism before publication were severe and unmerciful, there would be little left to criticize once the book appeared in print. Time proved this to be correct.

Many of the criticisms were almost devastating. In his eagerness to get the textbook off the ground, Harrison had written most of the chapters now being criticized. Some had been written rather hastily and without sufficient study of the more recent publications. Consequently, the bulk of the criticism was directed at his chapters. His initial reaction was one of slight pique and a desire to protest against unjustified criticism. However, it soon became clear that, in the main, Resnik and Beeson believed that the comments of Wintrobe and his Utah wolves were right.

These strictures concerning what had been written were motivated not by malice but by a desire to aid in the production of a first-class textbook. Therefore, Wintrobe was thanked by his fellow editors and told to express their appreciation to his colleagues. Of the many contributions Wintrobe would make to the book, none would be more important than his sponsorship of this free and frank criticism. To some extent, his procedure was subsequently followed by other editors in securing comments from their own colleagues. But the credit for initiation of this method properly belongs to Wintrobe and the Utah faculty.

In June 1948, the AMA met in San Francisco. Of the editors only Wintrobe and Harrison attended. Ted Phillips invited them to dinner at Trader Vic's in Oakland. Other guests were Becky Wintrobe, Eunice Stevens, and Tinsley's brother, Groce Harrison Jr. Neither the Wintrobes nor Harrisons had previously sampled Polynesian food, which on this particular occasion was superb. No doubt the scorpion punch which preceded the food enhanced the taste, as well as the discussion. Although no official activities concerning the book were undertaken, the excellent fellowship elevated the already high morale.

There was much discussion and correspondence concerning the choice of a site for the first long meeting which was to be held in the summer of 1948. Once again the suggestion of Wintrobe prevailed. Signal Mountain Lodge, near Jackson Hole in the Tetons, some miles south of Yellowstone Park, was selected. The meeting was especially important for several reasons. It would be the first discussion that George Thorn would have attended. All final decisions concerning the first edition would need to be made because the schedule called for delivery of the full manuscript to the

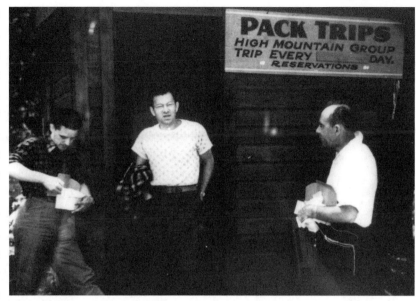

The editors of **Principles of Internal Medicine** *met at a lodge in the Teton Mountains of Wyoming, 1948. From left, three of the original editors, Drs. William Resnick, Max Wintrobe, and Tinsley Harrison.*

publisher within the coming year. Likewise, the wives and some of the children of the editors would attend. Thus, depending on circumstances, the morale within the group might be elevated still more or might be compromised.

It was decided that the mornings would be devoted to work and the afternoons to play. Paul Beeson came, but it was not possible for Barbara Beeson and the Beeson children to attend. At the last minute Ted Phillips had to cancel. Eunice Stevens came in his stead. The other adults in attendance were Bill and Lorraine Resnik, Max and Becky Wintrobe, George and Doris Thorn, Betty and Tinsley Harrison. The younger generation included Kate and Paul Resnik, Susan and Paul Wintrobe, Wesley Thorn, Betsy and John Harrison. Each family was housed in its own small cabin, all joining for meals at the Lodge.

Thorn and Harrison decided to meet each morning for a before-breakfast swim. Upon the first such occasion on the following morning Harrison emerged from Lake Jackson in a semi-congealed state because the water was the coldest he had ever encountered. This was his last venture into the lake. However, Thorn, being made of sterner stuff and accustomed to the water off the coast of northern Massachusetts, continued the morning dips.

The Wyoming gathering was the most fruitful meeting the editors would ever have. The final details concerning arrangement and chapters that had been written were reviewed. Many were returned to the authors with sometimes minor but more often major comments and suggestions for revision. Rarely was a chapter deemed satisfactory as submitted, meaning that all the editors considered it to be first-class; such a chapter was called a *dead pigeon*, which soon became *DP*. Toward the end of the meeting Beeson remarked that *DP* was the sweetest sound in the English language.

The day's schedule usually began with breakfast at 7:30 to 8 a.m. followed by intensive work until 1 p.m. After lunch, most of the group would follow a guide for a long ride into the mountains on horseback. Some were fair riders while others were neophytes who were assigned to the less-spirited horses. Even so, Bill Resnik will never forget the trip to Lake Solitude which included some narrow passages where one could look down 2,000 to 3,000 feet, if one dared. It was his first time on a horse and he kept saying to himself, "How did I ever get into a mess like this." Nevertheless, before the meeting ended even Resnik and the other neophytes were reasonably adept at managing their mounts.

At twilight the group, now relaxed and pleasantly weary from their exertions, assembled for cocktails at one of the cabins. The food was not sumptuous but was tasty. Appetites were stimulated by the rides, the mountain air, and by the feeling that after three years of effort the book was a not-too-distant reality.

As the editors came to know each other better the discussions became even more frank. Even temporary slights were rarely felt, and no editor ever took lasting offense at another. The rides together and the cocktail gatherings stimulated deepening friendships while the meetings, no matter how stormy, engendered growing respect of each editor for his fellows.

Initially the arguments were usually brief and between Resnik and Harrison. The latter, knowing from their long association that Resnik was usually right, ordinarily retreated without contesting the point. The infrequent argument between Resnik and Wintrobe commonly ended differently. Wintrobe was far less likely than Harrison to make a rash statement. When Resnik disagreed with Wintrobe he expressed himself explosively. However, Wintrobe kept his emotions under control and never raised his voice. Thus, he usually won the support of the other editors in his disagreements with Resnik.

In the earlier meetings Beeson had been the main peacemaker. Now he was joined by Thorn, a born diplomat. These two had the rare quality of expressing their views, even if they disagreed, in language that was so soothing and tactful as to be convincing. This quality was conspicuously lacking in the other three editors.

Had the various stormy arguments been concerned with "who is correct" their effects on morale would have been disastrous. It was obvious to all of us that each was concerned rather with "what is correct" and was endeavoring to boost, not his own ego, but the quality of the book. Thus, the debates tended to raise morale.

A notable feature of this meeting was the cordiality of the wives toward each other. The result was enthusiasm for future long meetings, which in turn stimulated interest in the preparation of future editions.

It was at the Wyoming meeting that friendships crystallized and that strong feelings of respect of each editor for his colleagues developed. Wintrobe, Beeson, and Thorn were admired for their clear style of writing, their deep knowledge of their own fields, and their strong interest in the entire field of internal medicine. Thorn and Beeson were admired and indeed envied, at least by Harrison, for their diplomacy and peacemaking ability. Wintrobe and Resnik were respected for their devotion to the intellectual quality of the work and their willingness, if need be, to let the chips fall where they might as a means to this end. Resnik's fellow editors were gratified and at times amazed at the breadth of his knowledge of internal medicine and at his capacity to recall information gleaned from reading years earlier. Harrison was acclaimed for his initial ideas concerning the arrangement of the book, for his suggestion that it be called *Principles of Internal Medicine*, and for his successful efforts toward morale building. (Although in the latter respect, Harrison believed that he was given credit which actually should have been shared by the group as a whole as well as by the Wyoming environment; all the other editors believed that by far the lion's share of the credit belonged to him.)

. . . In retrospect, after two decades, it is clear that the Wyoming meeting contributed more to the success of the first edition and possibly to that of several subsequent editions than did any other event.

During the subsequent year the chief responsibility of the editors involved reviewing the manuscripts of contributors and modifying their own manuscripts along the lines agreed upon at Signal Mountain Lodge. One of the chief difficulties involved neurology. Prior to the Wyoming meeting the decision had been made to omit neurology at least from the first edition. However, Thorn urged that we have a section on neurology and that we give serious considering to adding a neurologist to our editorial group. His views, although stated with his usual tact, were firm and adamant on this question. Subsequent events have confirmed his position.

The last minute decision to include neurology created a problem. Houston

62. Especially Mr. Derek Jeffers, 1980, who had worked in management in both companies.

63. Years later Dr. Ryals, born and raised

Merritt agreed to write the section provided he could be aided by his associate Daniel Sciarra. Their chapters were necessarily written hastily and arrived late. Thus, there was no time for detailed editorial suggestions. The blame was attributable to the editors who were rescued from a disastrous blunder, that of omitting neurology entirely, by the sound judgment of Thorn. Neurology was given too little time and too little space. It was a mistake that was not to be repeated in later editions.

The final meeting prior to the appearance of the first edition was held at the Philadelphia home of Ted Phillips (May 1949). The manuscript had been completed, the proof had been corrected, and the presses were rolling. The meeting was largely concerned with plans for a second edition, some years later, in case the first edition should prove to be a success.

Wagers were laid concerning the sales of the first edition during its first year. The editors, having strong faith in the quality of their book but believing that the new arrangement would be slow in attracting sales, were pessimistic. The guesses varied from 3,000 to 6,000 volumes. They believed that Ted Phillips's guess of 8,000 copies represented wishful thinking. When the tallies were available more than a year later, all the estimates were wrong. The actual sales during the first year were somewhat above 14,000.

This meeting, which was the final one in Ted Phillips's home, had several delightful aspects. Once again it was spring, and the flowers were beautiful. Again Phillips wore his high chef's hat and proved himself a master at cooking steaks on his backyard grill.

The Kentucky Derby was being run that day. Each of the group paid a dollar and in turn drew from a hat the names of horses until all had been drawn. There then ensued a period of exchanging, purchasing, and selling horses. Only when the radio was turned on to listen to the broadcast of the actual race was it realized that somehow or another Thorn now owned not only all the horses but also all of the dollars. Thus a lesson was learned. The others would never again engage in wagering or bartering with that sharp New England Yankee.

THE FIRST EDITION OF what is now known as *Harrison's Principles of Internal Medicine* finally appeared in 1950, and it continues into the 21st century as a leading textbook of internal medicine. It stands as one of the best-selling medical textbooks in all of history. Harrison began working on the book soon after he accepted the position of chair at Southwestern Medical College in Dallas, Texas, and the first edition was published as he was leaving to build a new school in Birmingham in 1950. In that sense, it was a transition on both ends, and it marked perhaps the ultimate in Harrison's balance between scholarship and clinical practice.

The second edition of *PIM* was published in 1954, but Tinsley considered it the poorest of all the editions, especially because the index had been prepared by literary people who knew little about medicine or what people in medicine were interested in. Later preparation of the indices was led by Miss Minnie Mae Tims, his faithful assistant since the Vanderbilt days, and others familiar with medicine and what interested doctors, as well as with medical publishing. All this also took lots of time, attention, effort, and energy. But he was doing what he loved. The book was increasingly successful. By 1964 *PIM* was successfully challenging Cecil's *Textbook of Medicine*. Several people who had worked in both McGraw Hill, which published *PIM*, and Saunders, which published Cecil, said that the former had overtaken the latter in numbers of sales.[62]

At the time Robert F. Loeb, chair of medicine at Columbia, was editing *Cecil*. As the graduating medical students prepared their 1965 yearbook with all their photos, and so on, Dr. Jarvis Ryals added a photo of Tinsley looking straight into the camera with his eyebrows raised and a quizzical look. The caption read, "Cecil and Loeb? Oh, I always throw those pamphlets away."[63]

Tinsley said of the success, "I'll give us [the editors] six months off after a new edition, then we have to go to work on the next edition." They stuck to this schedule for many years, publishing new editions every four years through the seventh edition in 1974. Then, perhaps spurred by the increasing explosion of new information as the last quarter of the 20th century came, the eighth edition came out in 1977, only three years after the seventh. By then Tinsley was 77, a full-time VA employee, and no longer directly involved in editing the book. Later editions appeared after intervals of either three or four years.

PRINCIPLES
OF
INTERNAL MEDICINE

T. R. HARRISON
Editor-in-Chief

EDITORS

PAUL B. BEESON   GEORGE W. THORN
WILLIAM H. RESNIK   M. M. WINTROBE

Philadelphia · THE BLAKISTON COMPANY · *Toronto*
1950

The title page of the first edition, 1950.

in Lowndes County and a good friend of Tinsley's friend Jack Kirschenfeld, presented UAB with a gift of millions of dollars for the construction of a large building for the School of Public Health, named in honor of his parents.

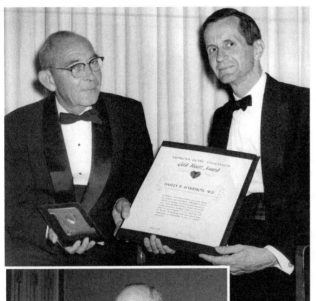

IN THE HEAT OF the cold war in 1960, Tinsley was called back into service by the U.S. Army as a consultant and lecturer to physicians based in western Europe, especially West Germany. On May 7, 1960, he became a member of the "Society of Medical Consultants of the Armed Forces." His old friend from the Mass General Hospital was also a member, and they saw each other in Germany. While there he also lectured to a group of medical students and young physicians in Heidelberg. At the outset he asked whether they would prefer that he speak in good English or bad German, and they replied loudly, "Schlechtes Deutsch! Schlechtes Deutsch!" So he gave the entire lecture in German.[64]

As America was experiencing cultural explosions in the 1960s, Tinsley continued what he knew and did best, teaching medicine to younger physicians and inspiring them with mature clinical judgment. In 1961 he was given the Gold Heart Award by the American Heart Association, presented by his old friend Oglesby Paul.

In 1963, the Alabama medical school, on the suggestion of the former chairman of biochemistry, Emmett Carmichael,

Top, Dr. Oglesby Paul, presenting Tinsley with the AHA's Gold Heart Award, 1961. Above, Tinsley giving the first Distinguished Faculty Lecture, UAB's highest honor for medical faculty, 1964.

started an annual Distinguished Faculty Lecture to be given at an evening dinner by a faculty member selected by the faculty. That year Tinsley was selected and gave the first DFL on "Witches and Doctors."[65]

In 1964, Tinsley received the Honor Award of the American Medical Writers' Association for Distinguished Contributions to Medical Communication. As Tinsley's retirement as chief of cardiology came in 1965, it became a bounty year, with the Distinguished Service Award of the American Heart Association, a House Joint Resolution of the Alabama legislature for his contributions to medicine in the state, an honorary doctorate from the University of Alabama, and a resolution from the state senate for "Contributions to Science."

In 1966 Tinsley was elected a Master in the American College of Physicians, the highest rank of the clinicians, after Associate and Fellow. In 1967 the popular magazine *Modern Medicine* selected him with some students for their cover photo on the June 19th issue. The pose was typical. The group is standing beside a patient lying in a bed, and Tinsley is standing with one hand raised as though gesturing. There are four onlookers: W. Crawford Owen, M.D., chief medical resident of 1966–67, Joe Allen, M.D. 1967, David Gaillard, M.D., 1967, and J. Michael Straughn, M.D., 1966. Within the magazine is a complimentary article under the heading "Contemporaries."

BY THE MID-1960S, ISCHEMIC heart disease was recognized as an epidemic in the United States and most of the western world, with its high fat diets, smoking, increasingly sedentary life, and other invitations to heart attacks and strokes. In 1965, Tinsley himself had a myocardial infarct. One side effect of this heart attack was discussions between Tinsley and his protege T. Joseph Reeves, resulting three years later in a book that would be Tinsley's last major publication, *Principles and Problems of Ischemic Heart Disease.*[66] Joe Reeves had interned under Tinsley at Parkland Memorial Hospital in Dallas. In 1954, Tinsley recruited Reeves, by then a respected cardiologist, to the faculty in Birmingham. Reeves then managed most of Tinsley's medical care during his infarct episode, even though it was done diplomatically through the local practitioners.

Tinsley was a classical bedside clinician, but Reeves was at the beginning of the technology takeover of clinical medicine, having done the first aortic pressure-pulse curves while working with Donald McDonald in Edinburgh and at Hammersmith in London. He and L. Thomas Sheffield in Birmingham produced the first data showing that heart rate correlated best with cardiac oxygen consumption,

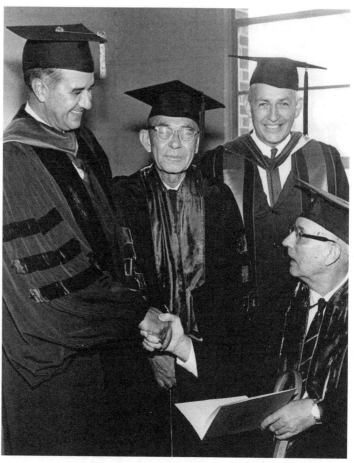

Champ Lyons (seated) and Tinsley Harrison receive honorary degrees from the University of Alabama, presented by President Frank Rose (left) and Dr. Joseph F. Volker (right), October, 1, 1965.

64. Audiotape interview with T. R. Harrison, UAB Archives.

65. The next year it was given by his surgical colleague Champ Lyons. The DFL lecture series became extremely successful and has continued each year without interruption except for 1988, when Dr. Ricardo Ceballos, about to introduce Basil I. Hirschowitz, M.D., inventor of the fiberoptic gastroscope, dropped dead at the podium. J. Hecht, *City of Light: The Story of Fiber Optics* (New York: Oxford University Press, 1999).

66. T.R. Harrison and T. J. Reeves, *Principles and Problems of Ischemic Heart Disease* (Chicago: Year Book Medical Publishers, Inc., 1968). Tinsley had for some years been an editor of two of the many annual yearbooks by this publisher, the cardiovascular portion of the *Year Book of Medicine*, and the *Year Book of Cardiovascular and Renal Diseases*.

67. J. T. Reeves and L. T. Sheffield, "*O2 Consumption with Exercise.*"

68. Examples: "The physician who fails to

thereby paving the way for the "Bruce Test" of cardiac fitness widely used in later treadmill exercise tests.[67] Tinsley considered himself clumsy and never did cardiac catheterizations.

Reeves later generously said that "he did about 30 percent and Harrison the rest of the book," but it seems probable that though Harrison's vast experience with and knowledge of ischemic heart disease was likely unequaled in any other physician of the time, especially in its bedside manifestations and courses, Reeves was much younger and still vigorously active in producing more data and probably did at least half the work and assured that the project made it into print.

Both authors show through in the text. For example, the first chapter, "The Problem of Fear," is reminiscent of a talk Tinsley later gave about "anxious fear" before the AMA convention. This first chapter discusses not only the patient's fear, but also that of the physician and of the family. The attempt at balance is also evident in the preface:

> During our life span, clinical medicine has changed from a mainly rule-of-thumb affair to a reasonably respectable branch of biologic science. . . . To decry of even to belittle the impact or the importance of scientific medicine should automatically label the detractor as not only a spiritual descendant of Cassandra but also as a candidate for the madhouse. But this does not mean that the meticulous labors of a hundred generations of Hippocratic physicians can be casually dismissed because they were not based on quantitative measurements and were therefore, "unscientific." Careful bedside observation is sometimes nonscientific but, unlike quackery, is never unscientific.

Some of Tinsley's favorite dicta[68] are also in the text, and, in an incident that coincidentally occurred while they were working on the book, Reeves proved himself a diligent pupil by diagnosing a mysterious ailment of Alabama's former governor, James E. "Big Jim" Folsom. He was bothered by a persistent and bothersome ringing in the ears—tinnitus. On EKG examination he was also found to have a prolonged QT interval. The house officers and junior faculty did not know what was wrong but supposed the two findings were unrelated. It was Tinsley's long-time pupil and colleague Reeves who took a more careful history and followed Tinsley's dictum: "The answer is often in the history alone." Reeves noted that Folsom, famous for his alcohol habit, was drinking multiple gin-and-tonics every day. He had cinchonism:

quinine poisoning. He was advised to change to bourbon. He did, and the manifestations disappeared.

The reviews of *Principles and Problems of Ischemic Heart Disease* were generally favorable. The main objection revolved around the book looking too much to the past and not enough to the future. However, there are excellent discussions of the outlook for various methods of attacking IHD, including mammary artery implantation and coronary artery bypass using veins, endocardial punch resections by Vineberg, Kazei, and others, endarterectomy alone by Longmire, DeBakey, Effler, and others, as well as other methods just being tried in the mid-1960s as this book was being written. While it was not the classic of the 1935 book *Failure of the Circulation*, it was a very respectable work.

become the master of laboratory medicine is destined to be its slave. . . . The scientific method involves both deduction and induction. The former poses the problem and the latter seeks the solution. Thus, the *validity* of one's work depends on the controlled experiment, but its *significance* stems from the question that is asked. . . ."

8

Bowman Gray School of Medicine

Winston-Salem, North Carolina, 1941–1944

As the Great Depression receded and a new decade opened, life in Tinsley Harrison's world was good. The war in Europe was far away, and America First speakers were abundant. General Motors was producing 50 percent of U.S. cars. Tinsley spent much of late 1940 and early 1941 in discussions and negotiations with Bowman Gray officials and with colleagues at Vanderbilt. He was excited about taking a senior position at the founding of a new school. He had been at Vanderbilt when the new school opened; he knew about the progress at Duke so richly endowed by the other great North Carolina tobacco (and electric power) fortune; and he had visions of similar developments at Winston-Salem. Meanwhile, though they did not want him to leave, Tinsley's Vanderbilt associates saw the opportunity that awaited him and were enthusiastic in their assessments of his readiness for the post.

On November 26, Tinsley wrote Archie Woods of the John and Mary R. Markle Foundation in New York. "I have just been approached in regard to the chair of internal medicine at the Bowman Gray School of Medicine," he said, which "may become one of the best in the country and for this reason will give the matter very serious consideration, in case they later decide to formally offer me the position. However, at the present time there is no prospect of there being immediately available funds in the research budget of the Department of Medicine to carry on my problem on the large scale required at the moment." He asked Woods if the foundation would permit him to move the $7,500 allocated for the work of July 1941 to July 1942 and said he would like to visit with him in New York soon.[1]

1. T. R. Harrison to Archie Woods, November 26, 1940, VUMC Archives.

Woods replied, ambiguously, about moving the Markle money to Bowman Gray. While the Markle Foundation was commendatory about his work and would continue his grant until July 1942, support after that was uncertain. Tinsley wrote Coy Carpenter in mid-December telling him of this development but also expressing his conviction of the efficacy of his renal extract in lowering the blood pressure, not only in animals, but also in patients. Tinsley proposed going to New York to discuss this with Woods in person. He also thought it would be desirable to have some sort of commitment from Bowman Gray prior to talking with Woods, since the question of research support from the school had been brought up by the Markle people in connection with his work at Vanderbilt. As the board of the Markle Foundation would meet December 20th, perhaps he should go immediately rather than in January as previously planned. He asked that Carpenter wire or phone him his advice. Carpenter's answer, although unknown, seems clear; the trip was not made until January 1941.

In early December 1940 Carpenter wrote Vanderbilt Dean Walter Leathers to document for his later recommendations to President Thurman D. Kitchin and the Wake Forest trustees what he already knew about Tinsley. Leathers gave a good report. He said that Tinsley was "a conscientious and untiring worker and at the same time possesses a degree of brilliancy that is unusual"; that he was "eminently qualified for the position"; and that he had "unquestioned research ability." As for Tinsley's clinical abilities, Leathers said, "I regard him as a man of superior ability in dealing with clinical aspects of cardiac conditions. He has a consulting practice which covers a considerable range of territory." Tinsley's qualities as a teacher elicited the greatest praise: "The students tell me that he has remarkable ability as an instructor . . . In other words, he possesses marked inspirational qualities as a teacher."[2]

On December 16 Carpenter wrote Leathers thanking him for his report. "So far as I am concerned, your enthusiastic endorsement of him for the position of Professor of Medicine here settles the question," he said. "As I have told you personally, I have for several years gratefully acknowledged the debt we owe you and Vanderbilt for your cooperation in the development of our school."

There were also exchanges discussing arrangements for space, particularly research animal space, the laboratories and their equipment, the furniture, the decor and colors, and a host of other things. Tinsley arranged to visit Winston-Salem with his friend and younger coworker, Dr. John R. Williams, in conjunction with an otherwise unrelated trip to Duke in January and worked in a conversation with Dr.

2. W. S. Leathers to Coy C. Carpenter, M.D., December 14, 1940, VUMC Archives. Leathers also commented that he (Leathers) had been associated with Tinsley's mother's brother who has been Professor of Latin at the University of Mississippi for about 40 years.

George Harrell while there. He was enthusiastic at the prospect of Harrell's being in the department of medicine.[3]

Tinsley felt confident but also somewhat manic. He negotiated an unusual salary arrangement, based on his large family and the necessary moving expenses. During his first year at Bowman Gray, he would be paid $15,000 by the school. His second year he would make $14,000, and the third $13,000. Thereafter he would earn an annual base salary of $12,000. This was a substantial increase. At Vanderbilt, Tinsley had earned only $5,000 a year. Hugh Morgan's salary as a higher-up had been $10,000.[4]

Tinsley asked John Williams to move with him and Williams tentatively agreed; the move would mean an academic promotion and higher income. He also talked with F. Tremaine "Josh" Billings, who had trained at Hopkins, had worked with him at Vanderbilt, and was still on the Vanderbilt staff. Billings declined, which Tinsley took in good humor.[5] Arthur Grollman, who had visited Vanderbilt for several weeks on several occasions to work out the acetylene method for determining cardiac outputs in dogs, remained at Hopkins but was most receptive when Tinsley contacted him about moving to the new school. The pieces were falling into place. All it took now was money. Meanwhile, Tinsley received a letter from Emory University in Atlanta inquiring whether he would be interested in a professorship of medicine there.[6] It was exhilarating to be in demand and to be building a great department of medicine!

ON DECEMBER 20 CARPENTER and Tinsley had a detailed discussion of plans for the department of medicine over the coming few years. At the discussion's end, Carpenter suggested that Tinsley write him summarizing his "impression of the general conclusions which we had arrived at in our discussion of the future of the Department of Internal Medicine at Bowman Gray School of Medicine of Wake Forest College." Tinsley thought this was a good idea, not only because there were a lot of details and it would help to have them codified, but also in case the administration changed or Carpenter moved to some other position and be replaced by someone unfamiliar with the commitments. Therefore, on December 21, Tinsley sent Carpenter a 25-page typed letter.

After a preamble setting forth the reasons for recording these matters, Tinsley gave a paragraph titled "Aim of the Department of Internal Medicine": "To become the best department of internal medicine anywhere. This should be looked on not as

3. In one letter Harrison comments, "If one has to choose between inadequate research laboratories and inadequate outpatient facilities for the Department of Medicine I feel sure it is more important to remedy the former." T. R. Harrison to Coy C. Carpenter, December 14, 1940, VUMC Archives.

4. Morgan, Medicine Annual Report. Though this budget was for the previous year, the salaries from the school were probably about these amounts for 1940–41, perhaps 8 or 10 percent higher; but certainly not threefold higher! These matters are always somewhat tender, but perhaps it would have been wise for Dr. Carpenter to discuss this in a bit more depth with Dr. Leathers. On the other hand, the "base salary" was $12,000, and Harrison had already said that he did not want to do much practice in Winston-Salem.

5. F. T. Billings, Oral history transcription for R. H. Kampmeier, 1980, VUMC Archives.

6. The letter to Har-

just a praiseworthy Utopian dream but as an attainable although difficult objective. The velocity of progress toward this aim will naturally vary according to conditions, but the direction of progress should not be altered under any circumstances."

The letter goes on to discuss attaining the aim of the department (start small, but *always* select and appoint *only* the *very best person* for the position, especially when considering junior positions and younger people; there will be necessary expansion of the department in future years). Some sections of this portion of the letter, if known to other faculty members later, might have caused resentment: "It is the expressed purpose of the Dean to have a department of internal medicine second to none, and if possible better than any, and since it is the policy of the school that the department of internal medicine is the most important single department, this expansion of the budget would go on even if it interfered in some degree with the functions of the other departments of the medical school."

Tinsley hoped that the annual financial support of the department from school sources might reach $50,000. He was clear on the priorities for expenditures. The first priority would not be patient care, which would be expected to take care of itself financially and perhaps add money to the coffers of the school. And it would not even be teaching, which should follow along naturally in the wake of other activities. No, ". . . it is recognized that in a clinical department excellent teaching and excellent care of patients can be obtained at very little expense, and further, that the outstanding difference between a good department and a great department is in the quality and the volume of investigation carried out. Such being the case it would be the approved policy of the department to expend funds chiefly for investigation."

Tinsley discussed the desirability of building a dormitory for medical students to facilitate the fourth-year students' serving in "somewhat the capacity of rotating interns." Lectures and clinics would be "primarily to stimulate thinking rather than to teach facts. The second and third year students should be given thorough drilling in the basic techniques of medicine, that is, in history taking, physical examination and various laboratory procedures." Tinsley wanted to select the students from only the best applicants, and he wanted to build scholarship assistance funds to help attract the best students, regardless of their ability to pay. As he often said, he disliked "systems," and he certainly was not stuck in any particular system: "An experimental attitude of mind will be maintained toward medical education and various methods of training and instruction can be tried from time to time and those which do not prove useful will be discarded."

rison is now lost, but it appears to have been an offer, or at least an inquiry. In a December 27, 1940 letter, C. C. Carpenter wrote to Harrison: "I want to congratulate you on the letter from Emory. I am sending it to Dr. Kitchin [president of Wake Forest] and asking that he return it to me. I might say parenthetically that I heard while in Philadelphia that there was some discussion among the deans at the Ann Arbor meeting of the Association of American Medical Colleges last October about the possibility of your going to Emory. So it may be more generally known that you considered it than you think." This letter, which also comments that Dr. Grollman's salary of $6,000 "would be financed from outside sources for the first three years," has scrawled across the top in bold handwriting, "all looks O.K. to me. T.D.K." This is undoubtedly the endorsement of President Thurman D. Kitchin and was saved carefully by Carpenter for future reference, if needed.

An example of this experimental attitude would be placing fourth year students in the PDC, the private diagnostic clinic, where they could work with the practitioners and "revive some of the benefits of the apprentice system and yet . . . avoid the disadvantages of this system."

The house staff he felt would be critically important and "must be selected with utmost care," because they exert such a large influence on the students and serve as examples for the students. "It is clearly recognized that the members of the house staff are the backbone of any teaching institution, for they more than anyone else, set the example to the students." They are also important for any institution because it is from them that a large proportion of the junior staff and faculty may later come. The resident would be someone who gives promise of an academic career, and he would receive $1,000 a year, the three assistant residents $500 each annually, and interns no payments.

With regard to the PDC, Tinsley placed complete faith and complete control in the hands of Wingate Johnson, even to the extent that "in case of a disagreement between us [about faculty appointments to the clinic] his decision is to be final." Tinsley did not want to spend time and attention on the PDC; he had learned of his dislike of administrative duties and preferred the bustle of the doctor-teacher. It's clear, though, that Tinsley also felt Johnson was capable, trustworthy. Paragraph after paragraph ends with the qualifier: "Upon the death or retirement of the Clinical Professor all of his authority in regard to such matters will revert to the Professor."

Young doctors—mostly men in that era—who failed to perform well in research would be let down gently by gradually lowering the medical school component of their income over several years while giving them an opportunity to move into the PDC and build their private practice. Tinsley did not concern himself with how the increased costs would be covered when a replacement was recruited before the incumbent was completely off the school budget. He insisted on separating the money for his department from that of the PDC and that of the hospital, which would pay the house staff and provide for the costs of all laboratories other than the research labs and some of the teaching labs. The hospital would thus cover the costs of the student/house staff labs in the hospital, eliminating what had been a chronic bone of contention at Vanderbilt.

As for the responsibilities of Tinsley himself,

My primary functions would be two-fold. First, to assume charge of the public patients in the hospital wards and, in so doing, to train the house staff and the students. This function will occupy practically all the mornings for three or four days of the week during most of the year. The two Assistant Professors will aid in this task. My second chief function will be to encourage and stimulate research in the department. Since it is clearly recognized that the best way to encourage this is by example, I will be expected to devote a certain amount of time to actual research work in the laboratory in the hope that eventually I will be able to spend one quarter to one half of my time in this manner, although this will probably not be possible at first during the organization of the department. However, I shall make every effort to show an active interest in investigation and to carry on some investigation, both on the wards and in the laboratory. In order to stimulate the younger men it is my plan to spend at least one evening a week working in the laboratory personally, and whatever additional time that can be found from other duties in the afternoons. I . . . recognize clearly that my main function in investigation will be to help the younger men, to start them working on new problems, and then to leave them to their own initiative.

Tinsley's comments on his functions in more formal teaching are typical:

Aside from the training given the students and house officers in my regular ward visits I do not expect to do much formal teaching but plan to conduct one clinic a week and to conduct the clinical-pathological conference in association with the pathologist-in-chief of the hospital. In addition I shall organize and direct one weekly meeting of the staff, at which time patients displaying unusual or interesting problems will be discussed and shall direct the weekly meeting of a "Journal Club," at which time one member of the department will report on recent developments in medical literature.

He insisted over and over: "My most important function will be that concerned with the selection of personnel for the department." For his personal clinical activities, he planned (and apparently with Carpenter's approval) to do no office practice of any kind,

. . . [and] not to assume personal charge of any private patients in the hospital, except for such members of the medical faculty and their families who desire me

7. "Expense for the purchase of reprints of published works and for preparation of photographs, drawings, and lantern slides" is excluded. Presumably the dean will be grateful enough for the good publicity to provide the money.

to care for them. . . . I shall however, be available to any physician for consultation either in the hospital, in the city of Winston-Salem, or elsewhere. Judging from my previous experience a large part of such consultation work will deal with the families of physicians and there will of course be no remuneration. However, when patients are seen who may properly be charged a consultation fee, this fee will belong to me personally.

He reiterated his personal salary arrangements, with the initial $15,000 decreasing over three years to the base salary of $12,000. After five years, the dean would review his performance, at which time a raise to $15,000 would be considered. "However, the Dean shall be under no obligation to grant this increase in salary," and if the decision is against any raise, "I agree to feel no resentment whatever in case he declines to grant it." Tinsley also outlines conditions for his removal in case he turns out "to be a decided failure as head of the Department of Internal Medicine." The arrangement would be moving into the PDC with a gradual reduction of his medical school salary, as with other faculty.

The remainder of Tinsley's letter is occupied with details of the functions and funding of Grollman, the research professor, research and clinical laboratories, bed assignments in the hospital, equipment and furnishings, overall budgets and expenditures, specific exclusions from his department's budget, and a promise that Tinsley will be placed on the search committee for a new dean should Carpenter leave that post.[7]

Having gone on for two dozen typed pages containing many details of paying for the electricity, telephones, and other mundane details, Tinsley concludes:

After having spent a good many hours thinking the situation over it is my firm conviction that you are going to start with a medical school which will be fairly close to the top. If the support which looks so promising at present really materializes on a large scale in the future I think that you have an excellent chance to build the leading medical school in the country. However, as my final word in this very wordy letter, I would like to have you know that it is not primarily this prospect which was the decisive factor in my decision to join with you. Although the opportunity to start from the beginning and build a new department has always seemed to me to be the best opportunity one can have, this likewise has not been the deciding factor. My decision has been based rather on my complete faith in your own sincerity and sound judgment and in the aims and ideals of Dr. Wingate Johnson.

With expressions of the deepest appreciation for the honor you have done me and for the opportunity you have afforded me, and with expectations of many years of happy work together, I am,

Sincerely yours,

Tinsley R. Harrison

All this talk about expenditures from the medical school's budget made Carpenter nervous. He was one of the few who knew how limited the funds really were, and there were no plans to start the third-year teaching right away. When the Wake Forest School of Basic Medical Sciences, the two-year school near Raleigh, moved to Winston-Salem in 1941, the upperclassmen would go on to other medical schools as they always had.[8] Only the freshman medical students would move with the school, and clinical teaching at the new four-year school would start in 1942. Perhaps, Carpenter thought, it would be better if Tinsley, having accepted the position, would remain another year at Vanderbilt.

Professor Hugh Morgan at Vanderbilt was not impressed by the wisdom of this idea for his department. On January 3, 1941, Tinsley wrote Carpenter,

> Dr. Morgan was out of the city during all of December and only returned yesterday. I discussed the situation with him then and rather gathered the impression that he is uncertain as to whether this will be a wise thing from the standpoint of his Department. Although he is a devoted and loyal friend of mine he naturally has to consider the business in the light of whatever plans he may have for getting someone to take my place.

Tinsley went on to say that he would prefer to move soon because of an "epidemic of rat plague" which was killing nearly 90 percent of his experimental rats and disrupting his research. He felt that starting in a completely fresh setup, in newly constructed quarters with newly manufactured cages, would solve this problem. He wondered whether moving in July 1940 would cause a space problem, since now he had commitments from Drs. John Williams and Robert Finks[9] and hoped to bring Grollman as well. Finally, there was the problem of his own salary and "whether by any possible means you could take care of this by July 1, 1941, instead of taking

8. Meads, *Miracle*. The background is also explained at some length in "The Two-Year Medical School at Wake Forest College" at www.newsouthbooks.com/thmd_supplement.

9. Kampmeier, *Recollections*, 80. Robert Finks was completing his residency in 1941 and was known to Harrison to be an excellent physician and very bright individual, as well as a good teacher. Probably he was interested in research as well. Dr. Allan Bass later quoted him as telling interns and medical students, "Never believe a diagnosis on the chart at the time of admission of a patient. Always examine the patient as if you expect the diagnosis to be wrong."

10. Note that the above budget gives Harrison $15,000 for two years, 1941–42 and 1942–43. This is so obvious that it must have been an honest mistake in tabulation, but it was corrected by Carpenter in a July letter, together with his recording of a concession from Harrison to include any earnings from medical consultations "on budget" and reduce the school's commitment for the bonus by those amounts. Carpenter allowed Tinsley to keep honoraria from speaking engagements, but he negotiated a concession in that Tinsley's bonus (of $3,000 the first year) above his regular $12,000 would be reduced by the amounts he earned from practice, including consultations. Coy C. Carpenter to Tinsley R. Harrison, July 3, 1941.

care of a little more than half at that time." Carpenter's request had backfired.

This final item alludes to Tinsley receiving his whole annual salary for 1941–42 at the time of his arrival in the summer of 1941. Carpenter may not have been surprised at this request, in view of the unusual salary arrangements Tinsley had already negotiated. No record has been found of whether the request was granted. Perhaps it was. Tinsley was expensive, as many good people are, especially in medicine.

ON JANUARY 14, 1941, Betty and Tinsley met in Durham during Tinsley's visit to Duke, where he gave a lecture, probably on congestive heart failure. He also met George T. Harrell there, whom Carpenter had already signed as an assistant professor in the department of medicine. Harrell was studying sarcoidosis and would soon become well known for work with rickettsial diseases and their treatment, especially Rocky Mountain spotted fever.

On the 15th, the Harrisons took the train to Winston-Salem, where they met John Williams and his wife. Tinsley spent the day with Carpenter and others at the medical school, while Betty looked for a house—the usual tradition. During the day, Tinsley handled logistic details concerning the laboratories and other matters, then in the evening he gave a talk to the Winston-Salem Medical Society. This was probably the first time he met the other doctors, certainly as chairman-designate for the new department coming to town. The next morning he took the 9:55 train to Baltimore for talks with Grollman about the developing arrangements, "to get his approval to the tentative plan which Dr. Williams and I have."

Tinsley sent Carpenter detailed annual budgets for the department for the years 1941 through 1945. The totals expected from the school were: $27,900, for 1941–42, $15,500 for 1942–43, $27,900 for 1943–44, and $27,900 for 1944–45.

In the first two of these years Tinsley's personal income from the school amounted to more than half the school's expenditure for the department, and was nearly half the total for the last two years. On the other hand, Tinsley's efforts resulted in $14,000 from extramural sources the first year, and the Bowman Gray Fund contributed another $13,200 in recognition of the importance of bringing Tinsley to the new school. The dean's contribution that year to the department was $10,400. This small amount might have been a signal to Tinsley, but if it was, he did not notice.[10] Tinsley kept pushing. Could John Williams come about April 1 to establish residence there and get the research started? Mr. Woods had given approval to move the Markle money for Williams's salary from Vanderbilt at that time. Would it be better to have the new rat cages fabricated in Winston-Salem? And a host of other details.

In February, Tinsley traveled to Indianapolis with Arthur Grollman to visit officials of the Eli Lilly pharmaceutical company. Here they were guaranteed $1,500 annually for three years for Grollman's salary and "a few hundred dollars to take care of John Williams' problem when he gets ready to move, together with a small bonus for him to begin July 1st, and to continue until such time as the private diagnostic clinic opens." The exchange was that Grollman would fall under the existing agreement for Lilly to have priority on any discoveries of blood pressure-lowering agents.

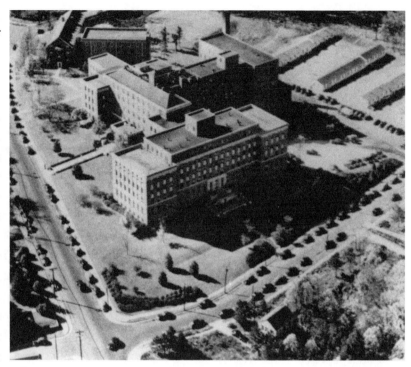

North Carolina Baptist Hospital, 1941.

Carpenter congratulated Tinsley on his success, but he also asked that Harrison write President Kitchin at Wake Forest and apprise him of the budget details for the coming years that he had sent Carpenter. He said, "I have gone into this with Dr. Kitchin, but I am afraid that I am not able to get it properly summarized, and I am very anxious that he be entirely acquainted with all of the details."

THE SPRING WAS SPENT in more discussions and negotiations with biochemistry chairman Dr. Camillo Artom, and others, in much worry about the best cages for the rats, and in more trips (now paid for by Bowman Gray) looking for money. And, of course, the annual ritual of the spring clinical research meetings was at Atlantic City on Tuesday and Wednesday, May 6 and 7, 1941.

Atlantic City that spring was indeed enjoyable. The main meetings were held, as always, in the huge auditorium on the Steel Pier over the sea. In the evenings there was dinner at Hackney's, the restaurant on the north end of the boardwalk famous for its lobster and oysters. In the early mornings, before the meetings started, there

11. Tinsley did not present a paper this year, but he asked a question on glomerular filtration in patients with impaired renal function and variable urea clearances dependent upon urine volume (*Trans. Assn. American Phys.*, 56:297, 1941). It was particularly pleasant that he now, as a member of the AAP, was permitted to sit in the restricted "members only" area in the front of the room and to speak without the necessity of being introduced by a member then granted specific individual permission by the chairman of the session.

12. Tinsley Harrison to Coy C. Carpenter, December 11 1940, VUMC Archives. This letter discusses details of space assignments, location of the teaching amphitheater, animal quarters, and similar matters.

13. Coy C. Carpenter to W. S. Leathers, December 16, 1940, VUMC Archives.

was walking south along the boardwalk with the morning sun and the surf to the east. The hotels were top-notch: the sumptuous Marlborough-Blenheim Hotel or the elegant old Traymor Hotel with its marble-trimmed fireplace, large enough to stand up in. Time was spent talking with friends from throughout the nation and world about medical politics and personnel changes—and about the war raging in Europe. The Nazis had just swept through the Balkans, overrun Greece, and sunk five ships attempting to evacuate British troops from the area. The Greek capital had been moved to Crete. Moscow had signed a non-aggression pact with Tokyo, thus permitting movement of Soviet troops from Siberia to the defend against possible attack by the Reich.

In the United States there were fewer than 80 medical schools, thus fewer than 80 chairs of medicine total. The chairmanship of a department of medicine was the peak of academic success in the profession. For Tinsley, his new major job ready for the occupancy, and the talk of all his friends and of the medical politicians, it was a very pleasant conference.[11]

After Atlantic City, Carpenter and Harrison traveled to New York, where the morning of May 8 was spent discussing strategy. In the afternoon they met with Alan Gregg, head of the Rockefeller Foundation division of medicine, to discuss methods of medical education. Tinsley's hope was to obtain money for a dormitory attached to the hospital to implement his plan for fourth-year medical students to act as rotating interns.[12] Tinsley had already discussed some ideas with Dr. Frank Fremont-Smith of the Macy Foundation in New York.[13] Late that afternoon, Harrison introduced Carpenter to his friend from the Brigham and Hopkins, Bill Resnik, now in practice in Connecticut. Resnik had known Harrison since their internships at the Brigham in 1922, and they had kept contact over the years. Resnik had initially published as much as Harrison, or more, and in similar areas. But when he found some doors closed and his academic progress slow, he became disenchanted with academic medicine and withdrew to private practice, where he was considered an outstanding internist. Harrison liked to keep in touch with outstanding people, especially those in private practice, as a counterweight to the academic pressures he always felt.

After what must have been a productive day in New York and dinner with Resnik, Carpenter and Harrison departed by train for Winston-Salem.

THERE IS AN UNSIGNED and undated detailed outline, 16 double-spaced typed pages, apparently from Harrison to Carpenter, in Harrison's files at Vanderbilt with 1941 correspondence and written very much in Harrison's style. Harrison did most of his writing, including scientific papers and textbooks, by dictating the first draft then polishing subsequent drafts. The relative lack of commas is therefore probably as much the style of Miss Tims as of Harrison.[14]

Tinsley wrote another long letter—16 typed pages—which detailed the curriculum for medicine including neurology and dermatology, and perhaps psychiatry. Neurology was to be taught "as an integral part of internal medicine." Tinsley's curriculum had some very modern aspects. All students were required to take a one-hour weekly course throughout the third and fourth years, "Bedside Problems in Family Practice: A discussion illustrated by case demonstrations and case histories of the common problems encountered by physicians in caring for patients at home. Emphasis will be put not only on major diagnosis and treatment but on the management of minor symptoms and on the physician's relation to the patient's family and to other physicians." Patients were to be presented to the first-year class at weekly conferences held throughout the year to enhance correlation of their basic science studies with clinical applications. Tinsley emphasized nutrition and prevention. A course titled "Biochemical and Physiological Aspects of Disease" was to be given during the fourth year. All in all, Tinsley's proposed curriculum would look good 50 years later, and did.

WINSTON-SALEM WAS ALWAYS THE loveliest city to the Harrisons. A small town dominated by the Reynolds Tobacco Company and the Hanes textile industry, Winston-Salem in July was beautiful. The growth was lush, and the town was leafy green. Many places were still ablaze with blossoms when the Harrisons arrived on the first of July. There was only one hotel: the Robert E. Lee. There were no small places to eat lunch, so the faculty routinely went home for lunch or brought a brown bag. Tinsley skipped lunch most of the time, subsisting on black coffee and cigarettes. Tinsley must have been pleasing to the Gray family. He smoked at least one pack of cigarettes a day. He wasn't alone.[15]

Tinsley's arrival in Winston-Salem was different from his arrival in Nashville 16 years earlier. In both cases, friendly, helping hands assisted in getting settled. In Winston-Salem, however, those hands included the senior pillars of the community. The Harrisons now were a family of five children, and they had sufficient money to live in a much more pleasant style. They bought a large house in a fashionable part

14. T. R. Harrison to Coy C. Carpenter, December 21, 1940, VUMC Archives. In this outline, page 12 is missing, and the missing page is in a place which would have been appropriate for psychiatry.

15. Katherine Davis, audiotape, April 15, 1993, UAB Archives. To conceal the stench of the gross anatomy dissecting laboratory, medical students encouraged each other to smoke strong cigars while working. Since the Reynolds Tobacco Company did not make cigars, it is surprising that officialdom did not insist they switch to Camel cigarettes, their popular brand which continues into the 21st century.

16. *N. Carol. Med. J.* 3 (1942): 515, 534. For example, she joined the Auxiliary of the state medical association, in which Mrs. Wingate Johnson was chairman of the Public Relations Committee.

17. George B. Walden to Tinsley R. Harrison, July 2, 1941. Dorothy Carpenter Medical Archives, BGSM.

18. T. R. Harrison to W. Groce Harrison Sr., July 14, 1941, 1. Dorothy Carpenter Medical Archives, BGSM.

19. T. R. Harrison to Alfred Blalock, Aug. 2, 1941. Chesney Archives, JHMI. This and approximately 100 other letters to Blalock from Harrison and vice versa are in the Chesney Archives of the Johns Hopkins Medical Institutions, Baltimore, Maryland.

of town, and Betty settled down to homemaking and getting to know the wives and families of faculty and town physicians.[16]

Tinsley worked hard with John Williams organizing the laboratories, equipment, animals, and logistics. There were no medical students in town during the summer except those few who had jobs around the hospital. Tinsley worked diligently on the curriculum, impinging on the dean's responsibilities in these activities, promoting his ideas on organization of the school and faculty, negotiating teaching hours and schedules with various other chairmen, inserting a course in the history of medicine—to be taught by his father—and another in "broader aspects of medicine": ethics, legal and social aspects, and philosophy of medicine, taught by Wingate Johnson. He prepared for his teaching of the first- and second-year students, which was limited to weekly clinics the first part of the first year, the Saturday noon sessions, the CPCs on Monday evenings at 7, and perhaps helping a bit with George Harrell's course in laboratory diagnosis.

His main teaching activities were directed to the house staff, with whom he made daily rounds on the ward patients. He probably had a few private consultations, but, consistent with his prior agreements with Carpenter, essentially all his practice and most of his teaching at this time was limited to working as attending physician on the wards. He continued to pursue external funding. In July he received a check for $5,000 from Eli Lilly for support of his search for a naturally occurring blood pressure-lowering agent, some sort of molecule which would be to hypertension what insulin was to diabetes.[17] Grollman arrived on July 13.[18]

In general, things were going well. In August Tinsley wrote Blalock to work out a brief golfing vacation together, perhaps at a club at Roaring Gap, some 60 miles west of Winston-Salem.[19] Blalock favored the beach (nearer Baltimore) and Mary Blalock did not like the mountains but did like the beach. The effort ran aground when other friends from Nashville said they had unchangeable plans, and Betty did not want to go if Mary brought her children. "With the children, it's no vacation," she said. The final coup was Tinsley's realization that he could not leave Winston-Salem until October or later, since the grand opening of the school would be held in mid-September. Over the next 24 years of the abundant correspondence between Harrison and Blalock, a large proportion is occupied with attempts to work out vacation times together with their wives, even during the war, usually to include several of their former Nashville golfing partners of years past, the Frank Lutons (one of the few psychiatrists Tinsley ever trusted) and the Joe Hibbetts.

Tinsley's July 14 letter to his father indicated the press of current activities and hinted at reasons for both optimism and concern. Tinsley was working on the curriculum and expected that there would be "a lot more instruction in internal medicine [at Bowman Gray] than in any other one I know about." He mentioned that Dr. Carpenter expected Groce to give a series of medical history lectures in the fall (and in future years) suitable for both medical students and lay people in the community. And he hinted at some developing tensions with local physicians over part-time teaching and ward service responsibilities, both areas the local men had controlled but that Tinsley was now pulling under his wing.[20]

Trouble with the local physicians was worse than he thought. Two weeks later, on August 1, 1941, he wrote the dean that he was aware of the criticisms of Bowman Gray's takeover of the charity medical services. But, he said, charity patients had in the past received inadequate care because some local physicians were too busy and others were mediocre practitioners—Tinsley cited the case of a patient who had been hospitalized for several months for a supposed coronary thrombosis but who actually had an undiagnosed gallstone. Further, Tinsley told Carpenter, some local doctors had been sending bills to charity patients, "contrary to the regulations of all good hospitals." Tinsley generally praised the nursing service but noted that "all the kindness and all the good nursing will not atone for errors in diagnosis which inevitably lead to improper treatment." In short, he said, he would have to keep charge of the charity service "until a proper house staff is obtained . . . and perhaps until a general house cleaning has taken place."[21]

No response has been found to this letter, but after receiving it Carpenter probably rejoiced in private. Here was a physician leader who was not afraid to state the case for excellence in patient care and to put his new job on the line to promote it. Carpenter must have felt then that he had, in fact, chosen the right man for the job.

Tinsley was in many regards the academic spirit and soul of the medical school, as well as its most visible leader to colleagues in other schools across the country. There is sometimes discussion of whether Tinsley or the first chief of surgery, Howard H. Bradshaw, a thoracic surgeon from Jefferson Medical College, brought more prestige to the school.[22] Bradshaw was undoubtedly a talented surgeon and had participated in the developing field of thoracic surgery, and he was doubtless a good teacher. Carpenter later wrote, "He was best known for his leadership in surgical education and the training of interns and residents in surgery. He had wide connections and served on many boards and committees in medical education."[23] About Tinsley,

20. T. R. Harrison to W. Groce Harrison Sr., July 14, 1941. Dorothy Carpenter Medical Archives, BGSM. See full letter at www.newsouthbooks.com/thmd_supplement.

21. T. R. Harrison to Coy C. Carpenter, August 1, 1941. Dorothy Carpenter Medical Archives, BGSM.

22. Joseph B. Hankins, audiotape, luncheon, April 15, 1993, UAB Archives. Attended by Dr. Manson Meads, Dr. Joseph Hankins, Mrs. Dorothy Carpenter Howard (formerly wife of Dean Coy C. Carpenter), Mrs. Hankins (former Miss Nola Reed, assistant to Coy Carpenter from June 1940 and functionally fiscal officer for the school in its early years), Miss Katherine Davis (secretary and assistant to Dr. Herbert Vann, director of anatomy and chairman of the admissions committee — and functionally the committee in many cases; started work at Bowman Gray in 1942).

23. Coy C. Carpenter, *The Story of Medicine at Wake Forest University* (Chapel Hill: The University of North Carolina Press, 1970), 36.

24. Ibid., 35. Carpenter gives the date of Artom's joining the faculty as 1937, but Paschal in a tabulation which looks as if it were taken directly from old records gives 1938. G. W. Paschal, *History of Wake Forest College*, vol. III (Wake Forest: Wake Forest College, 1943) 517.

25. Addison Scoville, M.D., interview, VUMC Archives. Scoville says on the transcript: "My acquaintance began with him [Harrison] in 1939 when I arrived at Vanderbilt to begin an internship in Medicine. I had come from Cornell and when I arrived the only person that I had ever heard about on the faculty at Vanderbilt was Tinsley Harrison."

26. Meads, *Miracle*, 24.

27. Coy Carpenter, manuscript in private holdings of Dr. Manson Meads, Dorothy Carpenter Medical Archives, BGSM.

Carpenter said, "The election of Dr. Tinsley Harrison as the first professor and chairman of the Department of Medicine, like the election of Dr. Artom, brought the institution a national image that was greatly needed at the time." TDr. Camillo Artom, chairman of biochemistry, was Jewish and had been forced to leave his position at the University of Palermo by the oncoming conflicts in Europe. When Carpenter turned to Dr. Emmett Holt Jr. at Hopkins in his search for a new head of biochemistry, Holt, who also had an interest in lipid biochemistry and knew of Artom's problems in Europe, immediately suggested him, and he joined the two-year school at Wake Forest in 1938.[24]

In fact, Artom and Bradshaw were the only other faculty members who had even a shadow of a national or international reputation when the school opened, though of course many faculty had friends in other schools and on committees. There was no one in Tinsley's league of solid research and publications, so important in academic visibility and standing. Even at Vanderbilt several years earlier, interns sometimes arrived having heard of only Tinsley Harrison among all of the much more luminary faculty at the time.[25]

Dr. Manson Meads, who became dean of the Bowman Gray School of Medicine and vice president for health affairs, later wrote, "Among this group [i.e., the whole original medical faculty in 1941, including Bradshaw and Artom], only Dr. Harrison had an established academic and scientific record."[26] Finally, there is a private, but recorded, statement from Carpenter written years later: "Tinsley Harrison was the most dynamic, inspiring medical teacher I ever knew, and one of the most exciting medical scholars this country has ever produced. He is due more credit than any other person for leadership that produced high academic and professional standards in Wake Forest University medicine."[27]

Tinsley continued to work on the curriculum and educational infrastructure. He sent copies of the curriculum not only to his father but also to C. Sidney Burwell, his former colleague and chief of medicine at Vanderbilt and now in 1941 dean at Harvard Medical School. Burwell responded on August 12 that he thought Tinsley's curriculum was "on the whole, not particularly radical but good," that he liked the plan to have students living in the hospital, and suggested that "somewhere in a course in physical diagnosis there ought to be an appropriate series of exercises relating to the fact that the human organism is actually a series of organisms: that the fetus, the infant, the child, the adolescent, the young adult, the mature adult (middle age is 10 years older than you are), and the geriatric patient can never be included under the same description either from the point of view of morphology or function." Burwell concluded, "I am sorry to be less destructive than customary but I think your outline is really swell and I am all for seeing it go into effect. I am sure it will work well if you have good teachers."[28]

Thus, Tinsley had the endorsement of the dean of medicine at Harvard to bolster and back up his curriculum. He also wrote others for advice. Late in November he wrote Goodpasture noting that Jim Dawson had sent pathological material from Vanderbilt for use in CPCs at Bowman Gray and that Wingate Johnson, editor of the *North Carolina Medical Journal*, would like to publish some of those CPCs in the journal. Tinsley wanted to be sure this was okay with Goodpasture, "as the material is derived from Nashville. Dr. Johnson and I would appreciate your letting us know whether you would have any objections to our doing this."[29]

There was no objection. Clinical-pathologic conferences had been a part of the *North Carolina Medical Journal* since it reconstituted and resumed publication in 1940.[30] Some of the CPCs came from Duke and others from the City Memorial Hospital of Winston-Salem. After Bowman Gray began in 1941, CPCs regularly appeared from that source, often with Tinsley or George Harrell as clinician discusser, sometimes Grollman, sometimes with two CPCs in the same issue.[31]

In October 1941, the *North Carolina Medical Journal* announced that Bowman Gray had begun "its first year of instruction on September 10, 1941. Seventy-two students were registered, 43 students in the first-year class and 29 in the second-year class."[32] In the same item, the *NCMJ* announced "establishment of the Bowman Gray Institute of Medical Research, which will operate as an integral part of the school . . . made possible through the generosity of Mrs. Benjamin F. Bernard, who gave to the school a group of buildings occupying the southwest corner of the Bowman Gray Estate. Plans have been completed and work will begin immediately on transforming these buildings into research laboratories."[33]

As noted earlier, students who had just completed their second year at the old two-year medical school at the town of Wake Forest did not move to Winston-Salem that year but proceeded on to other established four-year schools in the North as they had since the earliest years of the school. The Philadelphia schools were favorites among such students. Since there were 29 students in the second year, Tinsley's real clinical teaching of medical students would not begin until 1942.

Not all the laboratories and equipment were in place yet. One student recalled that they took pathology and bacteriology with no water for the labs, as the plumbing

28. C. Sidney Burwell to T. R. Harrison, August 12, 1941. Dorothy Carpenter Medical Archives, BGSM. See full letter at www.newsouthbooks.com/thmd_supplement.

29. T. R. Harrison to Dr. E. W. Goodpasture, November 25, 1941.

30. The *N. Carol. Med. J.* existed in the 19th century but ceased publication after the 1899 volume. It resumed with the same name but as a new journal in 1940 with well wishes from Dr. Morris Fishbein, editor-in-chief of the *J. American Med. Assn.* and others.

31. The Goodpasture letter of November 1941 is important because of implications by some that Harrison "cheated on CPCs" by using material already published in the *New England J. Med.* However, it is obvious that Harrison was looking for material from Vanderbilt, and probably from Boston as well. In any case, if Harrison did look at published CPCs in advance of their presentation and discussion (and this is simply an assertion many years later), there is no reason why

any other physician should not also have read the *N. England J. Med.* and been aware of the discussion; G. H. Harrell, personal communication, April 24, 1993.

32. Meads, *Miracle*, 25. One of these students was apparently in some kind of academic limbo, as Meads says there were "42 freshmen and 30 sophomores." Only 27 graduated with the class in December 1943. *N. Carol. Med. J.* 5 (1944): 32.

33. *N. Carol. Med. J.* 2 (1941): 570. Mrs. Benjamin Bernard was the remarried widow of Bowman Gray Sr., whose bequest had created the medical school. However, there was no additional money with the gift of the buildings for their renovation into laboratories or their operation afterwards, and this effort finally came to naught.

34. Hankins, audiotape.

35. Davis, audiotape.

36. C. Daniel, ed. *Chronicle of the 20th Century* (Mt. Kisco, N.Y.: Chronicle Publications, 1987), 527–28.

had not been completed.[34] There was also some interdepartmental bickering over "unnecessary luxuries" being purchased by some departments, such as electric fans to help ward off the heat. There would be no effective air conditioning for another 15 years, and it was exceptionally hot that September, so hot that the faculty tried at first to delay gross anatomy until the cooler months "to avoid the odors."[35] Anatomy was later taught first in recognition of the necessity of a natural sequence for learning physiology and medicine, regardless of the heat.

There were some difficult spots, like those with the attending physicians on the ward services. But in general the laboratory work with Drs. Grollman and Williams was moving ahead. Papers were being submitted, teaching was going well, and the patients were interesting and abundant. The outlook was bright.

HOWEVER, TWO MAJOR PROBLEMS beyond Tinsley's control were about to assert themselves. The first was America's formal entry into World War II, 13 days after Tinsley's letter to Goodpasture. The United States had maintained diplomatic relations with Germany despite the news of persecution of Jews and the bombing and sinking of U.S. ships by German forces in October.[36] Although the U.S. had instituted its first peacetime draft, mobilized physicians for the armed forces, approved lend-lease for Britain, assumed protection of Greenland, and taken many other actions in preparation for war, it was only after Pearl Harbor that the country formally declared war on the Axis powers and started active fighting.

The profound effects on U.S. society would include restrictions on the availability of money for anything other than the war, medicine and medical education not excepted, which thus exacerbated Tinsley's second major problem: the emerging desperate financial situation of the new Bowman Gray medical school. Recall that the Rockefeller Foundation and its ancillary organizations had pumped at least $17.5 million into the creation and early sustenance of the Vanderbilt medical school, with $4 million going to the initial physical plant alone. That does not count the $1 million from the Carnegie Foundation and assorted other gifts. The 1924 gift of James B. Duke, the other large North Carolina fortune initially based on tobacco and therefore probably thought by some to be at least in the same rough category as Bowman Gray's, provided $10 million to Trinity College (which became part of the new Duke University), $4 million of which was for construction of the medical buildings. But the residual estate was even larger and eventually contributed even more, since 90 percent of the income from that residual was committed by the will to medicine.[37] For example, when the first dean of medicine at Duke, W. C. Davison, needed money to buy books for the new library, he asked George G. Allen, chairman of the trustees of the Duke Endowment, for a special appropriation of $100,000 and obtained it without hesitation, since "both of us knew that Mr. Duke had designated in his will that 90 percent of the income from the residue of his residual estate, which was larger than the original Duke Endowment, should be used for hospitals and had left the remaining 10 percent 'to and for' Duke University." When Davison requested the $100,000, Allen asked whether the medical library was a university library or a hospital library.

Davison answered promptly, "Hospital library, of course."

"There's more when you want it," Allen said.[38]

Davison was clever. He took this money, and more, to Germany, where he bought whole medical libraries for very little, with the mark much devalued by the recent hyperinflation. In fact, the General Education Board of the Rockefeller Foundation had given $3 million in 1920–23 for a joint effort of Trinity College, the University of North Carolina, and Watts Hospital (of Durham) to establish a medical school. So the initial amounts of money for Duke approached those available for Vanderbilt.

It would have been natural for Tinsley and others to assume that Bowman Gray had left about as much for the establishment of the Bowman Gray School of Medicine—at least several million, probably $10 million to $12 million. The first meeting between representatives of Wake Forest College and the executors of the late Bowman Gray occurred on November 11, 1938.[39] At that meeting, James A. Gray informed the Wake Forest group, including Carpenter and President Kitchin, that the fund amounted to about $600,000. "Mr. Gray sensed a fall in Dr. Kitchin's enthusiasm and asked him why, on learning the amount of the fund, he appeared less certain that it could be done," Carpenter said. "Dr. Kitchin replied that he had understood that the fund was much larger and that the actual amount made him hesitate. Mr. Mull,[40] Dr. Kitchin, and I were under the impression prior to that time the fund available amounted to over $5 million."[41]

Wake Forest University appears to have developed early on a tradition of building shoes around shoestrings—a sort of cliff-hanger approach to progress.[42] For example, the initial vote in the state legislature granting the charter for establishment of Wake Forest College in 1833 had come only after the suspicious legislature had amended the charter with restrictive phrases, such as "for the purpose of educating youth,

37. Davison, *Duke,* 1–11.

38. Ibid., 1–11. Davison had been a young physician at Hopkins when President W. P. Few of Trinity College/Duke University asked his friend Dr. Wickliffe Rose "(the head of the Rockefeller Foundation campaign against hookworm in North Carolina)" to write his friend William H. Welch, to find "the best possible man" to become dean of the new school. Welch had unambiguously endorsed Davison. The pervasiveness of Hopkins and the Rockefeller money in establishing good U.S. medical schools in the early part of this century, and the informal collegial fashion in which things progressed, is impressive.

39. Carpenter, *Story,* 26.

40. Mr. Odus M. Mull, a lawyer active in North Carolina politics and a key figure in obtaining the Gray money for Wake Forest.

41. Ibid., 26.

42. Meads, *Miracle,* 28.

43. Paschal, *History*, 60.

44. Meads, *Miracle*, 9.

45. Davis, audiotape.

46. Harrison, audiotape. There may have been considerable self-deception here. Harrison clearly enjoyed the travel and the adulation he received as the center of attention at these meetings, especially when he was a featured or the only speaker.

47. *N. Carol. Med. J.* 2 (1941): 628. One suspects the hand of his New York friend Bill Dock in these invitations, though he was certainly well enough known to be invited by people unknown to him.

48. Ibid., 570.

and for no other purpose whatever." Even then the vote was a 29–29, requiring the Speaker's yea for passage.[43] A century later the two-year school was saved from being closed by the AMA in 1935 only by a counterattack by its dean, Thurman D. Kitchin. It was placed on probation in the late 1930s and given until June 1939 "to correct its deficiencies."[44] In part because of the pressures against it as a two-year school, it had accepted the Gray money to convert to a four-year school. Now it was struggling, supported by flimsy finances.

Tinsley must have become aware of the poverty of resources at Bowman Gray at some point early in his career there, but no records have been found to indicate when—or indeed even if—he did so. He behaved as if he considered himself the Canby Robinson of the new school, though he was much more careful spending money than Robinson and never ran Robinsonian deficits, perhaps because he was aware of the school's precarious financial state.

CARPENTER'S OPTIMISM MUST HAVE been infectious. Tinsley's buoyant energy left no time to stop and fret about the past. He rushed ahead in his customary fashion, with the tails of his long white coat streaming out behind as he hurried about his business, and perhaps everybody else's as well.[45]

He traveled a lot, which he later attributed to the urgings of the Grays, who felt this would make their new school known throughout the nation.[46] The first day the students attended school, Wednesday, September 10, 1941, he and Grollman drove to Anderson, South Carolina, to speak at the Piedmont Postgraduate Clinical Assembly. Tinsley spoke on "Cardiovascular Emergencies"; Grollman talked about "Some Practical Aspects of Endocrinology." On Sunday, September 28, Tinsley took the train to Emporia, Kansas, to speak at the Kansas Medical Society's annual postgraduate course on heart disease. In early October he traveled to New York to be the "honor guest at a banquet . . . given by the New York Academy of Medicine on October 4, at which time he delivered a paper on 'Effects of Renal Extracts on Hypertension.' "[47] He returned to New York on October 24 to speak at the New York Academy of Medicine's Annual Graduate Fortnight on "Effects of Renal Extracts on Hypertension."[48]

On the way back from New York he dropped in on Blalock. The visit resulted in a series of letters in which they discussed work and compared schedules trying to arrange visits. On September 5, 1941, Tinsley had written Al that he would be in the East in late October and hoped to get his friend's ideas about "the organization of the medical service and would like to have an opportunity to spend a couple of days observing Dr. Longcope's setup." On October 14, he wrote that he and Betty would be in New York on the 25th to see a show and would take the train to Baltimore the next morning. Al replied on the 20th that he and Mary were looking forward to the visit and gave Tinsley cab instructions to the Blalock home.[49]

After the visit with the Blalocks, Tinsley went directly to Richmond, probably still accompanied by Betty, where he joined Carpenter for the annual meeting of the Association of American Medical Colleges. The dean of the Harvard Medical School, his old friend and mentor C. Sidney Burwell, also attended. Afterwards, they hurried back to Winston-Salem by train.

On Halloween of 1941, "Dr. Sidney Burwell, Dean of the Harvard University School of Medicine, held a medical clinic for the students and faculty" in the morning. "On the afternoon of the same day he addressed the faculty, students and invited physicians, and in the evening he gave an address on 'The Role of a Medical Center in Community Progress,' to which the public was invited."[50]

Such visiting professorships were fun, as Tinsley knew because he also did a lot of them over his career. But they involved hard work. Giving speeches and clinics forced doctors to gather and organize their thoughts. Tinsley learned from the exposure to others distant from his home base. Speaking engagements offered a doctor a chance to swell the size of his bibliography, that sacrosanct measure of academic accomplishment (Harvard faculty have always been most adept at getting virtually every syllable they utter rapidly into print somewhere).

Tinsley wrote the Blalocks on November 7 with thanks for their hospitality the week before. He mentioned that Sidney and Edith Burwell had accompanied him and Betty back to Winston-Salem and that "Sidney gave us a great deal of useful advice and valuable suggestions about the medical school. Since then I have been trying to get the problem of the house staff for next year settled. . . . Since leaving Baltimore I have thought a good deal about Al's advice to 'stop running around the country and making speeches and to go to work in the laboratory.' I am reasonably certain this is good advice and insofar as I can am planning to take it."

On November 29, at a Wake Forest alumni banquet in Charlotte, W. S. Rankin, O. M. Mull, Howard Bradshaw, Tinsley, and Coy Carpenter gave speeches. Though it was not a long drive from Winston-Salem to Charlotte, this trip prevented Tinsley from seeing his father, who was at Bowman Gray from the 23rd through the 30th giving the public lectures on the history of medicine. Groce's topics were "Animal

49. Copies of Harrison's original letters and carbon of Blalock's replies were obtained from the Chesney Archives at the Johns Hopkins Medical Institutions, Baltimore. Much of Harrison's files were destroyed by fires or lost during his multiple moves, including the letters received from Blalock.

50. Ibid., 628.

51. Ibid., 678.
52. Ibid., 362.
53. Ibid., 362.

Medicine," "Folklore in Medicine," "The Dawn of Medicine in the East," "Early Greek Medicine," and "Classical Greek Medicine."[51]

Other faculty members also traveled and spoke. Bradshaw had attended the annual meeting of the American College of Surgeons, where he participated in a discussion of spinal anesthesia, and he spoke to the Lenoir County Medical Society in October on "Surgical Treatment of Suppurative Diseases of the Lung." Harrell and John Williams spoke at a meeting in the Veterans Administration facility at Mountain Home, Tennessee. Wingate Johnson spoke in Chicago on "How Can a State Medical Journal Best Support Organized Medicine?" And J. P. Rousseau, professor of radiology, addressed the annual meeting of the Radiological Society of North America in San Francisco, December 1–5. His topic was "The Value of Roentgen Therapy in the Treatment of Pneumonia Which Fails to Respond to Sulfonamide Therapy."

Tinsley was in a different league.

ON DECEMBER 7, JAPANESE planes bombed Pearl Harbor. On Monday the 8th the United States declared war. The nightmare in Europe had been going on for more than two years. After a treaty with Germany, Russia had been attacked in June 1941, and the Soviet government had reestablished relations with the exiled Polish government in London. The Japanese, Italian, and German armies struck decisive victories against the French and British.

In June 1941 the War Department announced "an extensive program to provide for the procurement of Doctors for the Army of the United States during the next few years."[52] The program assured that junior and senior medical students, as well as interns, could complete their medical training before being called into the service. (The draft was already in existence.) All male medical students in their last two years, if in good standing and good physical condition, would upon application be appointed second lieutenants, in the Medical Administrative Corps of the Officers' Reserve Corps. They would then be classified 1–C by their local draft boards, and they would not be called into active duty until after their internship.

Notices stressed that such applications and appointments were "absolutely voluntary." However, it was pointed out that if such an opportunity were declined the student would be subject to draft into the army as a private. If they volunteered, at the end of their medical training they would be transferred to the Medical Corps Reserve, given the rank of first lieutenant, and "ordered to active duty as an officer in the army of the United States for a period of one year."[53]

The military and the war recast the medical schools in drastic ways. The medical schools' academic year was shortened to nine months. Soon the internship was also shortened from 12 to nine months. Summer vacations were eliminated. New classes began every nine months, and senior classes graduated every nine months. Before the war was over, there were doctors who took only five calendar years to move from high school diploma to M.D. degree, a regular possibility if one could be accepted into medical school after only two "years" of college (which could be calculated by the number of hours completed, thus completed in far less than 24 calendar months), plus four nine-month "years" of medical school, or 36 months—a total of less than 60 months.[54]

During the two decades prior to America's entry into the war, medical education in the United States had become routinely organized along the Hopkins model: completion of high school and entry into college; completion of four years of college and entry into medical school; completion of four years of medical school, two basic science and two clinical, then entry into an internship; completion of a one-year internship, then residency training in a specialty. There were rare exceptions to this routine, such as admission of occasional outstanding students after only three or two years of college.

The postdoctoral residency training was less routinely followed. By the late 1930s most medical graduates entered general practice after one year of a rotating internship, but many took no internship at all. Rather they simply entered practice upon receiving the M.D. degree and gaining a license, though as time wore on this was a decreasing proportion of the graduates, since the individual states, the licensing entities in the nation, increasingly required at least a one-year internship for licensure. Twenty-two states required an internship as a condition for licensure in 1943.[55] Some states later required two or more years of postdoctoral residency training to qualify.

Most of the major medical specialties were established before World War II, and this tended to encourage residency training in order to qualify for examination by the certifying board.[56]

In the 1930s and '40s, and even into the '50s, if you flunked your board examinations, not all was lost; you could still present yourself as board qualified—specialty trained in the requisite number of years of residency. These were not entirely theoretical or academic distinctions, as salaries, for example in the Veterans Administration, and promotions, in the armed forces, were influenced by them.

54. Edwin G. Waldrop, M D., personal communication, August 9, 1993. Dr. Waldrop started college in September 1941 and received his M.D. degree in October 1946. In the 1970s, when a variety of shortened and otherwise "unorthodox" medical curricula were encouraged by federal grants, similar "short-circuited medical educations" were possible. Dr. Waldrop, despite his abbreviated time in the formal curriculum, was one of the most respected practitioners in Birmingham, Alabama, at the time of his retirement.

55. *N. Carol. Med. J.* 4 (1943): 522.

56. James A. Pittman, "U.S. Academic Community and Foreign Medical Graduates," *The United States Academic Community and the Training of Foreign Medical Graduates for Careers in Asia* (New York: The American Bureau for Medical Advancement in China, Inc., 1983). Of the 23 primary boards, 11 are surgical disciplines, and 10 are separate from the board of general surgery, though they may require one or more years of general surgical residency

before beginning the discipline, such as orthopedics or urology. In a different approach, the American Board of Internal Medicine beginning in 1972 coordinated the administration of examinations in subspecialty boards, which are certifications in the subspecialties of internal medicine, such as endocrinology, infectious diseases, rheumatology, nephrology, hematology, oncology, and so on. The medical subspecialties of cardiology, gastroenterology, pulmonary diseases (originally known as TB), and allergy had developed earlier, but all except allergy joined in the subspecialty route. More recently pediatrics has tended to follow the path of medicine, with special certification in pediatric infectious diseases, and so on. The splitting continues as specialized knowledge and techniques multiply and as groups using them define themselves in formal organizations. Hence, orthopedics has specialists in hand surgery, among other specialties. There are also other special cases, like psychiatry and

The designation, or self-designation, "board qualified" has gradually disappeared from use and is now virtually gone.

American medicine had been quietly specializing, especially during the decade before the war, when 14 of the major specialties were created.[57] In some cases it happened almost unnoticed by the participants themselves. Tinsley, for example, as noted earlier, was grandfathered in for certification by the American Board of Internal Medicine in 1936. And he certainly was a general internist, as he claimed and as his teaching of medical students and residents demonstrated. However, his research work and public lectures at medical gatherings were nearly always about cardiology, or cardiovascular diseases. In a 1943 listing of fellows, or senior members, of the North Carolina state medical association, Tinsley was designated as a specialist in cardiovascular disease.[58]

The social forces impelling specialization are complex, and perhaps the economic situation of the 1930s was an important force driving their creation. However, the most essential requirement is specialized knowledge and techniques, without which a specialty is spurious and ephemeral. So Tinsley, despite himself, was a factor forcing the fragmentation of medicine into the multiple specialties which he so decried, and which communicate among themselves with only variable amounts of success. He was part of the problem he identified and abhorred.

ON THE FIRST OF January in 1942 the PDC (Private Diagnostic Clinic) began operations on the first floor of the medical school building under the overall supervision of Dr. Wingate M. Johnson.[59] Four physicians were listed for medicine: Johnson, Harrell, McMillan, and John Williams; and three for surgery: Bradshaw, William Sprunt, and Arthur DeTalma Valk; plus 12 other physicians in other specialties. A total of 63 physicians had originally responded to Carpenter's original offer of a faculty appointment to any physician in town who wanted one, and they were duly appointed by the board of trustees in May 1941.[60]

Although the trains ran less reliably than before the war, Tinsley seems to have been unimpeded by this or other difficulties.[61] Domestic travel, though now less convenient, continued. The main problem in traveling by automobile was staying under 40 miles per hour so as to save gas.

Shock again was an important topic of investigation, and early in 1942 Herbert Wells, chairman of the Bowman Gray Department of Physiology and Pharmacology, "visited the laboratories of surgical research at Johns Hopkins, the University of Pennsylvania, and Wayne University to observe studies being carried out on burns and traumatic shock" and the use of a method of "clinical measurement of peripheral blood flow recently developed at the Bowman Gray School of Medicine."[62] Tinsley addressed the Medical Officers of Camp Davis on January 9.[63] He spoke on the "Differentiation Between Structural and Functional Disorders of the Heart"—the "soldier's heart" of the first world war.[64] Dr. R. L. McMillan, a physician from Winston-Salem who had joined Bowman Gray as a "geographic full-time" faculty member[65] and was interested in cardiology, joined Harrison at this time and gave a lecture on "Treatment of Heart Disease in Young People." Bradshaw gave a series of 10 lectures on chest wounds to local physicians who expected to enter the service soon.[66]

One day George Harrell went to Tinsley's office to talk about a problem. As he entered the office for the scheduled appointment, the telephone rang. Tinsley answered, asking Harrell to wait outside while he took the call. It was from Boston, probably from his friend Sam Levine. The newly appointed chief of medicine at the Brigham Hospital, Soma Weiss—young, brilliant, the Hersey Professor of the Theory and Practice of Physic—had suddenly died from a ruptured berry aneurysm. When the conversation ended, Harrell, who had been standing just outside listening to Tinsley's side of the conversation, started again to enter the office, but Tinsley again asked him to wait a moment. Tinsley then placed a telephone call to Boston (probably to Harvard Medical School dean Sidney Burwell) and asked to be considered for the job, to replace Weiss.[67] Nothing further is known about this exchange, and no written records have been found of it. In any case, George W. Thorn, the young endocrinologist at Hopkins, was chosen for the position.

Tinsley had been urging Henry Valk, a young Bowman Gray student, on Blalock for surgical training at Hopkins, and Blalock accepted him. Because of the shortage of manpower, Blalock asked that Valk be released early to start work at Hopkins several months before the usual time of July 1. Late in the senior year, the young student had no more required courses or topics, just electives. Perhaps even these were optional and not required for graduation. Blalock wrote Tinsley on February 18, 1942, to bemoan that the war requirements made it difficult to make any definite plans involving young men who might be called into service at any time. He mentioned that the National Research Council expected him to interview John Williams and George Harrell, but that he had not heard from them. And he asked after Betty and mentioned that he had not played golf in a

neurology, originally and still a single board, but with two divisions, the practitioners of which tend increasingly to do one or the other, neurology or psychiatry. The complications continue. Nuclear Medicine is a "conjoint board" sponsored by internal medicine, radiology, and pathology. The more recent specialty of geriatrics is co-sponsored by internal medicine and family medicine. And so, on and on.

57. "Creation" of a specialty is always difficult to date with precision. Is it when a group forms and declares itself a specialty?—Usually an early step in the process. Is it when an examining group or "board" constitutes itself? Is it when medicine in general (e.g., as represented by the AMA) recognizes the specialty? Is it when third party payors begin reimbursement "as a specialty"? This became especially contentious in the case of emergency medicine, which accounts for the broader dates there.

58. *N. Carol. Med. J.* 4 (1943) : 315, 321.

59. *N. Carol. Med. J.* 3 (1942): 47.

60. Meads, *Miracle*, 23.

61. Alfred Blalock to Tinsley Harrison, June 2, 1942.

62. *N. Carol. Med. J.* 3 (1942): 103.

63. Ibid., 103.

64. Paul Oglesby, *Take Heart, the Life and Prescription for Living of Dr. Paul Dudley White.* (Boston: The Francis A. Countway Library of Medicine, 1986), 43.

65. "Geographic full-time" refers to physician faculty members who receive no salary from the school but limit their practices to (or base them at, since they may make house calls or consultation visits at other hospitals or clinics) the facilities of the school, Bowman Gray in this case; and in this case it refers to the PDC, the Private Diagnostic Clinic.

66. *N. Carol. Med. J.* 3 (1942): 209.

67. Harrell, personal communication.

68. *N. Carol. Med. J.* 3:373, 1942.

69. *The Daily Times Herald* (Dallas), March 22, 1942, Part 4, 1.

70. *The Daily Times Herald* (Dallas), March 22, 1942, Part 4, 2.

while but that it seemed less and less important.

However, there were staffing problems everywhere. It was so difficult to obtain physicians to help staff the hospitals and do the work that, despite his urgings for Blalock to take Valk into his program, Tinsley felt he could not release Valk even a few weeks early. He finally wrote Al on May 29 to say that he had had to keep Valk to help prepare wards to receive students for the first time; Valk would arrive at Hopkins in mid June.

Bowman Gray would start its next class that year on June 29, with 50 new students in the first year, 36 in the second year, and 33 in the third year. Instruction in the third year of medicine was being offered for the first time.[68]

IN MARCH TINSLEY MADE a trip which may have been fateful for him, though there is no record to prove it. He went to Dallas to speak at the annual meeting of the Dallas Southern Clinical Society, which expected 800 doctors.[69] He was one of 13 "distinguished surgeons, physicians and research workers" from throughout the country—Colorado, Chicago, Boston, Emory, Vanderbilt (Barney Brooks)—who spoke at the four day meeting beginning Monday the 23rd. Each morning there was a plenary session in the Hotel Adolphus at which the speakers gave general talks. Tinsley spoke on "Some Common Causes of Recurrent Attacks of Weakness."[70] After the plenary session the group broke into smaller specialty sessions for more specific talks followed by roundtable discussions of clinical problems and lunch, with additional split sessions later and buffet suppers or dinners in the evenings. Since this meeting had organized in 1929 "under the direction and sponsorship of the Dallas County Medical Society," Tinsley probably could not help comparing the size, vigor, and high quality of medical coverage at this meetings with ones of the smaller societies in Winston-Salem and Nashville. Despite its obvious Southernness, Dallas seemed more cosmopolitan. He probably met there his old Michigan friend Walter Bauer—now Colonel Bauer in the Eighth Army Command and responsible for military continuing medical education in the southwestern United States. Bauer, as a medical leader based in Dallas, would almost certainly have known Edward H. Cary, past president of the AMA and medical leader in Dallas. Cary was also chairman of the National Physicians' Committee, thus also a friend of Wingate Johnson. He was a major force in the development of medical education in Texas and president of the newly formed Southwestern Medical Foundation, the function of which was to raise money to save Dallas's financially ailing Baylor medical school. In fact, negotiations between the Foundation and Baylor were ongoing as the medical meeting was occurring in Dallas.

THE U.S. ARMY STILL needed doctors. Officials from the Roosevelt administration in Washington told the doctors what would be required in terms of manpower.[71] The problem was that there simply were not enough doctors. "The medical profession will be expected to send one-third of its membership into service."[72] Two-thirds of those going to the service (Army and Navy combined; the Air Force did not yet exist as a separate service) would come from those doctors under the age of 45, and most young doctors who had completed a nine-month internship were expected to go immediately into the service.[73]

In this situation the AMA pledged that it would give "all out collaboration," but some worried about the effects of the federal government's entering into arrangements for medical education and practice. They emphasized the corresponding commitment from the government. "Let us hope that . . . officials of the Administration will [not] forget two promises made the House of Delegates at Atlantic City. The first was that 'All out collaboration does not involve any theoretical assaults on, or support of, any theory of medical practice.' The second promise was that if organized medicine does its duty in obtaining enough physicians for the Army and Navy, and at the same time allocates men to important positions in industry and in civilian life, 'the profession should certainly have no fear of any drastic change in medical practice after the war.' "[74]

By July the *North Carolina Medical Journal* announced that it had received word "that North Carolina is one of the first states in the Union to reach its 1942 quota of doctors for military and naval service. While anyone who feels the urge to volunteer may still do so, it is probable that Uncle Sam will not demand any more medical officers from North Carolina this year."[75] Even this early in the war effort, however, there were concerns about the immediate effects on medical education and hence the long-term effects on doctors and patients. There was concern about the adequacy of training and staffing:

> The war has brought a new and subtle danger to medical education. Young graduates are denied more than one year of intern training, a restriction which is said to be a military necessity, and one, therefore, in which the profession gladly concurs, although recognizing it as a misfortune for the future of American medicine.

71. Paul V. McNutt, *JAMA* 20, June 1942.

72. *N. Carol. Med. J.* 3 (1942): 367.

73. Meads, *Miracle*, 33. Actually, one-third of those completing the nine-month internship were permitted to proceed directly with residency training of an additional nine to 18 months.

74. *N. Carol. Med. J.* 3 (1942): 367.

75. "In Defense of Mr. McNutt," *N. Carol. Med. J.* 3 (1942): 367.

76. "Medical Education and The War," *N. Carol. Med. J.* 3 (1942): 366.

77. Meads, *Miracle*, 33.

78. Ibid., 36.

79. Ibid., 21.

80. Carpenter, *Story*, 45.

81. Ibid., 30.

82. Meads, *Miracle*, 22.

83. Ibid., 25.

84. Ibid.,15.

85. Carpenter, *Story*, 43. The income of the school for 1941–42 was $181,774.70, including the $33,209.32 from student fees. In 1944 when Harrison left, these figures were $338,820.28 and $108,004.51, respectively. The endowment income was "approximately $44,000 per year," according to Carpenter.

86. Meads, *Miracle*, 20–21. "A satisfactory agreement with the City Hospital System [City Memorial, 225 beds; Kate B. Reynolds for Negroes, 190 beds; and their associated clinics] was negotiated, which included the statement that any expense or cost incurred from using any part of the system for teaching

Now, however, great pressure is being brought on the medical schools to strip their teaching staffs to the point where good medical training will become impossible, and this at a time when the schools have increased their enrollments materially, and are teaching continuously throughout the year.[76]

Many others, in academic medicine and private practice, agreed "that the accelerated program lowered the quality of training."[77]

Meanwhile, the financial advantage to Bowman Gray School of Medicine was minimal; overall tuition revenue increased less than $20,000 a year as a result of the accelerated curriculum.[78] At the same time, the medical school was having its own private crisis. Recall that the initial gift of the Bowman Gray bequest was Reynolds Tobacco Company stock worth about $600,000, which together with accumulated dividends brought the total to $720,000.[79] An additional gift of $10,000 came from Mrs. Ida Charlton and was used to purchase 300 more shares of Reynolds stock.[80] Early in the planning when President Kitchin had visited Alan Gregg at the Rockefeller Foundation to seek help, Gregg had strongly advised against the idea of a four-year school and suggested the new money go to improve the two-year school; however, that was an impossibility because of the conditions of the gift.[81] Rather than spend the money outright, Kitchin and Carpenter used the stock to secure a loan of $444,881 from the National Shawmut Bank of Boston at 1.5 percent interest. "A year later Mr. James Gray arranged for the loan to be moved to the First National Bank of Atlanta at 1 percent interest."[82] However, the school was barely scraping along, and "only interest payments were made during the first five years."[83] The bank was worried that no payments were being made on the principal.

Then something worse happened. The value of the Reynolds stock declined unexpectedly, and it was no longer sufficient to cover the loan, which required a 25 percent margin. As the Grays had promised Tinsley when he originally considered the job, they came through with help. "Bowman and Gordon Gray loaned the medical school 6,000 shares of Reynolds stock and $22,800 in cash to satisfy" the bank's requirement. The Duke Endowment was also helping, with the "$1 per day for each charity patient in hospitals in North and South Carolina" and, stimulated perhaps by Watson Rankin, with other gifts as well.[84] The parent Wake Forest College continued to provide its $22,450 annually, which it claimed was the maximum it could under an agreement nobody could find.[85]

Apart and largely independent from the school, the North Carolina Baptist Hospital was expanding to provide facilities for clinical teaching. Initially there had been plans for using all the hospitals in the Winston-Salem area, especially the large city hospital for the indigent. However, the city hospital wanted excessive payments for its cooperation and was initially lost from participation.[86] As a result, Baptist Hospital spent $647,246 to expand to a total of 270 beds plus 50 bassinets. The Baptists themselves worked hard throughout the state, but especially in Winston-Salem, to raise this money. The saving assistance came from R. J. Reynolds Jr. and the Duke Endowment, which each contributed $150,000. The expansion was completed in November 1941, but a year later some Baptists were still trying to raise $150,000, but other Baptists (including President Kitchin) were engaged in a major fundraising effort to expand and improve the campus at the original Wake Forest site.[87] Later Kitchin was converted to moving the whole university to Winston-Salem, but this only aggravated the fundraising problems, since even more money was needed.

When the war began, money became available from the federal government for hospital construction relating to civil defense, and it was suggested that Baptist Hospital should obtain help there. The idea of "assistance from this source was rejected on the principle of separation of church and state, [and] this event sparked a denominational debate concerning the acceptance of federal funds for facilities, a debate not resolved until almost two decades later."[88]

In November 1943 the trustees of the hospital "authorized a major expansion of the three-story nurses' home. It was to be financed by a federal Works Progresss Administration grant related to the nurse cadet program and by loans. The grant award of $63,000 was accepted by the trustees 'in the public interest' with three dissenting votes; however, the Baptist State Convention met in Winston-Salem in 1943 and soundly rejected the acceptance of this grant, authorizing the hospital to borrow $110,000 for the project."[89]

The hospital's religious affiliation troubled Tinsley. During the financial turmoil, Tinsley told Carpenter that he felt bound by his conscience to announce that he was an atheist.[90] Carpenter expressed dismay and talked him out of it. One can imagine the conversation. We do not know Carpenter's response. Tinsley's reply is recorded in Carpenter's confidential manuscript. Tinsley said that it was "a matter of intellectual honesty." This could have been a major problem for Tinsley's career. Tinsley most likely thought that by making such a dramatic announcement he could

would be paid for by the medical school. Just before the agreement was presented to the Board of Aldermen for approval, Dr. J. B. Whittington, superintendent of the City Hospital, added a qualifying paragraph which stated that the added costs due to teaching would be those over and above the average cost per day per patient, which was to be calculated as the average for the last five years. The record showed a steady increase in costs during this period, and Dr. Whittington refused to present the agreement to the aldermen without this statement. Negotiations were discontinued, and Dr. Carpenter indicated that the wisdom of this decision was borne out in that, if such a condition had been agreed to, it would have cost the school 'the almost unbelievable sum of $300,000 per year' over the ensuing five years."

87. Ibid., 21.
88. Ibid., 21.
89. Ibid., 33. The construction was completed in 1945 at a cost of $131,500, "with the help of approximately $21,500

confront the issue directly and bring it to a head. But Tinsley again was saved by a friend from a disaster he was about to create.[91]

THERE WERE OTHER, MORE serious problems than those of the Bowman Gray School of Medicine. In 1942 and into 1943 German submarine warfare was terrifying Americans. Rumors circulated of submarines putting spies ashore in small boats off the east coast of Florida. Apparent German submarines surfaced in sight of Florida beaches.[92] One man from Morehead City, North Carolina (near the Cherry Point U.S. Marines base), "remarked that he did not have to go to war; the war came to him. He has more than 200 casualties to treat as the result of the submarine activity off the Atlantic Coast."[93]

On May 5–6 came the Atlantic City rites of spring, the Old Turks meetings.[94] A paper from Tinsley's lab on renal extracts had been accepted for presentation at the major meeting on the Steel Pier, and Harrison made this presentation on Tuesday afternoon.[95] After the presentation there was discussion about the species specificity of the responses and whether dogs would respond in a manner similar to rats. They had early tried the extracts in dogs and had obtained responses, Tinsley replied, but those extracts were crude and it was uncertain what caused the response, the extract itself or the ammonium salts. Preparation of the extracts was so laborious and expensive that they preferred to continue working with rats, which required smaller amounts and which they assumed would respond in a fashion similar to man.

Tinsley enjoyed the rest of the meeting. It was announced that in 1943 the AAP's highest honor, the Kober Medal, would be presented to Vanderbilt pathologist Ernest Goodpasture, Tinsley's old friend. Hugh Morgan was at the meeting and was a councillor of the AAP, and Youmans gave a paper on nutrition. It was a Vanderbilt reunion. It was also a Brigham reunion with Sam Levine and Bill Dock, as well as a Massachusetts General reunion (with Tinsley's old classmate Walter Bauer, soon to become chief of medicine at the MGH, now pursuing synovial fluids and Reiter's syndrome; and the MGH gastroenterologist Chester Jones, who had spent a year at Vanderbilt while Harrison was there), and a Boston Beth Israel reunion (Herrmann Blumgart, A. Stone Friedberg, Munroe Schlesinger, all cardiologists and Harrison's friends, interested especially in coronary atherosclerosis and its treatment), and a Boston City Hospital/Thorndike Laboratory reunion (Bill Castle).

Bill Dock was president of the Young Turks (ASCI) at this meeting and presented a paper—on hepatic arterial flow in patients with cirrhosis and portal

generated from government funds received from housing for nurse cadets." The Baptist argument was that these government funds were simply a regular commercial exchange, money for facilities, and therefore not a "gift" or grant likely to bring with it government control.

90. Carpenter, manuscript.

91. Manson Meads, personal communication, August 10, 1993. On the other hand, this was Carpenter writing many years after the fact, and it may be that he was trying to justify some of his own dealings with Harrison by this story. Carpenter appears to have been pragmatic on these issues. Dr. Manson Meads tells of how in the early 1950s Carpenter was trying to recruit someone from Maine and telephoned him from Winston-Salem to ask him his religion, which he needed to complete some form. The man answered that he really had no religion. "Fine," said Carpenter, "I'll just put down 'Baptist.' Is that all right?" The recruitee must have needed the job, for he is reported to have as-

hypertension— at the Old Turks meeting as well. Tinsley's Hopkins classmate Chester Keefer, soon to become famous with antibiotics,[96] was on the council of the Young Turks.[97] Canby Robinson gave the after-dinner address at the annual dinner of the AAP Tuesday evening. The attendance was down somewhat, and the atmosphere was more somber than usual, but the surf, wind, sun, huge hotels, good meals, and companionship were still there.[98]

The following week, Paul Dudley White (who had not been at the Atlantic City meetings) went to North Carolina to speak on recent advances in cardiovascular disease at the state medical society meeting in Charlotte. Mr. Charles Dollard, assistant to the president of the Carnegie Corporation of New York, visited the school in March, but it is not recorded that he provided any money.

On the afternoon of May 5, as Tinsley was presenting his paper in the pleasant and stimulating surroundings of the Atlantic City meetings, Japanese troops were pouring into Yunnan Province in southwest China via the Burma Road, thereby threatening Kunming, to which much of academic Beijing had earlier escaped to form the Southwest China Associated Universities.[99] The Battle of Coral Sea was raging, where the American carrier *Lexington* was sunk and the carrier *Yorktown* was badly damaged. During this battle, the U.S. also lost 60 planes, a tanker, and various other smaller craft and equipment, while the Japanese lost a carrier and several cruisers and destroyers. On May 6, as the Atlantic City meetings continued after the evening talk by Canby Robinson, the island of Corregidor fell to the Japanese, just three miles across the water from Bataan Peninsula which had fallen April 9. Some 42,000 American and Philippine soldiers were captured by the Japanese, who also held Singapore and were bombing Ceylon in an attempt to reach the Persian Gulf. Near Ceylon they had just sunk the British carrier *Hermes*, and British forces were landing on Madagascar to defend the western Indian Ocean against attacks. Along the west coast of the U.S., Japanese-American citizens were being rounded up and herded into internment camps. As Tinsley discussed cardiovascular disease with Paul White in Charlotte, Rommel's tank corps were pushing out of Libya toward Tobruk and into Egypt, the Suez Canal, and points east.[100] The war was going badly for the Allied forces.

In July, Tinsley wrote Carpenter that he had obtained a volunteer to help with the lab work, thus releasing the $600 allocated for that purpose. He now wished to add that to George Harrell's salary (then $2,400) for teaching preventive medicine, at least temporarily. Tinsley also asked that, since they still had $118.62 in the Gray

sented without further discussion.

92. J. A. Pittman Sr. to J. A. Pittman Jr., 1942. These sightings seemed more prevalent around Cape Canaveral, which jutted out away from the smooth north-south curve of the Florida east coast and out into the Atlantic.

93. *N. Carol. Med. J.* 3 (1942): 366.

94. T. R. Harrison, A. Grollman, and J. R. Williams Jr., "Separation of Various Blood Pressure Producing Fractions of Renal Extract," *Trans. Assoc. Amer. Phys.*, 62 (1942).

95. Ibid., 187. Acceptance of this paper was itself an accomplishment in a situation where perhaps only 70 or 50 percent of those submitted were accepted for presentation. At this particular Old Turks meeting papers by Henry Christian, Reginald Fitz, Max Wintrobe, Hobart Reimann, Stanley Cobb, Emmett Holt, and many others were "read by title" only; i.e., the titles and authors were printed in the program, but there was no presentation. *See also xxxvii.*

96. Ibid. A sign of the

times was in the title of a paper at this meeting: "A Comparison of the Results of Treatment of Pneumococcic Pneumonia (1939–42) with Hydroxyethyl-apocupreine and with Sulfonamide Derivatives." Antipneumococcal antisera and even external X-ray therapy were used in serious cases.

97. Record of the officers of the American Society for Clinical Investigation ("Young Turks"), provided by Andrew Schafer, M.D., Secretary-Treasurer, 1993.

98. Means, *Association*, 201.

99. Cha Liang-Cha: audiotape of Drs. J. A. and C. S. Pittman, Taipei, Taiwan, May 12, 1981, UAB Archives.

100. Daniel, *Chronicle*, 534–538.

101. Harrison to Carpenter, July 17, 1942. Dorothy Carpenter Medical Archives, BGSM. Harrison had earlier written Carpenter (May 18) saying: "We are both naturally disappointed that the emergency facing the nation has forced a temporary abandonment of some of the future plans for the school. However, the

Fund, checks for $50 each be sent to Drs. Harrell and Williams, plus whatever support was possible to help Grollman with his expenses for the Boston trip in April. He had hoped that the school would cover some of his own expenses for the trip, as well as those of Drs. Johnson, McMillan, and MacMillan of the department of medicine, but there just wasn't enough money.[101]

The departmental report for the first year (1941–42) lists six publications for Tinsley, three from the lab, and 15 out-of-town speaking engagements. He rejected six other invitations to speak. There were also four CPCs published that year in which Harrison was the principal discusser, but these did not appear on his bibliography.[102] He had been appointed chairman of the AMA's Section on Experimental Medicine, was associate editor of *Advances in Internal Medicine* (an annual book which reviewed recent topics of interest), and was a member of the American Heart Association's board of directors and its certifying committee for cardiology.[103]

Tinsley and Carpenter also discussed and corresponded about plans to inaugurate teaching medicine at the County Hospital in March 1943.[104] Tinsley thought this would require that they obtain quarters for the senior students at the hospital, not only to implement his plan for the students to actively provide care on the wards, but also because "in view of the rubber and gasoline situation it is highly improbable that the students will be allowed to drive their own cars by next spring. Hence, the school will need to have a bus large enough to hold about 20 men," 14 medical and five or six surgical. Proper authorizations would have to be obtained for tires and gasoline. If quarters could be found the bus would have to take them from the Bowman Gray campus to the County Hospital by 8 A.M. and return them at 11 P.M., to return again to the hospital before 8 the next morning. There was also the problem of a library at the County Hospital; Tinsley suggested that $150 be allocated for this to purchase "about 25 books."

Tinsley's discussion of the problems of teaching medical students in an outpatient area (the PDC) still sounded modern at the start of the 21st century. How can we utilize those private offices and patients without interfering with the doctors' practices and reducing the income? Can we find other space for this? And, even if we can, how will the patients react to having to spend additional time with a student? The regular outpatient clinic might do, but then we do not have the advantage of having the teaching faculty of the PDC, unless we pull them out of the PDC, which again reduces income. No fully satisfactory answers to these questions emerged.

Wingate Johnson was fighting another battle, against socialized medicine, or "state medicine." The very first article in the newly reconstituted *North Carolina Medical Journal* in 1940 was on this topic, and concerns continued as the Roosevelt administration seemed determined to extend government-aided sickness insurance to the whole population. The North Carolina State Medical Society had established a "Committee on Socialized Medicine," but there were worries that if this became politically active, the medical society might lose its tax-exempt status. Similar worries existed among physicians around the nation, so in 1939 a separate organization was formed, the National Physicians' Committee (NPC) for the Extension of Medical Care; Dr. Edward H. Cary of Dallas, a past president of the AMA, was chairman of the NPC board.[105]

At its June meeting in Atlantic City, the AMA gave formal approval of the NPC, thereby encouraging support from individual doctors.[106] Wingate Johnson was a member of the NPC board, and his position as secretary of the AMA's new Section on General Practice gave him an added podium from which to spread the word against state medicine.[107] At that same AMA meeting Tinsley gave a paper on "Some Puzzling Aspects of Pain in the Chest."[108]

Back in Winston-Salem, the days continued to pass with sick patients and teaching. Work in the lab seemed bogged down. The tides of war seemed to be turning a bit in favor of the Allies. In October, Tinsley again accompanied Carpenter to the AAMC's annual meeting, this time in Lexington, Kentucky. In December he chaired the section on experimental medicine at the AMA's interim meeting in Chicago (the winter meeting was smaller than the annual session in June), then he attended the annual conference of section secretaries with the Council on Scientific Assembly.

Tinsley planned a trip in December to meet with Alan Gregg of the Rockefeller Foundation to discuss an idea for promoting research among the Bowman Gray faculty and at the same time providing financial support during a five-year probationary period. Rockefeller would add funds for salary support,[109] and the school would provide a $1,000 a year base for research. At the end of the fourth year, the foundation and the school would evaluate the individual faculty member and his research progress and potential. If the assessments were positive, the school would be obligated to keep the faculty member in a more permanent capacity. Though Tinsley was vague on the point, presumably the foundation would continue some research support. The school would agree "that it would undertake to see that such individual had approximately 70 percent of his time free for research work," thus precluding private practice except possibly for occasional consults or old patients.

Department of Medicine is not only willing but anxious to do its bit toward helping tide over the immediate difficult future." He then discussed the increased duties of Harrell and Grollman and his hopes for their return after the war, confidently expecting that then the planned expansion will resume.

102. *N. Carol. Med. J.* 3 (1942): 93, 202, 399, 566.

103. Tinsley Harrison, Department of Medicine Annual Report, 1941–42, Dorothy Carpenter Medical Archives, BGSM.

104. Harrison to Carpenter, July 17, 1942. The county hospital was different from the city hospital. The city hospital consisted of two institutions, the "City Memorial Hospital," for indigents patients but also for town physicians and their white private-paying patients, and the Kate B. Reynolds Hospital, the city's counterpart for black patients. The county hospital was primarily for long-term patients with chronic diseases.

105. *N. Carol. Med. J.* 4 (1943): 449.

106. *N. Carol. Med. J.* 3 (1942): 366.

107. Ibid., 373.

108. Harrison, Medicine Annual Report.

109. Annually $1,000 for single men, $1,500 for married men without children, and $2,000 for married men with children.

110. Tinsley Harrison to Coy C. Carpenter, December 8, 1942. Dorothy Carpenter Medical Archives, BGSM. Typically, Harrison proposed that he be included in the plan and, if he did not perform well, fired at the end of the five years: "I told Dr. Gregg that in order to avoid any misinterpretation of my own motives in attempting to help you secure the adoption of such a plan, that I would prefer to be put on the plan in the same way as the younger men, but with the exception that I should receive no increase in salary, such funds simply going into the research budget of the department. I trust that you will not think that this is simply an insincere or quixotic gesture on my part. It has long been part of my philosophy concerning medical schools to believe that the chief thing wrong with them is the profes-

This 70 percent would apply during the probationary period and, presumably, later. Harrison did make the trip, and Gregg promised to give the proposal consideration, but nothing further was recorded about it.[110]

So the year ended much as it began, with Tinsley writing Al on November 19 to inquire about a visit, saying he would be in Washington the next week and hoped to spend the evening with the Blalocks before taking the 11 P.M. train on to Boston. And on December 17 he traveled to Florence, South Carolina, to address the 94 annual session of the Peedee Medical Association on "Treatment of Congestive Heart Failure."[111]

The Tinsley–Al correspondence continued on into 1943. On March 6, Al wrote that his surgical staff was "terribly depleted" with "no full-time men on the staff at present." He praised Henry Valk, asked after Betty's health and Woody's status, said he was sending "reprints of mine which I do not expect you to read." And he enclosed a photograph—the 1901 Johns Hopkins University faculty. "Knowing of your admiration for President [Daniel C.] Gilman, I thought that you might be interested in this. I doubt if ever there has been such a celebrated group of men on a single faculty. I wish that I could think that it could be duplicated at Wake Forest or here."

The Hopkins photograph obviously pleased Tinsley, who wrote back the next week, March 13, to proclaim that Gilman "did more for American medicine than any man who ever lived." He added that Bowman Gray was beginning its fourth year and, like Hopkins, was "so short of personnel." Tinsley said he was getting really busy teaching and also had been made chairman of a committee to plan 250–300 new beds for the hospital. Even so, he was spending an hour or two a day in the lab and was keeping up except in his reading. "I don't get to read the journal of Physiology, of Biochemistry and the foreign journals the way I did ten years ago. However, I am thoroughly pleased with the whole business and think things are going pretty well when one considers the double handicap of [Bowman Gray] being new plus the war. There are about four people in the department who are carrying on a very active research program and half a dozen others who are doing useful things." Tinsley followed up on Al's mention of Henry Valk, saying he was "one of the finest lads I ever saw and it the kind of fellow you can always put your finger on. He is not brilliant but he is so solid and has such fine personal qualities that I believe he ought to go a long way." The letter was signed "Tinsley T."[112]

ON MARCH 22, 1943, Bowman Gray "began its first session as a complete four year school," with 51 freshmen.[113]

The little correspondence there was in 1943 between Tinsley and Carpenter concerned a familiar problem from the Vanderbilt days. How does one divide the responsibilities between the medical school and its main teaching hospital? In an expansive, philosophical letter to Carpenter on May 9, 1943, Tinsley wrote that he felt that the school was carrying more than its fair share of the financial load and that there were "inequities . . . between the hospital and the medical school."

The laboratories were supervised by the senior staff of the medical school, which paid the salaries of those supervisors. All technicians' salaries, operating expenses, supplies, and equipment were purchased by the medical school. The medical school was paying the salaries of the senior faculty who supervised and worked in electro-cardiography, basal metabolism, blood chemistry, bacteriology, parasitology, clinical microscopy, and so on. Yet the hospital took half the income, while the medical school experienced a net financial loss. Tinsley argued that the hospital would have to provide these functions itself if there were no attached medical school.

Tinsley estimated he spent one-third of his days caring for service patients, one-third devoted to administration, one-sixth teaching students, and one-sixth doing research work. He also estimated that of the third devoted to administration, about 60 percent was hospital administration and 40 percent medical school. This was also true, Tinsley argued, of the administrative duties of other faculty, for whom the school provided the salaries, offices, secretaries, heat, and lights "entirely from the medical school" funds. Tinsley continued for five single-spaced pages citing matters "in which the hospital seems to be profiting at the expense of the medical school." Contributions of medical students to laboratory and scut work, the library (supplied by the school), the white coats supplied by the school, the house staff's laundry expenses, and on and on.

After acknowledging that the medical school should bear the brunt of some of these loads, he suggested that Bowman Gray had to decide if it wanted to be a third-rate, second-rate, or first-rate hospital, and that it could never be first-rate until "research is considered as just as important a function of the hospital as of the medical school." He also observed that "in this way it becomes possible for a hospital to contribute not only to the care of the sick within its walls but to care of the sick throughout the world" and that such an "attitude would seem particularly appropriate for a hospital belonging to the Missionary Baptist Church, a religious

sors, who it seems to me often try to spur the young men on to investigation without setting the proper example. I do not believe that any professor of medicine who fails to make significant contributions to the field within a five-year period is fit for the job and shall be very happy to be replaced, in case the agency for the Foundation feels that after five years I have failed in this respect."

111. *N. Carol. Med. J.* 4 (1943): 33.

112. Miss Tims, whom they had come to call "Timmie," became adept at mimicking Harrison's signature.

113. At that time there were 32 seniors, 31 juniors, 46 sophomores, and 51 freshmen, for a total enrollment of 160. The increased number of students, with assurances from the army's ASTP (Army Special Training Program) and the Navy's V-12 program that the students' tuitions would be paid, helped somewhat with the school's finances.

114. Tinsley Harrison to Coy C. Carpenter, May 9, 1943. Dorothy Carpenter Medical Archives, BGSM. [see

www.newsouthbooks.
com/tinsleyharrison/
supplement for the
full text of this letter].
This letter, which
contains a mix of, first,
accounting details to
convince readers that
the hospital should
contribute more to
academic activities
and, second, broad
statements of philoso-
phy about hospitals
and medical schools,
is signed "Tinsley R.
Harrison" rather than
"Tinsley," as he would
have signed a personal
letter not intended for
further distribution
and readers. It also has
attached three pages of
budget data for the de-
partment of medicine,
presumably to support
his arguments. The
first of these pages,
"Expenditure of Funds
for the Department of
Medicine 1941-42,"
lists salaries for medi-
cine's personnel plus
"Research Supplies" at
$5,000 and "Business
& Miscellaneous" at
$1,000, for a total of
$37,600. The second
page, titled "Special
Funds, Department
of Medicine; January,
1942 to July, 1943,"
lists amounts from
various private sources
(no government
sources readily avail-
able), though several
of these extend beyond

organization which has always taken the attitude that goodness and beneficence should be distributed on a world-wide scale." If that was not the goal, he concluded, "there is serious question of the wisdom of attempting such an expansion."[114]

One facet of academic support that Tinsley neglects to mention in his May 9 letter—hospital support for indigent patients kept in the hospital solely for investigation—he had discussed in an earlier letter to Carpenter in which he had complained about needing to have discussions with the hospital administration and make particular arrangements for each patient. He suggested that a general plan for patients undergoing special studies might work better and be more efficient:

> 1. It would be understood that no service would have at any given moment more than ten percent of the service beds used for this purpose.
>
> 2. It would be understood that during a given year no more than five per cent of the beds be used for such purpose.
>
> I believe if there were such an arrangement and the house staff were informed of it, the privilege would never be abused. Obviously the hospital cannot be expected to keep a large number of patients in the institution for investigation. On the other hand it is also obvious that we will never have a first-rate institution unless a few patients are being intensively studied at all times. In the long run such studies will not only benefit the hospital in terms of prestige but will actually be worth dollars and cents to the hospital. . . ."[115]

Before condemning Tinsley as hopelessly naive about hospital budgets, we should remember that the per diem costs then were only several dollars a day, and the medical school handled many of the ancillary costs, especially the laboratories. In accordance with tradition, he appealed to quality to defend his argument.

DESPITE THE WAR, MEDICAL school continued as before. As 1943 began, doctors desperate for effective therapy were still using external X-ray therapy for clearly infectious diseases as such as erysipelas and carbuncles.[116] As the year ended, it was apparent that penicillin and other antibiotics would soon revolutionize the treatment of these conditions.[117] The year also ended with a slightly more optimistic view of the course of the war for the Allies, though the situation remained so perilous that the U.S. government requested cancellation of the AAP's annual Atlantic City and affiliated meetings.[118]

The country kept functioning, a necessity to support the war effort overseas. The Office of Civilian Defense approved a grant of $1,610.65 to Bowman Gray to help establish a blood and plasma bank in the hospital, and the medical students voted to give "up to two pints of blood for a reserve of 300 pints in the Blood Bank to be used in war emergencies."[119] In mid-January, the Nathalie Gray Bernard Lecture was a series of three addresses by Lieutenant Commander A. R. Behnke of the U.S. Navy medical corps, who was interested in undersea and aviation medicine. The first two of his evening lectures were on "The Military Environment Primarily in Relation to Changes in Barometric Pressure," and the third was titled "Fitness for the Military Environment in Relation to Changes in Barometric Pressure." Behnke, a physician working on human physiological reactions to the low pressures of high flight in airplanes and the high pressures of a dense atmosphere deep under the sea in a submarine, was to meet Tinsley on the same topics a decade later.[120] On the 14th there was a series of sessions, including special clinics by Tinsley and Wingate Johnson and by Bradshaw and others. In February Carpenter attended a special meeting of the Association of American Medical Colleges to discuss wartime medical education measures, and Harrison traveled to Rochester, Minnesota, to give two talks at the sectional meeting of the American College of Physicians, one on "The Interpretation of Pain in the Chest" and the other "Recent Advances in Hypertension."[121]

In February Tinsley traveled the short distance to Duke to give a clinic in the morning on "The Differential Diagnosis of Pain in the Chest" and an evening lecture on "Cardiac Dyspnea." In March as the complete medical school was beginning for the first time, Carpenter traveled to Atlanta for a meeting on Army-Navy Training Programs, George Harrell to a number of cities and countries abroad (Honduras, for example) to learn and talk about tropical diseases, tuberculosis, and other infections, and Wingate Johnson to New York for a meeting of the National Physicians' Committee to fight socialized medicine. Tinsley went to New Orleans that month to give several talks on heart disease before the Seventh Annual Meeting of the New Orleans Graduate Medical Assembly and, at home, continued CPCs with his friend the pathologist Robert P. "Moose" Morehead. Before the month was over, he had given his Cardiac Dyspnea talk again at Chapel Hill to students and faculty of the University of North Carolina's two-year medical school. So the year continued.[122]

Despite cancellation of the Atlantic City meetings, Tinsley had persuaded his friend Bill Dock, now professor of pathology at Cornell Medical School, to serve

the time limits of the title: Markle ($3,500), Macy (for John Williams, $2,000), Werthan (his friend in Nashville, $1,000 for 1942 and $2,000 for '43), National Life and Accident Ins. Company ($1,000 for '42 and another $1,000 for '43), Dazian [foundation] ($1,500 for '43), and McCanless ($500, buffer, no time limits). The three listed here for '43 were scheduled to expire 1/1/44. These total $12,500. The third budget page lists regular support from the school for the department and includes a "contingent item" of $2,000 for Harrison, with a note, "This will not all be needed and possibly none will be needed." Apparently he was bringing in enough money from patients to relieve Carpenter of most or all of the "bonus" he had negotiated for himself. While Harrison did not save the school money (he did, as he claimed, save the hospital money), and in fact cost it dearly, he certainly brought money to the school and enriched it in many other ways as well.

115. No mention of

"informed consent" or anything resembling it was found in material examined during the preparation of this book. Harrison's last research paper containing original data appeared in 1964. However, Faden, Beauchamp, and King, in their book *A History of Informed Consent* (New York: Oxford Univ. Press, 1986) point out that Germany had laws on their books throughout the Nazi period which required that German physicians do no harm to their patients or subjects and always obtain *informed consent* before any procedure or experiment, and guarantee that no harm will be done! Obviously, laws cannot guarantee this. Only a *good doctor* can do that.

116. R. J. Reeves, "Roentgen Therapy in the Treatment of Certain Inflammatory Conditions," *N. Carol. Med. J.* 4 (1943): 44. A. U. Desjardins, "The Action of Roentgen Rays on Inflammatory Conditions," *Radiology* 38 (1942): 274.

117. S. J. Crowe and A. T. Ward, "Local Use of Sulfadiazine, TyroThricin, Penicillin and Radon in Otolar-

as visiting professor at Bowman Gray June 10–18; they had a fine time together as they entertained and instructed students, staff, and faculty. Harrison was always stimulated by a colleague—not a foil, but a bright competitive fellow laborer in the vineyards of medicine—with whom to spar and duel in public contests over who knew more medicine or had greater skill in physical examination or the interpretation of data or understanding diseases.

Tinsley and Dock knew and liked each other, and both were devoted and competitive scholars of medicine, so it must have been quite a spectacle as they challenged each other with questions of anatomy (which vessel supplied the branch which supplied this part of that organ, or what was the central representation of a particular dermatome or motor function), physical diagnosis ("What?! You didn't hear that loud murmur?") or laboratory data ("Of course a *pathologist*, being interested only in *dead* things, would know nothing at all about *functional* tests in the living, like creatinine clearances!") or diseases and their treatment ("Well, penicillin probably won't cure rheumatic fever.").[123] Dock brought material for a CPC down from New York, which they presented with Tinsley as the clinician-discusser and Dock as pathologist.[124] It was a case in a 59-year-old somewhat hypertensive woman with symptoms and signs of congestive heart failure, a paradoxical pulse, lymphadenopathy, intermittent fever, and edema but no hepatomegaly. Tinsley thought scrofulous tuberculosis with pericarditis unlikely in a woman of this age, and, with the intermittent fever, diagnosed Hodgkin's disease with constrictive pericarditis. He was puzzled by lack of hepatomegaly with the congestive failure, but he had to start somewhere.

He was wrong. She suffered from miliary tuberculosis with constrictive pericarditis. The lack of hepatomegaly was explained by the presence of multiple fibrous scars throughout the liver where there had been old gummas despite the negative serology. Interestingly, 1943 data from the Metropolitan Life Insurance Company showed that tuberculosis was still the fifth most common cause of death in school-age children in America,[125] and it had killed this older woman. Dock also recalled advice received 21 years earlier: "Dr. S. A. Levine of Boston pointed out to Dr. Harrison and me in our youth how rarely the hypertensive patient becomes tuberculous, and I think that fact may have helped to persuade Dr. Harrison that this was not tuberculosis."[126]

In turnabout Dock served as clinician-discusser for a CPC on a patient who had died at Winston-Salem, a 52-year-old hypertensive man with bouts of chest pain, variable diastolic and systolic murmurs, pulmonary edema, and finally sudden death in the Baptist Hospital.[127] His acute pulmonary edema was relieved satisfactorily by administration[128] of morphine, oxygen by tent, and "3 cat units of digitalis intravenously."[129] The pathologist, Tinsley's good friend "Moose" Morehead, confirmed that Dock had hit virtually every point and had predicted the pathologic anatomy accurately.

Dock also contributed an excellent review article "Arteriosclerosis" to the *North Carolina Medical Journal*, which appeared as the lead article in the November issue[130] and reveals him as an acute and critical scholar and an articulate writer. He was paid little or nothing for his visiting professorship other than expenses, but the local medical community was certainly well served by it, and he probably learned some things as well.

Transportation was becoming more difficult. The annual meetings of both the North Carolina Tuberculosis Association and the National Tuberculosis Association were called off in 1943 at the request of the Office of Defense Transportation, despite the continuing importance of that disease and the continued openings of new TB sanatoria.[131] Doctors working near the coasts were required to attach small but readily visible Civil Defense flags to the left front of emergency vehicles and to equip their cars with dim-out equipment, so as to avoid revealing their locations to enemy ships off the coast at night.[132] Medical journals carried advertisements like, "She swapped glamour for guns, but she's still a woman," and advised the use of diethylstilbestrol or other estrogens to keep her going on her job at home.[133]

There was also a program of Wartime Graduate Medical Meetings for military installations in North Carolina. Wingate Johnson was chairman of the committee for Region 6, which includes North and South Carolina. Carpenter was secretary. The meetings were cosponsored by the AMA, American College of Physicians, and the American College of Surgeons and were held throughout the country. Those in North Carolina began August 30 and continued through October 6. Tinsley was lead speaker for the group in Schedule 1 and spoke on "Military Problems in Cardiovascular Diseases." David T. Smith from the Duke medical school faculty accompanied him to speak on "Respiratory Diseases" as they traveled to military bases around the state. Harrell was a member of Schedule 2 and spoke on "Tropical Diseases," accompanied by Donald Martin of Duke, whose topic was "Fungus Diseases." Similarly, Grollman spoke on chemotherapy and Bradshaw on "Traumatic Surgery of the Chest and Abdomen." Since there were six visits for these teams,

yngology," *N. Carol. Med. J.* 4 (1943): 431; Gladys L. Hobby, *Penicillin, Meeting the Challenge* (New Haven: Yale Univ. Press, 1985).

118. Means, *Association*, 201.

119. *N. Carol. Med. J.*: 4 (1943): 33.

120. Ibid., 71.

121. *N. Carol. Med. J.* 4 (1943): 33, 71, 112, 152, 153, 181, 190.

122. A. Grollman, "The Treatment of Hypertension in the Light of Modern Experimental Investigations," *N. Carol. Med. J.* 4 (1943): 246.

123. These are all statements I have heard Tinsley make in similar situations.

124. Ibid., 266.

125. Ibid., 266. "The five chief causes of death among children of school age are, in order of numerical importance: accidents, appendicitis, influenza and pneumonia, rheumatic fever and tuberculosis."

126. "The Early Years at Bowman Gray," *N. Carol. Med. J.* 44 (1983): 805-6. Dr. George Harrell, who was at Duke in 1937–38, was asked to serve temporarily as pathologist and

director of laboratories at the Winston-Salem City Memorial Hospital from December '37 through June 1938. In this capacity he organized the city's first CPCs. Harrell later claimed with regard to the CPCs at the new school that "Harrison gave most of these, using cases already published in the literature." He has also claimed that Harrison sometimes cheated when he was not the primary discusser (and by implication perhaps when he was) by looking up the cases to be discussed ahead of time and "was found in the stacks at the library doing this." It is apparent from the text before you that they did need material as the school began (cf., for example, Harrison's letter to Goodpasture about material from Vanderbilt). However, the CPCs published regularly in the *North Carolina Medical Journal* give no indication of having been published earlier, and Harrison certainly missed diagnoses in some of these. Harrell also was strongly critical of some of Harrison's "disorganized" methods of teaching, particularly of holding

this work consumed most of late August in preparation, then September and early October in execution.[134] Tinsley seemed safe and satisfied. But he was neither.

EXACTLY WHAT HAPPENED IS not clear. Probably nobody wished it explicitly, even in their own minds.[135] It was a combination of the extreme shortage of personnel, space, and money, the war and the changes and intensification of medical education and care that it brought,[136] genuine uncertainties about how best to organize the new medical school under these circumstances, and perhaps most of all the particular time and place together with the personalities and personal histories of the participants.

As 1943 ended and 1944 began, Tinsley continued to teach vigorously with characteristic enthusiasm and enjoyment, and the research was continuing with the expert work of Grollman and Williams along with himself when he could spare the time. Publications were coming out despite the pressures. He was corresponding with Blalock about coming to Winston-Salem in the spring, and it was going to work out for April 1944. Blalock committed to the local Forsythe County Medical Society to come then, in letters as late as February 1944. Then, March 2, 1944, Tinsley was gone. What happened?

In March 1943 Carpenter had revised committee memberships for the coming year, creating an additional, new committee of senior faculty called the Advisory Council.[137] It consisted of seven senior people and met about once a month during that summer and fall, sometimes several times in a month, sometimes not at all. The council considered matters such as where and how money might be obtained for the support of a department of preventive medicine, the need for a scientific director in the dean's office, advice that the dean should relinquish the title of chairman (or director) of pathology and name "Moose" Morehead to that post (Harrison made the motion to do this, and it carried unanimously), advice that a lay administrator be found as soon as practicable for the hospital but that Carpenter retain the title of medical director with authority over the administrator; that a department of bacteriology be separated from pathology; problems with the clinical laboratory (seen as too slow and unresponsive, but also as underfunded and parasitized by the hospital, which took 50 percent of the income but contributed little to its support), and similar matters. The council obtained an hour-by-hour schedule of the dean's activities to see what tasks might be delegated to clerical assistants.

The council requested that it review all proposed appointments, promotions, and dismissals of the faculty. Tinsley and Artom pushed hard for high standards: "Dr. Artom and Dr. Harrison agreed we should be very critical of promotions and should set standards as high as are set anywhere."[138] The problems of how to deal with faculty appointments for volunteer staff of practitioners remained sticky, but the hospital was overcrowded and some of those initially appointed had to be removed. The faculty had to be limited to those who actually participated in the teaching. Later, Tinsley moved that "all new faculty appointments should be on a temporary basis, for a time to be specified in the agreement with the man. The title, duration of appointment and salary are to be left to the department concerned and to the Dean, but the duration of the appointment should not exceed three years."[139]

Another modern problem—"poor attendance of students of the third and fourth year classes at certain lectures and clinics"—was taken up in July, with a solution proposed by Harrison to number and assign seats to make it easier for the faculty to take roll.

On August 1, 1943, Tinsley sent Carpenter an identically worded (but retyped) copy of his memorandum of the previous year. "Dear Dr. Carpenter: Rumors from various sources tell me that I am being severely criticized by some of the physicians in the city because of my action in assuming personal charge of the medical service patients rather than continuing to have the physicians practicing in the city assume responsibility . . . as in the past." And, "The charity patients have received in the past totally inadequate medical attention." What prompted this resending of the letter to Carpenter is not clear, but it may have been related to the removal of some of the local physicians from the faculty. Inaccurate versions of the contents might have been leaked. The local physicians certainly would have been aware of it.

TINSLEY DEMANDED MUCH FROM his friends. He was often a friend in need of others; but he was also a friend to others in need. In the fall of 1943, the pediatrician so beloved by the Harrisons and the Blalocks had trouble. As is often the case in academic medicine, the trouble was caused by internal ambitions and insecurities combined with external changes and individual personal beliefs. The faculty members evaluated the situation to be the same as that of bacteriologists evaluating a culture of microorganisms: if you're not growing, you're dead.

Vanderbilt's chairman of pediatrics, Horton Casparis, had died suddenly, and "after much bickering" Katie Dodd was made "temporary head." Rivens said, "It is possible that she was denied the appointment as head of pediatrics because of her

clinical rounds with medical students and house staff of all levels together. Harrell felt they should be separated and offered graded instruction and that putting them together in one group wasted people's time. While they apparently remained cordial, it seems likely that Harrell was vocally critical of Harrison at Bowman Gray; and while Harrison tried to be fair (e.g., the $600/year, or 25 percent, raise in salary mentioned here), the two may have represented problems for each other at the time.

127. *N. Carol. Med. J.* 4 (1943): 391. It was commonly said in the 1940s that dissecting aneurysms of the aorta were very common in CPCs, and this may have helped Dock arrive at the correct diagnosis.

128. Or the "exhibition" of morphine, as the more pompous doctors often said then.

129. Grollman, "Treatment," 246. At that time digitalis leaf was standardized by bioassaying each batch in cats. In reading this CPC one is struck by how the physicians and staff stood by

helplessly as the patient's blood pressure remained at "218–230 systolic, 130 diastolic." There were, in fact, no effective treatments then. One simply watched, avoided salt and proteins in the patient's diet, and waited for the inevitable stroke, blindness from retinopathy, heart failure or other cardiac catastrophe, or death from end stage renal disease. Phenobarbital was sometimes given, or sometimes thiocyanates, weight reduction was attempted, and venesection was used in congestive failure. Sometimes the major procedure of surgical sympathectomy was used. But nothing did much good, and this patient's end, though from an infrequent complication, was otherwise fairly typical of hypertension in the 1940s.

130. William Dock, "Arteriosclerosis," *N. Carol. Med. J.* 4 (1943): 456.

131. *N. Carol. Med. J.* 4 (1943): 112. Apparently these requests from the Office of Defense Transportation to medical groups were not orders which had to be followed but requests "that

gender. When her colleagues talked in the hallways, some mentioned her brusque, outspoken manner and said that she was just 'too liberal.'[140] But all that talk about her politics was perhaps subterfuge; it was probably her gender that prevented her from getting the job."

Tinsley wrote their cardiologist friend Albert Starr to try to generate a job for Dodd in Oregon, and he wrote Blalock on October 16 to send him a copy of Starr's negative response. "If you have any possible chance of saying a good word or doing anything to help Katie," he said his letter, "particularly in one of the smaller schools, I know you will do it. Unfortunately, it seems likely that her problem is an insoluble one. If you have any suggestions to offer me in regard to it I shall be most appreciative."[141]

Blalock replied on October 23 that he agreed with Tinsley but that "it would be a terrible mistake for Katie to leave Vanderbilt and Nashville. There is no obligation on the part of an institution that the person next in line should be appointed." He went on, however, to say he had spoken to Canby Robinson about finding a place for Dodd and that he had written to Philip B. Price at the University of Utah in hopes that Dodd might find a position there. Blalock added that he had not heard from his friend Tinsley in a while but had noticed his speaking "all up and down the west coast. I am keeping a record of your various travels for I may want to use it in some future argument with you. . . . Please give my love to Betty. Would certainly like to see all of you."

At the end of October, William B. Castle of Harvard—Tinsley's friend of many years and colleague from their time together as officers of the Young Turks—spent three days in Winston-Salem to give the second series of Nathalie Gray Bernard Lectures. As he talked on "Some General and Particular Aspects of the Pathological Physiology of Anemias."[142] Castle also gave a public lecture at the Robert E. Lee Hotel the evening of the 29th with "colored pictures of Australia and the East in 1938."[143]

Tinsley was not there for the visit. He had left the 27th for California to give "a series of lectures on cardiovascular disease . . . to the American Heart Association in Los Angeles, to the Academy of Medicine in San Diego, and to the Stanford University School of Medicine in San Francisco."[144] On his way west he stopped by Alabama, where he gave a talk on "Cardiac Dyspnea" at the two-year medical school in Tuscaloosa.

Unfortunately, Wingate Johnson was also out of town during Castle's visit. He was in Chicago to talk about "Care of the Aged" to the Inter-State Postgraduate Medical

Association of North America. Many faculty were absent from Winston-Salem for Dr. Castle's visit. Harrell and Frank Lock, chief of obstetrics and gynecology, were in Cleveland October 25–27 attending the annual meeting of the AAMC.[145] The restrictions on professional travel were not handicapping Wake Forest physicians.

In November, as chairman of the AMA Section on Experimental Medicine and Therapeutics, Tinsley attended the meeting of the section chairmen and secretaries in Chicago as well as the Council on Scientific Assembly of the AMA. Then he was scheduled to go on December 8 to New York for a meeting of the executive committee of the American Heart Association, of which he was chairman.[146] He wrote Al on November 22 asking if he could spend the night of December 3. Al sent a reply telegram, and he must have asked Tinsley to conduct a clinic while he was stopping over in Baltimore.

On November 27, Tinsley wrote again, saying in effect that he would give the clinic unless unreliable train service prevented it. "I am coming to Baltimore from Cincinnati, not from Winston-Salem.[147] If you want me to give the clinic I will be glad to give it on either one of the following subjects: 'The Differential Diagnosis of Pain in the Chest'; 'The Abuse of Rest in the Treatment of Cardiac and Other Diseases'; "Disturbed Carbohydrate Metabolism as a Factor in the Production of Cardiac Symptoms'; or 'Hypertension.' I prefer not to talk about the latter subject because it is in such a confused state at present. However, if you think it best I will be glad to talk about it. Perhaps the most suitable subject would be the one dealing with abuse of rest, because it is applicable not only to medical but I think to surgical patients as well. However, I am not sure whether my train will arrive there in time for me to give a clinic. Hence, you had better be prepared to give it. When I reach Baltimore I will simply take a taxi out to the school and go at once to your office. I do not like to simply give a lecture to students but would much prefer to have a patient. Therefore I would suggest that if you think it wise you have a patient picked out who would illustrate one of the above topics, preferably the one on the abuse of rest, and that you also be prepared to give your regular clinic. It is not necessary to let me know ahead of time which of the various topics you would prefer I talk about because I can talk on any of them without trouble if I have about five minutes before the clinic to collect my thoughts."[148]

Tinsley went on to explain that he wanted to discuss a private family matter with Blalock and with another doctor at Hopkins. It was concerning his second son, Randolph, now 16, who had fallen in with some boys Tinsley considered a

travel be limited to the lowest practicable minimum." The medical organizations were simply doing their part voluntarily to help the war effort, this despite the fact that tuberculosis was still a plague and new TB sanatoria were opening in North Carolina. The new TB sanatorium (or "sanitarium") which opened in eastern North Carolina in January 1943 had a total bed capacity of 220, 110 white, and 110 negro.

132. Ibid., 112.

133. "Advertisement of the E.R. Squibb and Sons pharmaceutical company," *N. Carol. Med. J.* 4 (1943): 363.

134. *N. Carol. Med. J.* 4 (1943): 397–398.

135. W. F. Bynum and R. Porter, eds., *Brunonianism in Britain and Europe* (London: Wellcome Institute for the History of Medicine, 1988), ix. One is reminded of the statement about John Brown, the Scot of "Brunonianism" fame: The events of his life in Edinburgh "remain—and surely will remain—veiled in obscurity. His own papers have not survived, and most of what we do know of him is

anecdotal—indeed . . . consists of highly contested anecdote." Most historians might say, "Would that my anecdotes were contested—not successfully, but at least contested."

136. *N. Carol. Med. J.* 4 (1943): 450. Wingate Johnson said, "Since Pearl Harbor I have worked harder than at any time since the influenza epidemic of 1918–19, and I know that virtually every other doctor in civilian practice can say the same thing."

137. Minutes of Advisory Council Meetings, March 5, 1943 through 1944. Dorothy Carpenter Medical Archives, BGSM. The initial seven members were: Wingate Johnson (chairman; apparently chosen by the group), Artom, Bradshaw, Butler (pediatrics), Harrison, Vann (anatomy), and Wells (secretary).

138. Minutes of Advisory Council meeting of March 31, 1943. Dorothy Carpenter Medical Archives, BGSM.

139. Minutes of the Advisory Committee meeting of June 2, 1943. Dorothy

bad influence. They had taken a car and driven to the Variety Shades farm in Virginia without telling the parents, and Tinsley was worried about him. The older son Woody was in the U.S. Navy learning to fly. Tinsley wanted Randolph to visit Hopkins and see if he could turn the boy from a shaky path.

The visit to Hopkins went well, and young Randolph was sent to the Hill School in Pottstown, Pennsylvania, where he made a good record. He was large, a strong person, like his mother and her family; he excelled in athletics. Blalock helped set him on a course for a good life later in a medical discipline. Randolph's situation improved so quickly that just over a month later Tinsley was able to write a five-page letter to officials at the Hill School. He was happy for his boy about the progress being made, filled with advice and the suggestion that perhaps an occasional weekend with one of Tinsley's friends might act as a stimulus—"I would like you to feel that any invitation to spend a Saturday night at the home of Mrs. William Dock in New York, Dr. William Resnick in Stamford, Conn., or Dr. Alfred Blalock, Professor of Surgery at the Johns Hopkins Hospital in Baltimore, should be regarded as of the same nature as an invitation to spend a week-end with his parents."[149]

GRADUATION CEREMONIES FOR THE first class to finish at Bowman Gray were on Sunday, December 19. Olin T. Binkley at the First Baptist Church delivered the baccalaureate sermon. Mrs. Carpenter gave a tea for the graduates and their relatives and friends and the faculty in the afternoon. That evening there was a special music program back at the church. The next day there was a medical clinic in the amphitheater, an alumni luncheon at the Robert E. Lee Hotel, a surgical clinic that afternoon, then the graduation exercises that evening in the R. J. Reynolds Auditorium. The Honorable J. Melville Broughton offered the address. Thirty-one graduates received the Doctor of Medicine degree that evening, and one person received a Master of Science degree.[150] An honorary Doctor of Science degree was awarded by Wake Forest on the recommendation of the Bowman Gray School of Medicine to Dr. Frederick M. Hanes of Duke (related to the wealthy Hanes textile family of Winston-Salem).

The school was working. The gamble had paid off. Wake Forest Medical was a success. Hanes commented at the time in an un-Baptist fashion, "In 1941, I knew damned well that it couldn't be done . . . Now that it has been done, I don't believe it."[151]

This was to be Tinsley's only commencement at Bowman Gray.

The situation at the medical school was unsettled. On December 7, 1943, Carpenter sent a confidential memorandum to the faculty attaching a report on the October 1943 inspection of the medical school by Drs. Zapffe and Johnson and a report of the curriculum committee, which Johnson had chaired, of the University of Chicago School of Medicine. "Please study both of these reports carefully," Carpenter wrote. "It is essential that we as a faculty have the same aims and objects and follow the same standards if we are to have the school that we desire." He called a mandatory faculty meeting for the evening of Tuesday, December 14, to consider the Zapffe-Johnson report. "You realize, of course, that this report is confidential. Your copy should be kept in your permanent files, and it should not be discussed with anyone other than members of the faculty."[152]

The 21-page report made explicit the worries and fears of the faculty. It stated: that the facilities were inadequate for the program the medical school needed to develop; that inadequate space for offices and labs crowded the clinical staffs into space intended only for the basic science departments; that cooperation between City Memorial Hospital and the medical school was not what it should be for the best medical education; that a lack of understanding and trust existed between hospital superintendent Dr. James B. Whittington and the medical school administrators; that it was misleading for the medical school catalog to state that there were 1,225 teaching hospital beds when far fewer were used for teaching; that outpatient work was the weakest part of the clinical instruction and that the outpatient department was "extremely poorly planned"—deficiencies recognized by the school and slated for improvement in the building of a new hospital; that in the past year some faculty had been dissatisfied in the amount of authority vested in the dean and the lack of authority in the faculty (a matter which now seemed resolved); that basic sciences faculty seemed inadequate in the "amount and quality of research carried out" at the level desirable for "a high grade medical school," with "minimal" research in anatomy and bacteriology, "some" in physiology, and "several projects" in pathology, "largely under the inspiration of Dr. Tinsley Harrison of the department of medicine"; that any increase in class sizes should be "strongly" resisted; that the school's financial stability was not assured; that the endowment "will not permit the development of a first-class educational and research institution"; and that clinical departments were understaffed.

After commenting favorably on the admixture of basic science with clinical teaching in the curriculum (though saying also that it could be greatly improved),

Carpenter Medical Archives, BGSM.

140. Rivens, *Worthy Lives*, 39–41, 44–45. Katie Dodd was born into a wealthy Boston family, attended Bryn Mawr college, then applied to Hopkins for medical school and was given "the privilege of taking the examinations," which she passed; but she was denied admission. A similar situation the following year precipitated the threat of a lawsuit by her father, and she was admitted and obtained her M.D. a year before Harrison and Blalock. After her residency she worked for a time in Russia, where she "saw no terror, no disorder, but thought Lenin's government as autocratic as the Czars' had been. But she opined, 'It is interesting to see a government run in the interests of the working man, and I think lasting benefits will come out of it.' She hoped to return to when Russia was 'freer and saner.'" She had come to Vanderbilt at the beginning of the new school in 1925, but now, disappointed not to be named professor and chair of the department to which she had given 17 years,

she took a job in the Children's Hospital Research Foundation in Cincinnati, then moved successively to the departments of pediatrics in Arkansas, then Louisville, then Emory. At the time of her 70th birthday in 1962 the *Journal of Pediatrics* had a festschrift by her former students and trainees in her honor.

141. Tinsley Harrison to Alfred Blalock, October 16, 1943, VUMC Archives.

142. *N. Carol. Med. J.* 4 (1943): 488.

143. Ibid., 451.

144. Ibid., 488.

145. Ibid., 489. A common joke among the unpaid volunteer faculty was, "The full-time faculty are gone all the time; the part-time faculty are gone part of the time; and the volunteer faculty does all the work." It may have more true than the "full-time" academicians cared to admit. On the thesis that "full-time" means either 168 hours a week (24x7) or some arbitrary figure such as 40 hours a week, and is therefore meaningless, some medical administrators later advocated preference for the term "regular"

Zapffe and Johnson turned to internal medicine, finding that: clerkships at the Baptist hospital were well-conducted, with students always on call and promptly working up new cases; the students were successfully taught from the first that they had a professional responsibility to the patient; histories were "excellent" and patient workups were "good," with progress written by students being "the rule" (no other department received such praise); that surgery needed more beds when the hospital was expanded; that the hospital's pediatric material was inadequate though "good use" was made of such as was available; that pediatric clerkships were "well planned and supervised"; that the medical school library, "one of the weakest departments," had 6,101 volumes and received 217 periodicals and would have to be greatly expanded for the school to "achieve the position it seeks in medical education and research."

IT WAS CRITICAL THAT the school be formally accredited. Otherwise the medical students might not be protected from the draft.[153] Despite the criticisms, the accreditation continued without even the mention of probation. The school was facing a crisis. The accreditation report served as a catalyst to a series of letters within the department.

On December 10, 1943, addressing him as "Dr. Carpenter" rather than "Coy," Tinsley wrote a more formal letter drawing on observations from his recent trip to Chicago and New York.[154] "I had occasion to see some of the problems which are confronting some of the other medical schools," he wrote, adding that he hoped his reflections would "help in preventing us from getting into the difficulties which seem to confront other institutions." Chief among Tinsley's reflections was that "many of the difficulties in medical schools are due to the tendency of the more senior members of the faculty to regard their positions as rewards for things accomplished rather than as opportunities for achievement." Another "cause of disagreement is the misunderstanding between individuals who are concerned primarily with rendering a service and those who believe that the function of a medical school is primarily to set a standard," and Tinsley made clear that he was among those who "hold the view that in the long run more can be accomplished, even in practical terms of actual service, by continuously concentrating on setting a high standard."

He then proposed that the Bowman Gray faculty consider two questions: Should the school concentrate on the "feet on the ground" approach or the "reach for the stars" philosophy? Depending on the consensus answer to the first question, then what should the organization be within the medical school? And he laid out three interesting possibilities, "each of which has certain advantages and certain disadvantages":

(a) The "state's rights" or "paddle-your-own-canoe" theory, in which "each man works to help the school, only through trying to build up his own department." This was the successful German method and, he said, the one in general use in the U.S. It gave department heads "great freedom to develop his own show," with minimum departmental conflict, minimum committee work, and maximum time for study and research. Its disadvantages were that it led to imbalance between the departments, "for the Dean . . . is naturally forced to aid most those departments which are accomplishing the most"; and it "almost inevitably leads to resentments and jealousies as the result of the competition between the various department heads."

(b) The "federalized" or "pull together" theory. This, Tinsley wrote, was "the only policy under which a well balanced, great school—outstanding in all departments—can be built." But there were serious disadvantages, including that "anybody's business is everybody's business" and that the concept cannot operate unless all of the department heads have common aims, common methods, and "a complete understanding of each other. Such a unanimity is theoretically possible but in practice one is not very like to find it."

(c) The "multiple confederated states" theory was, he wrote, "a compromise between the two previous concepts" that "had never been officially recognized but actually exists in many institutions." Under such a plan, department heads with similar aims and methods worked together, while those with a different shared set of aims and methods worked together. The obvious disadvantage was that politics might become more important than policies. However, he said, "it is perfectly possible to operate an institution with groups and cliques" if every department head understands the situation and is free to join any clique or to remain a "state's righter."

Tinsley noted that Bowman Gray had not deliberately adopted any organization type. "It seems to me that we would profit by having a settled policy in this regard, and I personally would be perfectly happy to proceed under any of the three types of organization mentioned."

Next Tinsley delved into another matter which he felt should be clarified—an institution's obligation to faculty members and vice versa. "It so happens that on my recent trip I had several long conversations with an intimate friend who has recently resigned his position at one of the leading medical schools.[155] We discussed

faculty, somewhat comparable to the term "Professor Ordinarius" in Europe. In essence the school pays the "full-time" or "regular" faculty a *retainer* to function as teachers, clinicians, investigators, and increasingly administrators, all of which involve considerable amounts of travel, thus stimulating the question, "Full time where?"

146. Ibid., 528.

147. Whether this trip had anything to do with Katie Dodd's upcoming move to Cincinnati is not known. Probably not, but no other records were found regarding this trip in Harrison's files.

148. Tinsley Harrison to Alfred Blalock, November 27, 1943. Chesney Archives, JHMI.

149. Tinsley Harrison to James I. Wendell, January 9, 1944. Chesney Medical Archives, JHMI.

150. *N. Carol. Med. J.* 4 (1943): 528.

151. Meads, *Miracle*, 28.

152. Morris Fishbein, *A History of the American Medical Association 1847 to 1947* (Philadelphia: W. B.

Saunders Co., 1947),
913. The inspection
was one of the first
carried out by the new
Liaison Committee
on Medical Educa-
tion, formed in 1942
by the cooperative
efforts of the AMA
and the AAMC. Dr.
Fred C. Zapffe was the
long-time secretary of
the AMA. Dr. Victor
Johnson was secretary
of the AMA's Council
on Medical Education
and Hospitals (488).
Zapffe had served in
the AAMC posi-
tion for many years
and was apparently
the exception to the
general severe criticism
leveled at Wake Forest
by leaders in medical
education for even un-
dertaking the project
to build the Bowman
Gray medical school
in 1940 (Carpenter,
Story, 29).

153. Meads, *Miracle*,
32.

154. Tinsley Harrison
to Coy C. Carpenter,
December 10, 1943,
Dorothy Carpenter
Medical Archives,
BGSM.

155. This was prob-
ably Bill Dock, who
never seemed to settle
down in one place for
long.

156. Advisory Council
Minutes, December
27, 1943, Dorothy

in considerable detail the general problem of the faculty members' obligations in this regard. One might perhaps adopt the attitude that a faculty member is justi- fied in resigning his position" when "his aim has been achieved"; when convinced that his aim can't be achieved under existing circumstances; when "he personally realizes that he is not filling his job"; when a better opportunity arises; or when personal issues intervene.

In any case, he told Carpenter, perhaps the school would profit by a "definite stand on the matters which have been discussed," especially before any large ad- ditional funding was forthcoming, lest such support prove an "Apple of Discord" rather than a "Horn of Plenty."

ON DECEMBER 27 CARPENTER called another meeting of the advisory council and recommended that it be enlarged to 12 members, including most department heads. This was approved. Dr. C. W. Sensenbach was added to the department of medi- cine faculty, and it was announced that the first meeting of the enlarged advisory council would be January 6, 1944.[156] In a separate memorandum Carpenter asked the enlarged council to meet at the Robert E. Lee Hotel at 6:30 for a "Dutch Din- ner," to expect to stay till 10 P.M., and to bring four categories of information: (1) a list of "the teaching personnel in your department, giving the exact assignment of each man"; (2) research projects actually under way; (3) articles published "last session"; and (4) "Outline briefly (not over one typewritten page) the ideas of your staff on things that should claim our immediate attention to improve our scientific, professional and educational program."[157]

Tinsley had dictated another long letter to Carpenter before receiving on the 31st Carpenter's memo of the 27th, again in formal language about distribution and use of private beds in the Baptist Hospital, a topic sure to be inflammatory. He reviewed for one and a half single-spaced pages the problems of obtaining adequate patients to give good teaching experiences to the medical students in the face of inadequate facilities and teaching personnel, now aggravated by the increased size of the fourth- and especially third-year classes.

He went on to detail the inadequacies of the long-term chronic patients in the county hospital, attempts at "more efficient use of the patients in the Medical Out-Patient Department of the Baptist Hospital," which he calculated could absorb only two students at most, and even then there were too few teachers for good supervision and teaching. Increased reliance on the patients in the PDC "was tried last year and proved to be entirely unsatisfactory both from the standpoints of the teachers and the students and I suspect from the standpoint of the patients." He would much prefer to have the senior students live in the hospital and function as rotating interns,[158] but he thought that only a few of their senior students as then trained would be capable of handling the clinical situations they would encounter, of supervising the junior students, etc.

The final possible source of clinical material for the fourth-year students in internal medicine is the private service. This plan has now been on trial for a full academic year. It has not only worked well but has worked far better than any of us had anticipated it might. It has been pleasing to the teachers and excellent for the students. Insofar as I know it has been also very satisfactory for the patients who are enabled by it to have more individual attention from men of professional status than they otherwise would have. Under this plan the students have had an intimate and almost preceptor relationship with one of our own teachers. However, we are now reaching a point where the supply of private patients is not adequate for the educational program of fourth-year students.

Tinsley then reviewed the hospital statistics, service by service, and noted that on average only 13 percent of the private beds were internal medicine's (16 of 123). His final paragraph asked that a fourth of private beds be assigned for medical cases at all times, but not on any rigid system. "In this way it will be possible, I believe, to meet more adequately the educational needs of the institution."[159] This must have been discussed with others, especially Bradshaw with regard to the surgical service and Frank Lock of obstetrics/gynecology. We can imagine the response: Did Harrison not realize that most of the private income of these doctors was from private patients, while he was fully salaried and did not even participate in care of the private patients on an ongoing basis—as "the doctor of record"—but only as a consultant?[160] And who would actually provide the day-to-day care of these increased numbers of private medical patients, if Tinsley did not participate but did so only for the service patients? For most of the staff, Tinsley's ideas were hard to take.

In any case, on December 31, Tinsley had dictated his letter about allocation of beds in the hospital, then he received Carpenter's request for information to be gathered in preparation for the advisory council meeting on January 6. To that memo, he responded that within a few hours he was going out of town for four to

Carpenter Medical Archives, BGSM.

157. Coy C. Carpenter, memorandum to Advisory Council, December 31, 1943, Dorothy Carpenter Medical Archives, BGSM.

158. Harrison did not seem concerned about the legality of medical students writing orders on patients. Perhaps he had a plan for such orders to be countersigned by residents, but none was discussed in writing. On the other hand, some medical schools (e.g., Northwestern) did not award the M.D. degree until completion of the internship in those days.

159. Harrison, December 31, 1943. He attached to this letter a chart of the hospital's patient data from October 1, 1942 through September 30, 1942. This chart of total private bed capacity of the hospital including all services shown was 123. When one considers the conventional wisdom and probable fact of those days that most of the patients seen by most of the doctors are those in internal medicine, Harrison would seem to have had a point. If one adds

together the surgical specialties (surgery, urology, orthopedics, and EENT), that totals 57 beds; or, with gynecology often considered a surgical discipline, 62 beds, or more than half in the hospital, even though medicine had the largest number of discharges. Obviously, without more details there were many ways to interpret these data. Perhaps the internists were hospitalizing trivial or investigational patients who did not really need to be hospitalized. More likely they were discharging them too quickly because of the lack of beds and pressures from the emergency room and outpatient department. From the standpoint of the doctors on other services, it was their income one was discussing. See "1942 Baptist Hospital Patient Data" at www.newsouthbooks.com/tinsleyharrison/supplement for a copy of this table.

160. Harrell, April 1993. It is also likely that the others had at least an inkling that Harrison's school-derived salary was much higher than theirs—in fact, twice that of the chief of

five days and thus could not compile the requested information but instead would send a letter setting forth his ideas "on things that should claim our immediate attention to improve our scientific, professional and educational program."

Further, he told Carpenter, he was asking Dr. John Williams to take his letter to each member of the department of medicine (Johnson, Grollman, Robert McMillan, Elbert MacMillan, and Harrell) and explain that each was not only free but had a duty "to express disagreement with these ideas, in case he feels such a disagreement. It is my urgent desire that each man in the Department express himself freely and frankly . . . it seems to me that all members of the faculty, including those in the Department of Medicine, should speak now or hold their peace forever on the question of what is needed to improve the institution." Tinsley's memo and the responses to it from the members of his department would then be submitted to Carpenter before the January 6 memo.

Having laid the groundwork, Tinsley then dictated his own response to Carpenter's core question. His first point was no surprise: "We should aim to become the best medical school in the world and thereby fit ourselves to be worthy of additional funds, if they are forthcoming, and of spending the available funds for the highest objectives, even if additional funds are not forthcoming."

He then goes on to list to list other points—to supply physicians for the region "to practice the medicine of 1970 rather than that of 1900," to train some to be leaders in medicine, to concentrate on doing a few things "superlatively well" rather than many in a mediocre fashion. He closes with two vital objectives:

(a) "To attract and train the ablest young intellects in American medicine for our faculty and the cream of the young men in the general locality for our student body."

(b) Excepting the dean and the registrar, who were largely administrators, "every single individual on the faculty should stimulate the students to study that which is known by setting a personal example in studying the unknown, i.e., by research." The quantity of research might vary, but the quality should be universally high and "no amount of teaching or administrative duties should . . . be allowed to interfere with this vital and primary function . . . The acquisition of new knowledge of the unknown, whether obtained by complicated laboratory methods or by simple clinical procedures, should be regarded as the first obligation of the faculty just as the acquisition of knowledge of the known is the first obligation of the student."

If those two simple principles were followed, Tinsley wrote, all other goals would follow "as the day follows the night."

OTHER MEMBERS OF THE department of medicine duly sent their letters. Grollman agreed except that he thought the dean and registrar should have experience in research, that there is a place on the faculty for some who "make no pretension at doing research," and that engaging in research is something that must come from within a person and cannot be coerced from without. John Williams's "Dear Tinsley" is a warm letter and is "in hearty accord with your desires to make this the best medical school in the world, and agree with you that in order to make it so every one in the school must have the scientific approach to medicine and be interested in research." Williams worried that their school at that time had low morale. With Grollman, he felt that the administrators, like the rest of the faculty, should have research experience but that research cannot be the sole criterion for selecting clinical teachers. But he, Wingate Johnson, and George Harrell—"no single factor would hinder the progress of our school more than a 'gag rule' on . . . the faculty"—worried that statements such as Tinsley's "speak now or hold their peace forever" were made in haste and contributed to low morale. Robert McMillan[161] agreed in general but worried that "the fact remains that our entering classes have not been up to the standard which we all desire. . . . a curriculum [should] be adopted and adhered to for a long enough period of time to allow the Faculty and Students to become accustomed to it, and so to determine its effectiveness."

Tinsley's tendency to push for changes and ad hoc solutions was even this early seen as perhaps excessive and leading to an erratic non-schedule. The neurologist/psychiatrist was concerned with a paralyzing lack of sufficient faculty for the tasks to be accomplished.

Harrell wrote a brief letter in which he agreed with most of Tinsley's objectives, but dissented "from the opinion that superior training for the students will automatically follow the extensive pursuit of research by the faculty. This is not the sole factor concerned in education.

The response of Wingate Johnson is interesting and marks him as the statesman he was considered. He agreed with Tinsley but qualified his response to define research more broadly—"I consider that any alert practitioner whose intellectual curiosity stimulates him to study unusual manifestations of disease or unusual reactions to therapeutic agents in his patients is engaged in research as well as the one who works in the laboratory. I believe that the men connected with our department, and the men that we want for it in the future, have this inquiring type of mind."

These responses were collected by Williams and taken to Carpenter's office

surgery. Harrell later claimed that "the dean didn't even know how much Tinsley made, since he did not have the data from the consultations." This seems possible, but, given Harrison's tendency to tell Carpenter these amounts (cf. previous letter on budget with "contingent" amounts), it seems unlikely that Carpenter was denied the data if he wanted it.

161. Robert L. McMillan was not a full-time faculty member, but he was "part-time" (i.e., in addition to being a member of the PDC he received a salary from the medical school for specific duties, including running the heart station). Elbert A. MacMillan held a similar faculty status and was the school's sole teacher for neurology and psychiatry.

162. Harrison's telegram was sent at 6:31 P.M. and arrived in Baltimore at 7:04, and it probably reached Blalock within a half-hour after that. Unless Blalock had a FAX in his house or read his e-mail at frequent intervals, this is better than could be accomplished in the late 1990s without using the telephone.

163. Riven, *Worthy*, 30, 32.

164. C. W. Sensenbach to Dr. J. R. Williams Jr., January 6, 1944, Dorothy Carpenter Medical Archives, BGSM.

165. Minutes of Advisory Council Meeting, January 6, 1944, Dorothy Carpenter Medical Archives, BGSM. Present in the preliminary meeting were: C. C. Carpenter, Dean (and Pathology); Frank R. Lock, Obstetrics/Gynecology; Robert P. Morehead, Pathology; John R. Williams, Medicine; Elbert MacMillan, Medicine; Edward S. King, Bacteriology; Herbert M. Vann, Anatomy; Wingate M. Johnson, Medicine (and PDC); Leroy J. Butler, Pediatrics; James P. Rousseau, Radiology; Howard H. Bradshaw,

on the sixth. Carl Sensenbach prepared answers to the first three of Carpenter's questions.

On the evening of January 3, 1944, Tinsley wired Blalock from New York: "Everything fine here will probably have supper with you Wednesday will wire later + T. R. Harrison."[162]

On Thursday the 6th, Blalock wrote Tinsley expressing pleasure at the previous evening's dinner and delight that Randolph's situation had improved, but cautioning that "I know that you have been under a tremendous strain and I hope that you will try to settle down now to a more normal existence with fewer worries. There is a limit to the time that any mechanism can withstand such high pressure."

Sam Riven, Tinsley's internist colleague and friend from Vanderbilt in the 1930s has made pertinent observations: "Harrison settled in at [Vanderbilt]—or rather, he unsettled things there, by the energy of his work and by the quirkiness of his personality. . . . Some people as unusually gifted as Tinsley adopt conservative outward habits . . . . Others, being perhaps less secure at some fundamental level of personality, create situations where they can take the lead, demonstrate their gifts, be seen and heard. For whatever reason, Tinsley was more like this last. If I did not always understand him, this I know: his eccentricity had a real innocence to it. In the end, he seems to me an extremely gifted, fundamentally good man, but one who was *sui generis*."[163]

This assessment seems accurate. Tinsley was certainly at times erratic, and he could be pettily demanding on occasion, but he was basically a decent person and man of good will who thought well and spoke well of colleagues, even those he criticized. While he may have recognized the political and financial realities around him, they obviously did not strike him as of first priority.

His ambition and his work ethic, his unwillingness to compromise, these things hurt him at Wake Forest.

On Thursday the 6th, Tinsley arrived later at the office than usual, around 7:30 A.M., and went about the day's work. He discussed with Sensenbach the proposed schedule changes for the fourth-year class and agreed that the students be permitted to remain at the county hospital the entire day on Tuesdays and Thursdays. He insisted that the students were "absolutely required" to attend the course in tropical medicine and Dr. Grollman's course in applied physiology and biochemistry, that the courses on Mondays, Wednesdays, and Fridays be given at certain specified hours, and similar matters.[164]

At 6:30 that evening he went to the Robert E. Lee Hotel for the meeting of the advisory council. Tinsley, probably without supper, waited outside Room 102 while the others had a "preliminary discussion." The minutes of that meeting[165] make it clear that the preliminaries, from which he was absent per mutual agreement with Carpenter, were about resentments which some faculty had built up toward Tinsley based on the belief that he had been given special privileges to develop policy, that he was too critical of the research of younger men, and that he interfered with other departments. Carpenter and Johnson responded that Tinsley had no such special privileges, with Carpenter saying he was "unalterably opposed to so-called one man institutions." Tinsley's December 10 letter was read on the three types of institutional organization, an institution's obligations to faculty, and when a faculty member could quit.

There was additional discussion and a motion was passed that "until such a time as a general policy is adopted, all members of the faculty should concern themselves only with the affairs of their own department and individuals of their department."

Tinsley was then invited into the meeting and the motion was read to him and the meeting opened to discussion of general school policies, including class size and the issue, raised by Dr. Wells, of "whether we really mean" it when "insisting we try to make this the best medical school in the world." This led to a response by Carpenter that "we do not expect to make this the best school in the world in one generation, but try to make it as good as we can."

Tinsley responded to that with a motion, seconded by Johnson, that "in [the] future every promotion or appointment be on the basis of aiming to make this the best medical school in the world." A motion to table Tinsley's motion passed 7–6. There were 14 present, including Dean Carpenter; so the 7 to 6 split must have seemed to Carpenter just the sort of polarized faculty mess deans dream of—in nightmares.

Then there was some drama, with Tinsley saying he would resign and getting up to leave, Moorehead and others insisting he return, which he did, Butler explaining that the motion to table was a sign of unreadiness, not opposition, and Tinsley apologizing for "intellectually" losing his temper.

The meeting then sputtered out. A Tinsley motion that the "policy of the school be that each department work for the school by the method of trying to develop

Surgery; George T. Harrell, Preventive Medicine; Camillo Artom, Biochemistry; Herbert S. Wells, Ph.D., Physiology & Pharmacology. All are M.D.s except for Wells. See "Advisory Council Minutes" at www.newsouthbooks.com/tinsleyharrison/supplement for Dr. Pittman's copy of this lengthy document.

166.　Carpenter, memorandum, January 12, 1944. "The following men are directed to attend a meeting in Room 404 at 4:30 o'clock this afternoon. I am asking Mrs. Smith to take this notice personally to each of you. Please sign your name to this notice if you will be present. If you will not be present, write me a letter giving me your reason." The memo was addressed to: Dr. Camillo Artom, Dr. Howard H. Bradshaw, Dr. Arthur Grollman, Dr. William Fishman, Dr. George Harell, Dr. T. R. Harrison, Dr. Edward King, Dr. Robert Lawson, Dr. Frank Lock, Dr. J. Max Little, Dr. Robert P. Morehead, Dr. James O'Neill, Dr. W. C. Thomas, Dr. Herbert Vann, Dr. John Williams, Dr. William Wolff, Dr. Herbert Wells. See www.newsouthbooks. com/tinsleyharrison/ supplement for the full statement.

167. A. Grollman and C. Rule, "Experimentally induced hypertension in parabiotic rats," *Am. J Physiol.* 138 (1943): 587. That is, two rats that have been joined surgically, usually along the

its own department according to its own department's ideas and ideals" failed to get a second. There was some unresolved discussion of a candidate for a position in anatomy, and an update by Carpenter on the possibility of purchasing the old Baptist Hospital and the potential uses of it. Then the meeting adjourned.

ON JANUARY 12, CARPENTER sent a memorandum to 17 of the faculty, including 10 who had been at the January 6 meeting, directing them to attend a meeting in Room 404 of the medical school at 4:30 that afternoon. He attached or handed out at the meeting a statement asking that they stop "the use of *supposition* as *fact*," stop gossiping, and get back to work.[166] Carpenter's statement seemed in some ways to support Tinsley's vision for the school, but he also emphasized the absolute need for teamwork, advised the faculty that they knew the "aims, objects and policies of the school" when they became faculty members, and said that if they now disagreed with those they should move on to other jobs. Tinsley must have felt this to be somewhat ambiguous but perhaps aimed at least in part at him.

Tinsley's department listed nine research publications for 1943, with him as author or co-author on five, including two on the renal pressor and anti-pressor factors. Grollman published a paper demonstrating experimentally induced hypertension in parabiotic rats,[167] thus demonstrating some factor circulating from the experimental rat to the one attached only by transplanted blood vessels and proving that a humoral factor is involved. Wingate Johnson published a paper on the use of niacin in treating Vincent's infections. This list did not include more than a dozen papers primarily of educational value or CPCs, and so on. It was a respectable performance and far better than that of any other department. But at Vanderbilt, Tinsley had never been aware of the sort of administrative verbiage now going on. His academic successes were being overshadowed by the interdepartmental infighting.

On January 14, Tinsley wrote asking Blalock to take Randolph into his house over Easter. He added a postscript relating to his and Blalock's earlier exchange about radiology: ". . . after talking the thing over with several faculty members we decided to try to get some information as to how much the average doctor in the state of North Carolina has occasion to interpret X-ray pictures before we make any decision as to the place of radiology in the curriculum. It will take a good many months, of course, to secure this information and will not be very accurate, with so many men out. However, I do have a strong feeling that radiology should be one of the really important clinical subjects and if you want me to write my own impressions about it directly and the reasons why I think it should be taught, I would be very glad to do so."

On January 19, Tinsley again wrote Blalock to say that he had been asked by the program committee of the local county medical society to invite him to make a talk at one of their meetings during the spring. Tinsley suggested April, as that was usually the prettiest month of the year in Winston-Salem, except for October.[168] He urged that Al bring Mary and stay a few days "to show you what is going on and to get your reaction and advice about a good many things." There was no mention of golf.

On January 27, Blalock wrote back accepting the April invitation to speak to the local medical society and to visit the Harrisons. But events were now moving quickly. In mid-February, Blalock expressed doubts about the visit planned to Winston-Salem, since perhaps "you will have changed your residence by that time." He also asked for a photograph—"one of those which make you look like Clark Gable."

Carpenter prepared an eight-page memorandum dated February 15 titled: "The Aims, Objects, and Policies of the Bowman Gray School of Medicine," to be read and distributed at a general faculty meeting on March 3. He discussed "Scientific Attitude and Attainment"; "Compensation for Achievement"; "Faculty Additions and Promotions"; "Salaries"; "Students and Scholarships"; and "The Kind of School We Want." With regard to the last he said: "It does not appear reasonable that any faculty member would want anything but the best. One can shoot low enough while aiming at the top. If the aim is lower, we may reasonably expect the shot to go lower."

But it was too late.

On February 22, Carpenter wrote President Kitchin about Tinsley's looking at a medical school position in Texas at the Southwestern Medical Foundation Medical School. He told Kitchin, "Of course, the first question you will ask and that I ask myself is what effect will Dr. Harrison's going have on us? We realize that it will be a loss from the standpoint of his ability and reputation as a physician. It will not hurt us as a school from the standpoint of education or our standing with other schools. I went over the matter with Zapffe, the AMA group, and other leaders in Chicago last week, and they all agreed that in the end we will be a better school by turning the direction of the Department of Medicine over to one of the younger men, although we will feel the immediate loss. From the standpoint of the school, further, we will save Dr. Harrison's salary and certain other expenses connected with the Department of Medicine. This money is very much needed at the present time

flanks, so that the two circulations become one.

168. Tinsley Harrison to Alfred Blalock, January 19, 1944, Dorothy Carpenter Medical Archives, BGSM.

169. Coy C. Carpenter to Dr. Thurman D. Kitchin, February 22, 1944, Dorothy Carpenter Medical Archives, BGSM.

170. Robert P. Morehead, audiotape. April 15, 1993, UAB Archives.

171. Tinsley Harrison to Alfred Blalock, March 2, 1994. Chesney Archives, JHMI.

in other places. So, we are all set to go right ahead if Dr. Harrison goes without adding anyone to take his place. You will, of course, be interested in knowing that Dr. Harrison assures us that his going is in no sense because of unhappiness here. He frankly says that he is very happy, and feels that this is one of the great schools of the country. His going is merely a matter of having an opportunity to do some things that he has wanted to do a long time in connection with radical changes in medical schools."[169]

Not everyone was as unconcerned about the loss as the dean. "Moose" Morehead, perhaps Tinsley's closest friend in the faculty aside from his own research colleagues, went immediately to Harrison's office on hearing that he might leave. Upon learning it was true and that he probably would leave, Moose, a husky ex-football player, could not control his feelings and broke into tears. "Why are you going? Damn you, don't go! Don't leave!"[170]

The morning of March 2, Harrison sent a telegram from Dallas, Texas, to Blalock:

> Thanks to you ten gallon hat wins write me South western Medical College = T R Harrison.[171]

9

Southwestern Medical College

Dallas, Texas, 1944–1950

Tinsley was indeed a teacher without peer, an outstanding medical investigator, and a superb clinician. But something about his personality enjoyed building a new program, and Southwestern looked like a place with promise, with better resources over the long haul, and a larger city and population base. Even so, Betty cried when they departed for Dallas,[1] as they both liked Winston-Salem and the friends and colleagues they were leaving behind. But the extreme lack of resources and the problems in organization and faculty seemed likely to continue at Bowman Gray for at least some years.

They packed their belongings, including Tinsley's library and papers, in two trucks for transportation to Texas. En route one of the trucks caught fire. The fire destroyed some of the papers and damaged some of the books. Many of the books were re-bound and saved. But the papers were gone, along with some of the furniture. These lost papers included much of the work that had gone into preparations for a planned third edition of *Failure of the Circulation* (see Chapter 7).[2]

As noted earlier, soon after he got to Dallas, Tinsley wired Blalock the news on March 2, 1944 (he had arrived the previous day). Al was not surprised and replied by post the same day. He wrote, "I knew all the time that you would accept this new position for it seems to me that it offers a tremendous opportunity. If you handle things properly, and I am confident that you will, I am sure that you can have the outstanding school in the South and probably in the country."

Al was in fact only a year older than Tinsley, but he wrote affectionately, "Since I am considerably older than you are, I am sure you will allow me to say that you

1. Hankins, audiotape.
2. Reichsman, personal communication.

223

should not act impulsively, that you should build slowly and carefully, that you should think in terms of having the best school not next year but ten years from now. This is some advice which Dr. Gregg [Alan Gregg of the Rockefeller Institute] gave me when I came to Hopkins and I am sure that he is correct.

"I know that you have a tremendous job with re-organization but I wish to continue to think of you as a Professor of Medicine and an investigator. Your two greatest talents lie in teaching and in research (particularly in stimulating research) and I hope that it will not be necessary for you to go for an extended period without carrying out these functions."

On March 8, Tinsley replied, on Southwestern Medical College letterhead from 2211 Oak Lawn Avenue, Dallas 4, Texas. Picking up on Al's age jibe, Tinsley began, "Dear Methusaleh: The very kind words of wisdom offered by the man with one hundred years of experience to the little infant embarking on an unknown sea are deeply appreciated."

He then leaped directly into the difficult demands facing him at his second new school in four years:

> At the moment I have three jobs, each of which is far more than I can possibly do. They are, respectively: Dean of the Faculty, which will be changed within a short time I hope to Chairman (There is a Dean of the Students working under me), Executive Professor of Experimental Medicine, and Professor of Medicine. I am now in the process of searching for an Executive Professor of Medicine, under whom I shall work. After two or three years have passed and I have managed to collect a good many professionals, I hope to be released from the job as captain and go back to pitching seriously in Experimental Medicine, which is my real love. However, you can be quite sure that I shall continue to do some experimental work come "hell or high water". . . .

However, Tinsley took prickly exception to Al's characterization of his "two greatest talents":

> While all this is going on you can be very sure that there is one thing above all else which will not be neglected—namely, contact with patients. I came into the medical picture originally as a doctor and expect to go out the same way. I resent strongly your statement that my so-called "greatest talents lie in teaching and in

research." What feeble abilities I may possess are much greater in the care of the sick than in any such relatively useless occupations as the ones you have mentioned.

Finally, Tinsley closed his somewhat manic reply to his lifelong friend and supporter by offering him a job—as assistant dean and/or resident in surgery.[3] What Al thought of this offer is not recorded, but he stayed put at Hopkins.

TINSLEY HAD SEEN THE physical facilities of the new medical school at Dallas during trips to the city, but they must have been a severe shock to the rest of the family. Their primitive condition was featured in a 1990 article in the British science journal *Nature*, which discussed the research excellence of the institution as the century closed.

If the facilities and resources at Bowman Gray had been constrained, those at Dallas were a calamity. They were plywood shacks hastily erected under the limitations of the war and scarcities of materials and equipment. The administrators had difficulties, for example, obtaining plumbing for the shacks and were able to do so only after special permission from the War Production Board.

The medical school buildings consisted of eight prefabricated military barracks-type structures 16 feet wide. Four of the buildings were 96 feet long and the other four 114 feet long.[4] In the winters, heat was inadequate and unprotected pipes often froze solid. In the summers, air conditioning was not yet even a consideration. Older physicians years later recalled "sweating over those greasy cadavers in the narrow little huts in the summer" when they were freshmen medical students.[5] The architecture was locally referred to as "hen house classic."[6] The plywood floors were only three-quarters of an inch thick, so fragile that within several years a heavy piece of equipment, or

3. Tinsley Harrison to Alfred Blalock, March 8, 1944. Chesney Archives, JHMI.

4. "Special Sunday Section," *Dallas Morning News*, May 30, 1943, SWMS.

5. T. J. Reeves, personal communication, January 10, 1993.

6. Chapman, *University*, 38.

The chairman's office at Southwestern when Tinsley arrived in 1944.

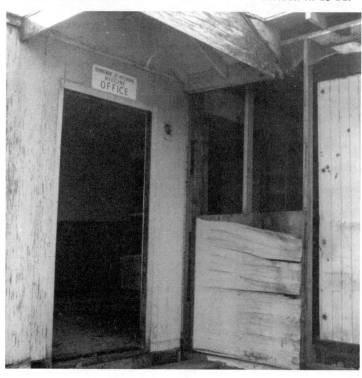

even the leg of a desk or chair, would occasionally pierce the thin floor and spill the occupant.[7]

While the prospect of adequate money may have looked bright in a future of uncertain distance, at Tinsley's arrival every scrap of resources was being consumed by the war effort, including money and people. The only source of funds was the Southwestern Medical Foundation, Inc., the local charitable organization formed in 1939 for the sole purpose of raising money to support the old Baylor medical school. Because of the newness of the foundation, and because it was the brainchild of the energetic Edward H. Cary, M.D., rather than based on wealth like the Rockefeller or Carnegie foundations, the SMF had to continuously fund-raise. Southwestern tried hard for Rockefeller money and support, but had not succeeded. Some of the faculty of the old Baylor medical school had left Dallas and moved to Houston to form the *new* Baylor medical school.[8]

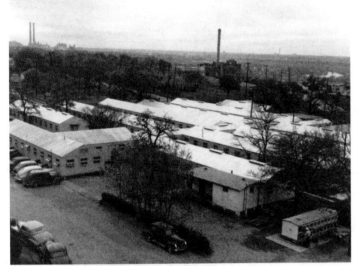

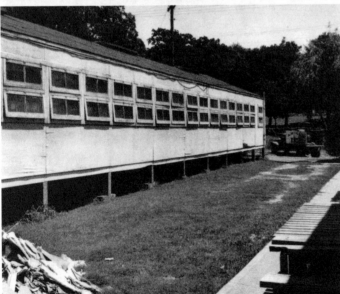

THE KEY FIGURE IN these developments was Edward Henry Cary. Born February 28, 1872, about four months after Groce Harrison Sr., at Chunnenugee Ridge near Union Springs in southeast Alabama, Cary's paternal family came from Bristol, England, via Virginia and Georgia to Alabama. They had a plantation in Alabama of more than 1,000 acres devoted chiefly to cotton—all destroyed in the course of the Civil War, or after it by marauding Union troops "traveling under the white banner of peace."[9]

During the Reconstruction years, Cary's father, a lawyer before the war, gave up law and moved the family to Missouri, Tennessee, Kansas, Georgia, and finally back to their old place in Alabama, where Edward was born. He was almost exactly the same age as Tinsley's father Groce and almost certainly had met him and might even have known him well, since Groce was president in 1938 of the state medical association, which worked closely with the AMA.

In 1891, Cary moved to Dallas to join his brother as a salesman of dental supplies, where he saved enough to get to the Bellevue Hospital Medical College in New York. After his M.D. in 1898 he interned at Bellevue then took special training in diseases of the eyes. Cary had suffered from vague eye trouble since childhood, and he wanted to understand what was wrong. He did not last long in his ophthalmology at Bellevue, because his brother died in Dallas and he returned to practice. He soon became dean at the University of Dallas Medical School. In 1903, at the AMA convention in New Orleans, he heard President Frank M. Billings say, "The vast majority of proprietary medical schools throughout the nation are doomed." Within five years, the AMA president predicted, no medical school could survive without university affiliation.[10] So Cary affiliated with Baylor College of Medicine, founded in 1900, the lineal ancestor of Southwestern. Chapman[11] and others[12] have described the situation in those days.

At the turn of the 20th century, medicine in Texas was as chaotic and splintered as elsewhere in the U.S.[13] There were dozens and dozens of schools, many underfunded, mismanaged, or under faulty leadership. "Dallas had its share of second-floor letter drops";[14] that is medical schools which were nothing but money-making diploma mills. One legitimate medical school, the University of Texas Medical Branch, at Galveston, had become part of the university in 1891, inaugurating a four-year curriculum in 1897. "By 1900 it was the single school in the state that could claim even modest distinction."[15] In Dallas alone there were at least eight medical schools founded during the first decade of the new century.[16] By 1910 Baylor Medical College had a four-year curriculum, a teaching hospital dedicated to its faculty and students, and most important of all a dean who knew the meaning of high standards and quality in medical education and had the intellect and personality to achieve it: Edward Cary.[17]

Supporting himself entirely from his growing medical practice, Cary guided the school through the Flexner review and report, obtained new facilities, achieved a Class A accreditation, and weathered the problems of World War I. In 1920 he gave up the deanship and turned entirely to medical practice, construction of a

7. Audiotape, meeting of medical students of the 1940s in office of George Race, M.D., Ph.D., Southwestern Medical School, January 25, 1993. Among those present were Drs. James Holman, Bryan Williams, and Howard Heuer.

8. Walter H. Moursund Sr., *A History of Baylor University College of Medicine 1900–1953* (Houston: Gulf Printing Co., 1956).

9. B. Mooney, *More than Armies: The Story of Edward H. Cary, M.D.* (Dallas: Mathis, Van Nort & Company, 1948), 20.

10. Ibid., 58.

11. Chapman, *University*, 3–8.

12. Moursund, *History*, 7–14. Samuel Wood Geiser, *Medical Education in Dallas 1900–1910* (Dallas: Southern Methodist Univ. Press, 1952).

13. Chapman, *University*, 5. "Texas Enjoyed One of the Worst Reputations in the Nation."

14. Ibid., 6.

15. Ibid., 5.

16. Moursund, *History*, 1.

17. Mooney, *More*.

18. James A. Pittman, "Meaning of the M.D. Degree from an Accredited Medical School," *Bulletin of the Federation of American Boards of Medical Examiners* (1994).

19. C. Schulze, "What Happened During 1943–1968," Dallas, Texas, 1971. Archives of University of Texas Southwestern Medical School, Dallas. Schulze's summaries are labeled as from the "Office of the Dean, 1948–71." It is not clear what her position was. Perhaps she was a secretary. If so, she must have been a wonderful one. Her summaries are superbly collected and arranged chronologically. Though they are telegraphic in style with few complete sentences, they are extremely well-written and apparently careful and accurate.

large doctors' office building in Dallas, and increasingly to the politics of "organized medicine"—the local medical society, the Southern Medical Association (based in Alabama and administered largely by Groce's close friend Dr. Seale Harris), and the AMA. Cary became president of the AMA in 1932. Above all else, Cary was a smart, energetic, and goal-oriented pragmatist. By the late 1930s he was wealthy, a director of an important local bank, and well established in the city of Dallas as well as in organized medicine. He saw his old medical school in trouble.

In 1938, perhaps as a result of the same pressures as had been applied to Wake Forest's two-year school, the Baylor medical school was under attack for low standards. It was placed on probation with the threat of withdrawal of accreditation. At this time state medical licensure laws had been strengthened to include two primary requirements: (1) graduation from an *approved* medical school; and (2) passing of the state licensure examination (often the National Board of Medical Examiners' test, which state licensing boards were increasingly accepting). If a school lost its AMA accreditation, its graduates could no longer obtain a license to practice, putting the school out of business.[18] Baylor/Southwestern's problems were largely financial, so Cary and a few friends established the Southwestern Medical Foundation.

DURING THE WORST OF the World War II deprivations, the Southwestern Medical College, though lacking in material resources, still had the essential ingredients of a four-year college, a teaching hospital, and a committed leader in Edward Cary. Now the school had hired a new dean and a new full time chief of medicine determined to establish the highest possible standards—Tinsley Harrison.

While Tinsley's move from Vanderbilt to Bowman Gray was anticipated by colleagues at both schools and was well-documented, much less is on the official record about Southwestern's offer and his acceptance.

Tinsley arrived in Dallas in March 1944, less than a year after the school was officially authorized by the Southwestern Medical Foundation—its only stable source of support. During that year, 1943–44, a great deal had been accomplished, spurred by the acceleration of the war. A campaign had been initiated to raise $1.7 million for a building fund on the outskirts of Dallas. Twenty acres of land had been acquired facing Harry Hines Boulevard. Sixteen members of the paid faculty, nearly everyone, all in the basic science departments, had remained despite the move of Baylor to Houston. The teaching faculty for the clinical departments had been private practitioners of Dallas and remained, as did the Baylor University Hospital, which simply dropped *University* from its title. Dr. Donald Slaughter, a pharmacologist, had been appointed acting dean and Cary had been appointed president. Parkland (the city-county hospital), Baylor, and Children's hospitals continued to be used for clinical training by practicing physicians. The prefabricated army barracks were erected and were being used for basic science teaching. On July 23, 1943, the first monthly payroll had been met ($10,621.90 for all 35 employees). Army and Navy contracts were prepared on August 17 to train doctors for the war effort and submitted immediately. The Army approved for all four years (due to the war, everything was done *imme-*

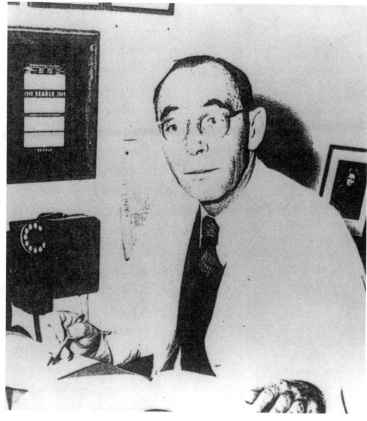

Tinsley in his Southwestern Department of Medicine office, 1944. The speak-through window is visible just above the telephone.

diately), and the unit (Army Specialized Training Program, or ASTP) was activated August 21. On the 27th, junior and senior students were inducted at nearby Camp Wolters and returned as Army trainees August 30. The Navy's V-12 Program was commissioned on September 27. These contracts afforded some measure of financial support for the school.

The school's organizational structure was beginning to look like traditional medical schools in northeastern and central parts of the country, as reflected in excellent summaries by Catherine Schulze in 1971.[19] Much of the material following was taken directly from those summaries, often verbatim. Additional full-time faculty members were recruited into basic science departments. Organizations were formed, including a Faculty Wives Club and six fraternities (one for women), plus one honorary scholastic fraternity. *Caduceus*, a student yearbook, was initiated. Edward H. Cary Lectureships were established "to bring outstanding scientists to Dallas each year to speak before the student body and the medical profession." A

20. The AMA had been the prime mover in making medicine more scientific since 1847, and especially after 1900—and in restricting the numbers of physicians produced in the U.S. We have met Zapffe before in this Harrison story, first at Wake Forest, then at Vanderbilt. This visit to Southwestern must have been one of the earliest made by the new LCME (Liaison Committee on Medical Education), formed in 1942 by appointees from both the AMA and AAMC, which unofficially merged into one body, previously operating separately. The LCME later was recognized by the federal government's Office of Institutional Eligibility for receiving grants, answering the question, What is a "medical school" or "college" eligible to be recognized financially? Thus, LCME recognition and approval became an instrument of the federal government.

Kellogg Loan fund of $10,000 was received, and a Markle Foundation grant was awarded for research on aging. In November the first full-time faculty member for the clinical departments was recruited, Dr. William Mengert, professor and chair of the department of obstetrics and gynecology.

All this effort and activity paid off. On December 15, 1943, the "Southwestern Medical College was given Class A accreditation on the basis of an inspection by Dr. Fred C. Zapffe of the Association of American Medical Colleges and Dr. Victor Johnson of the Council on Medical Education of the American Medical Association"—the 68th accredited medical school in the United States.[20]

On December 31 the Navy awarded its full approval for the V-12 program at Southwestern. Prior to this Navy program students had to move to Houston for their first two years, then back to Dallas for the third and fourth. By the beginning of 1944, with this problem rectified, the medical school was fully up and running. They just needed a dean and chief of medicine, among others.

It was in this atmosphere that Tinsley received the offer from Cary to become the dean and chairman and professor of medicine. His official title was "Dean of Faculty," and Donald Slaughter became "Dean of Students." Tinsley brought additional faculty with him from Vanderbilt and/or Bowman Gray: Arthur Grollman, a brilliant internist-biochemist-physiologist-pharmacologist, Morton Mason, a biochemist and clinical pathologist/lab diagnostics, and internists James Baxter, Joseph Crampton, and John Williamson.

Tinsley had been in Dallas less than a month when Southwestern held its first graduation exercise on March 20, 1944, at the nearby Alex Spence High School. Sixty-one students received M.D. degrees, 51 of whom entered military service. The commencement speaker was Morris Fishbein, M.D., editor-in-chief of the *Journal of the American Medical Association*, probably recruited by former AMA president Edward Cary.

IT IS DIFFICULT TO know what changes are attributable to the presence of Tinsley or to what degree, but they occurred. Tinsley remained Tinsley, and his fingerprints can be seen. Later that year, special public lectures were given jointly by the school and Parkland personnel. The home delivery program of Parkland Hospital was abolished. On July 1, Andres Goth arrived as assistant professor of physiology and pharmacology. New admission requirements and student selection procedures were adopted. The curriculum was revised, with bacteriology moved to the second year and lectures reduced in the clinical years with a concomitant increase in practical work with patients.

Harrison believed strongly in the admonitions of Thomas Sydenham, whom he often quoted, that medicine must be learned at the patient's bedside, not from books. Teaching programs were put in place in hospitals formerly used by practicing physicians solely for patient care, without interference from teaching. New procedures for student examinations and grading were put into effect. The overall effect was an upgrading of the standards of the medical school—higher standards—in all respects (except the physical plant). All these changes occurred before the end of 1944, despite family tragedies and disruptions at home and school, and the rationing problems of the war. Tinsley was certainly responsible for most if not all the changes aimed at increasing the quality and requirements for students, faculty, and programs. As the new, and first full-time dean of medicine, Tinsley held a lot of influence and control.

On the morning of Tuesday, October 24, 1944,[21] Tinsley had been working hard in Dallas for almost eight months. He left for work between 6 and 7, as usual. Around 10, back at home, Betty noticed two men in military uniforms approach the front door. They knocked, and she greeted them. They asked to enter, and she agreed. After they sat down, they broke the news: The eldest Harrison child, Woody, not yet quite 20 years old, had gone down at sea off the east coast of Florida while on a training mission in his Navy fighter plane, an F6F Grumman "Hellcat." There was nothing more to say. They had no further word; Woody was dead.

Betty telephoned Tinsley at work in the med school and broke the news. His response is not known, except that he stayed at work until that evening. Tinsley dealt with the immediate grief his way: he worked. Perhaps he was scheduled to give an important lecture for students with too little time to find a replacement, perhaps he

21. This date is not certain but it is family members' best guess today. Attempts to obtain details from the U.S. Navy have been unsuccessful.

Portrait of the eldest Harrison child, Lemuel W. "Woody," who was killed in a naval training mission in 1944

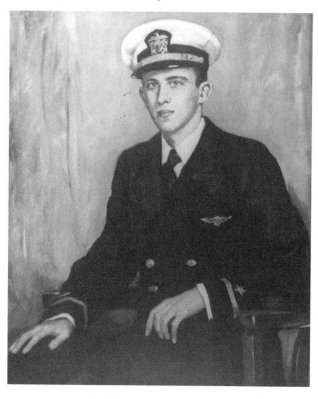

22. Emily Harrison to Tinsley Harrison, Nov. 6, 1944, UAB Archives.
23. Howard Rasmussen, M.D., personal communication.

worked an ongoing important dog experiment with scarce substances. Betty was left for the rest of the day to worry and grieve alone, and she never really forgave him for that.

Mimi, the oldest daughter and the child with a personality most like Tinsley's, was at that time a student at Rollins College in Winter Park, Florida. She flew, with Mrs. Ames, a lady friend and probably a school official, to Vero Beach, at the invitation of Woody's base commander.

She was treated with kindness. She met with other fliers, and Commander Harmer personally flew her out over the Atlantic on another search—fruitless as the others. On November 6, she wrote Tinsley to provide what details were known: Woody's squadron had been returning from a training flight to the Bahama Islands. A mere 15 minutes flying time from the base, Woody had radioed his wing man, Sullivan, that he was having engine trouble and was losing altitude. Sullivan saw Woody glide smoothly to a water landing—despite rough seas—climb out onto the wing, and inflate his life raft. Sullivan then flew for help and led some patrol boats back to the spot, but Woody was not found. Then and over the next few days, the Navy sent planes, blimps, and boats to search. But despite seven days' supplies on the raft, and three bottles of sea-staining yellow ink to aid in sightings, Woody was gone.[22]

The sea had remained rough for days after the incident, and perhaps the raft blew away from him before he could lash himself to it. He may have drowned minutes after he was last seen. It could have been sharks. We will never know.

This was a major blow to the family. Woody had always been the model child, always well behaved, an excellent student, a good athlete, the firstborn and probably the unconscious favorite. Shortly before he disappeared, he had told Mimi he thought he would try to enter surgery, which she felt would make his father very happy. Now he was just a memory, a void.

TINSLEY AND THE REST of the family carried on. There was a war going on, a medical school to build, students to educate for duty in the war, research programs to be built, money to be raised. Sad and disruptive as Woody's loss was to his family, he was one of a million American casualties, including more than 400,000 deaths. When Woody went down, MacArthur had only just made his promised return to the Phillipines. The Battle of the Bulge was still two months ahead, in which American GIs would stand in the freezing mud, diarrhea running down their legs,[23] as they watched their friends fall and die while hastening Hitler's last gasp.

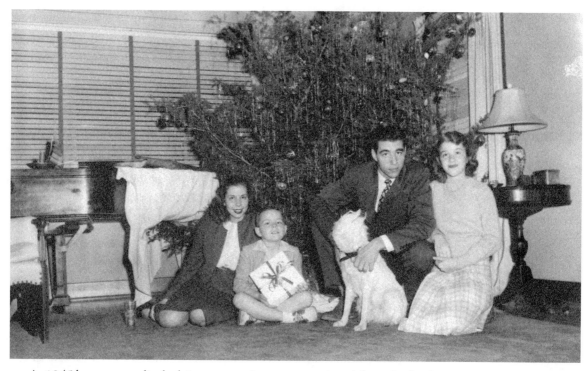

As 1945 began, a medical advisory committee was appointed from the faculty to advise the dean on such matters as private practice by full-time faculty. A business office building was completed (made from more "henhouse classic" Army barracks) in April, and starting in May salary checks were paid bimonthly. In April, policies regarding private practice were promulgated. Professors, associate professors, and assistant professors were permitted to see patients directly, by referral, or by consultation provided there was no interference with teaching, research, or service duties. There was to be an annual report to the dean of the income from this source, and the time was not to exceed a total of one day a week. As soon as facilities permitted, a total of 72 entering students was decided upon. The voters authorized construction of a new city-county hospital, to cost $7 million and be constructed after the war, but no site was designated and no funds were appropriated. Tinsley advocated a unified multidisciplinary center for the study of geriatrics, and $4,000 was received for the purpose from the Longview Foundation.

As usual, Tinsley was following his frenetic schedule of teaching, patient care, research, administration, juggling budgets, traveling to meetings, helping Cary raise funds, and generally trying to maintain the highest standards in the face of

The four younger Harrison children at Christmas, 1945. From left, Mimi, John, Randy, and Betsy.

24. R. H. Ferrell,
*The Dying President.
Franklin D. Roosevelt
1944–45* (Columbia:
University of Missouri
Press, 1998).

25. Hurst J. Willis,
"James Edgar Paullin:
Internist to Franklin
Delano Roosevelt, Os-
lerian, and Forgotten
Leader of American
Medicine," *Annals of
Int. Med.* 134 (2001):
428–431.

chronic shortages. Despite the limited resources and poor facilities, things were going reasonably well. Tinsley received the "Research Award" from the Southern Medical Association at its meeting in Cincinnati "in recognition of his outstanding contributions toward the elucidation of structural and functional aspects of cardiovascular disease and particularly of practical problems arising from failure of the circulation."

Meanwhile, FDR was desperately sick of a disease for which there was no effective treatment—hypertensive disease and renal failure.[24] On April 12, Roosevelt had a stroke while at his Warm Springs, Georgia, retreat south of Atlanta. Roosevelt's internist, James E. Paullin, chief of medicine at Emory, reached Warm Springs 90 minutes later and found Roosevelt's blood pressure to be more than 300/190 mm Hg.

> The president was in extremis when I reached him. He was in a cold sweat, ashy gray and breathing with difficulty. Numerous rhonchi in his chest. He was propped up in bed. His pupils were dilated and his hands were slightly cyanosed. Commander Howard Bruen had started artificial respiration. On examination his pulse was barely perceptible. I gave him an intracardiac dose of adrenalin in the hope that we might stimulate his heart to acting. However, his lungs were full of rales, both fine, medium, and coarse, and his blood pressure was not obtainable. There were no effects from the adrenalin except perhaps for two or three beats of the heart which did not continue. Within five minutes after my entrance into the room, all evidence of life had passed away.[25]

Vice President Harry Truman succeeded FDR. On April 28, Mussolini was killed by Italian partisans. Two days later, Hitler blew his brains out with a pistol. On May 7, Germany surrendered and the allied and Soviet troops bisected Germany. Meanwhile, the war with Japan continued.

On July 1, Southwestern held an open house for the first anniversary of its founding. About 2,000 attended and watched the first colored movies made by the department of medical art; the department had also designed a school seal.

On August 6, the atomic bomb was dropped on Hiroshima, turning thousands of souls into shadow and ash. Two days later another A-bomb was dropped on Nagasaki, and the Soviet Union declared war on Japan. On the 9th, Truman warned Japan, "Quit or be destroyed." The same day the Soviets attacked and invaded North Korea. On the 10th, Japan offered to surrender, and on the 15th, Japan formally did.

The war was officially over in both Europe and the Pacific. In New York, 100,000 workers were laid off as war contracts ended. Society now had to transition back to a peacetime economy.

AT SOUTHWESTERN, FURTHER CURRICULUM changes were made in all years, and correlation courses were emphasized. Teaching programs were developed at St. Paul and Methodist hospitals, and a master's degree in medical art was planned. In October there was an installation dinner for Sigma Xi, the student-faculty science society, and the Southwestern Medical Foundation announced a campaign to raise $1.3 million.

In November 1945, Southwestern decided to participate in the new medical care program of the Veterans Administration. Now that the war was over, personnel were more readily available to medical schools, including Southwestern. One of those released from the armed services was Ben Friedman, Tinsley's first research fellow at Vanderbilt in the early 1930s. Friedman had served in Europe with the 8th Army as a senior medical officer. After penicillin became available in 1943, he had been responsible for allocating the extremely limited supplies. His decision to give much of it to soldiers with gonorrhea or syphilis angered some of the regular army officers, but Friedman knew that if left untreated, these patients would spread the diseases to others and magnify the problem. After the war he returned to New York to resume civilian life in private practice with Dr. Oppenheim, but his old friend Tinsley had called him back to the academic life which was more to his liking. He became chief of medicine in the new McKinney Veterans Administration Hospital near Dallas, where he also held the position of clinical associate professor of medicine responsible for much of the teaching of third-year medicine—the first point when medical students assumed some responsibility for the care of live human patients. Friedman remained an excellent physician and exemplary teaching colleague for Tinsley and his steadfast friend as long as both lived.

Another full-time faculty member had arrived at Southwestern before Tinsley. This was William F. Mengert, the first full-time appointee in a clinical department, who arrived in November 1943 from Iowa, where he had been an associate professor. Mengert was also chief of obstetrics and gynecology at Parkland, the affiliated city/county hospital and an important clinical resource for students and residents. Upon arriving, he immediately encountered the turf and power struggles common in academic hierarchies. He had to compromise some of his own authority to begin

26. Schulze, "What Happened," 69.

27. J. D. Wilson, *Memories of Tinsley Harrison at Dallas*, video (2000; Birmingham), UAB Archives.

28. Moyer left after Tinsley in 1950 to further academic achievements as chief of surgery at Washington University School of Medicine and Barnes Hospital in St. Louis.

his work. "He learned at once that Dr. Lee Hudson, a local practitioner who had been chief of surgery and chief of staff at Parkland for many years, would have to be satisfied. Although Dr. Mengert had been appointed in charge of gynecology as well as obstetrics, he had to agree to take surgical residents for a three-month period of training in gynecology before he was permitted to assume his responsibilities at Parkland."[26] The Hopkins-trained Hudson was an able surgeon and politically amiable, but he had not been selected by the school administration. Hudson was not primarily a paid employee of the school; he regarded the school as something of a bother, an interference rather than a boon to teaching and elevating the quality of patient care. Hudson was not inclined to cooperate—especially when he could see no advantage to himself or his department of surgery. This slight clash with Mengert was a foretaste of more to come, mostly unrecorded except in the memories of old doctors.

After Tinsley arrived, Drs. James Baxter and Joseph Crampton, former students at Vanderbilt whom he had brought with him, devoted themselves primarily to improvement of patient care at Parkland and supervision of the students' clinical work there. At Tinsley's insistence, they also continued some research. Tinsley also brought from Vanderbilt Andres Goth, an M.D. from the University of Chile, as an assistant professor to help Donald Slaughter in pharmacology and physiology.

Dr. Franz Reichsman taught physical diagnosis to second-year students while supporting himself by helping in the care of aged and chronically ill patients in the city-county convalescent home, where he also lived. Reichsman's research was on pulmonary diseases in these days before antibiotics against tuberculosis.

Tinsley has been called a poor administrator. He certainly was disorganized, sometimes on purpose. He had little regard for schedules. He was prompt for his teaching and careful with his patient care duties. If he didn't like a schedule, however, he would change it arbitrarily to more to his liking, sometimes without warning those involved. He was willful and disregarded bureaucratic hierarchies. In the most important aspect of administration, Tinsley was truly outstanding: recruiting excellent faculty.[27] Tinsley was also skilled in keeping good faculty once they were recruited. He felt that loyalty is a two-way street: he was intensely loyal to his subordinates unless they were absolutely unworkable. He brought Carl Moyer from Michigan to become chief of experimental surgery.[28]

In late 1946, Tinsley, who had made clear his preference for the chief of medicine position from the beginning and did not enjoy the administrative fights with Parkland, resigned from the job of dean of faculty to devote himself entirely to clinical internal medicine, research, teaching, and the work he had now begun on what would become "his" book, *Principles of Internal Medicine*. His reputation in internal medicine and the budding specialty of cardiology was large. As was seen in Chapter 7, in addition to the demands of editing *PIM*, his time was also taken up by being repeatedly called on for other duties with professional and research organizations.

The constant pressures of deadlines and external obligations consumed Tinsley's attention, time, and energy through 1946, '47, and into '48.

There continued the hectic pace of daily patient care/teaching rounds on charity and indigent patients with the students and residents, CPCs, weekly or twice-weekly special patient presentations by students on the Chief's Rounds

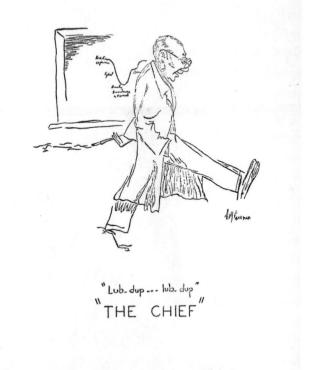

" Lub. dup ... lub. dup "
" THE CHIEF "

(FROM THE NOTE BOOK OF RAY FREEMAN-DALLAS-1948)

Med student Ray Freeman's sketch of Tinsley lecturing, with his characteristic vocalizations of a heart valve damaged by rheumatic fever sequelae, Dallas, about 1948.

(sit-down rounds more like conferences), endless administrative meetings often starting at 6:30 or 7 A.M. or during dutch-treat suppers at 7 P.M. or later, consultations on private patients, pushing the lab work as hard as possible, working with the research fellows and finding financial support for them, seeking private money for the lab itself in these days before much government funding, travel to national and local meetings, dealing with the presidency of the newly renovated American Heart Association and the new National Heart Institute, recruiting new or replacement faculty, lecturing to local medical groups, trying to balance the department's meager budget, trying to keep up on current literature and discoveries and medical opinions, and a myriad of other daily tasks, on and on, seemingly without end or respite. Everything had deadlines. Nothing could wait.

Southwestern was still on a flimsy financial and material foundation. The efforts to maintain and enhance it, along with the book, were draining Tinsley. He was exhausted. He never neglected a student, and only rarely his research. But he took

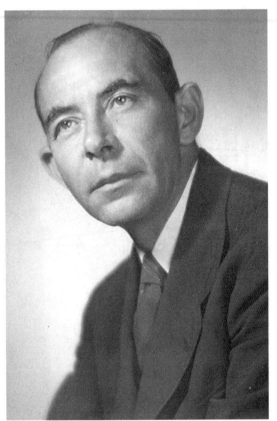

Tinsley Harrison,
about 1949.

his family for granted. After all, the family members were part of his life, part of him. His wife Betty felt alone. She found solace partly in the company of another, a certain Max of the Blakiston book company, which was to publish *PIM*. He was, unlike Tinsley, from New York, urbane, tall, and handsome. Tinsley increasingly sought relaxation in whiskey. Things became so strained that Betty proposed to move back to Nashville, where they had probably been happiest, and he talked of returning to private practice, perhaps doing part-time or volunteer teaching at Vanderbilt. He also talked of going to Knoxville, Tennessee, where the home campus of the University of Tennessee was located very near Oak Ridge. There he might be able to continue teaching, perhaps of residents only, in one of the excellent local hospitals, but especially he would be able to continue his real love, research, using the new atomic medicine at the medical division of ORINS, the Oak Ridge Institute of Nuclear Studies, headed by the hematologist Dr. Gould Andrews.

Meanwhile, his family was falling apart. In February 1949 Randy turned 21, inheriting $5,000. He immediately quit Hampden-Sydney College, bought a top-of-the-line Buick Roadmaster convertible, and drove it from Virginia to Dallas. On May 14, he married Evelyn Brown in Houston. As the turmoil in Dallas continued, 10-year-old John was sent in late August to Kennebunkport, Maine, to stay with Betty's oldest brother Ralph and his wife, Kay. There he entered (and completed) the fifth grade. In the fall, Betty moved to Nashville, rented an apartment, and enrolled 15-year-old Betsy as a day student in the Ward Belmont School, an upscale local private high school. Tinsley remained in Dallas in accord with his contract and lived in an apartment for the duration of 1949 and into 1950.

In addition to his personal problems, Tinsley had to contend with major problems and changes in the school, changes that would not have been to his liking even in the best of times.

As Southwestern's finances faltered toward total failure, Edward Cary and his colleagues saw their only salvation in the school's becoming part of the University of Texas, not an easy task in a state already skeptical that any good could come from government, and which in any case already had a state medical school, the University of Texas Medical Branch in Galveston, and the private Baylor medical school in Houston. Despite the odds, Cary's methodical political efforts succeeded. First he maneuvered passage, by a split vote, of a law by the Texas legislature to create another state medical school. Next followed a contest between various Texas cities each wanting the new school, to be determined by a vote of the House of Delegates of the Texas Medical Association. Again this was decided on a split vote, but by July 13, 1949, the matter was settled in favor of a second state medical school based in Dallas—Southwestern.[29] Though still a struggle, state financial support would be assured. The downside: the school would be required to accept classes of 100 students, which Tinsley said would make impossible the sort of intimate education between student and teacher which he advocated. It was just too many students, too big!

"Soon after Harrison learned that Southwestern would probably become a branch of the University of Texas with an entering class of 100, he submitted his resignation, stating as his reason that classes of 100 were simply too large. But perhaps of equal importance was the residential restriction that he very correctly anticipated."[30] Any personal problems, stemming largely from his near total devotion to medicine, were not mentioned in local announcements. But his decision to leave Dallas was firm.

The Dallas Southern Clinical Society expressed its admiration and appreciation for his service attempting to build a solid foundation for the medical school and to establish and maintain the highest possible standards by presenting him with "The Marchman Award for Outstanding Contributions to Medical Education."

Meanwhile, Tinsley gathered up his things, closed his office, and left. He was replaced by Charles Burnett as Southwestern's second professor and chairman of the Department of Medicine. Burnett was from Yale and soon recruited the young nephrologist, Donald Seldin, M.D., who would succeed him as the third chairman of medicine and would overshadow all other departmental chairs. Southwestern carried on, and over the years Tinsley was largely forgotten there.

29. Chapman, *University*, 52–53 & related notes.

30. Ibid., 53.

10

The Patient at Mid-century

The 1950s

Sometime in 1957, when the South was in racial turmoil and also the poorest section of the United States; a time when the first thing most wealthy citizens would do to get medical care was leave Birmingham, one of the nation's leading internists brought his wife to see Dr. Tinsley Harrison—now at the University of Alabama Medical School—for an examination concerning some obscure but severe chest pains she was having. This was Cecil J. Watson, chairman of the Department of Medicine at the University of Minnesota, one of the nation's leading medical schools. Why would Dr. Watson, originator of the Watson-Schwartz test for porphyria and knowledgeable about where the best medical care was to be found, bring his wife to Birmingham when he could have gone to Boston, New York, or even the Mayo Clinic just 80 miles away?[1]

The answer is that Tinsley was not only one of the world's greatest cardiologists of the time, but also a superb general internist, widely known to other internists to be one of the best anywhere. There was simply no better doctor to take her to.

This was the era of the Great Clinician, and Tinsley was one of the greatest. New procedures and tests were being developed, but they were not yet routine or standardized or reliable. A few years later, standardized exercise tests, cardiac angiograms, phonocardiograms, and the like would make the professor's murmur obsolete. But this was the time when the final word on whether the murmur was there or not was the professor. If he heard it, it was there. If he did not, it was not there.

Tinsley had several quirks in the way he practiced. He always liked to reproduce a symptom he could not explain. If a patient had faint spells with palpitations and

1. It is possible that the very last place he would take her was the Mayo Clinic, not only because of the competition between the two institutions, but also because neither would send patients to the other for fear of losing them—a common phenomenon among medical centers later.

shortness of breath, he would try to reproduce these by postulating hyperventilation syndrome, and making the patient breathe rapidly and deeply until something untoward happened or the symptoms were reproduced. Sometimes this required addition of a small amount of insulin, on the supposition that hypoglycemia might be involved. Sometimes a bit of atropine to speed the heart. If there was left upper quadrant pain, he might have a tube inserted to the splenic flexure of the colon then inflate that area to reproduce the pain. He was always careful and considerate, but he was famous for wanting to explain the symptoms.

Hospitalizations in the 1950s were less hurried, and much less expensive, than at the end of the century. When the time came for the discharge, Tinsley would take a few of his pupils from rounds—especially the house staff involved in the care of that patient, and seat himself on a chair beside the bed. He would then go over all the findings and test results with the patient, and perhaps the patient's spouse or children, and would give his opinions about the situation, what should be done about it—including medications, diet, activity, and other advice—all the while recording this on his dictaphone as a letter to the patient with a copy to the referring doctor. Sometimes he would dictate a separate letter to the doctor, with or without a copy to the patient. All this required time and a more leisurely pace than was possible late in the century with increasing masses of people.

ONE OF THE DISEASES conquered by mid-century was the malady that took the life of Susan Chambers, the woman in Chapter One near Talladega. She had coughed up blood and had not been well since her last pregnancy. She died after being taken by buggy to Birmingham; the autopsy had revealed a tumor throughout the lungs in which the tissue was very bloody. A the time, the pathologist (a part-time surgeon) had not known a name for it. Now in the mid-1950s the pathologists did have a name and knew the course of the disease—choriocarcinoma, also called gestational trophoblastic disease and by a variety of other names. The diesease was fatal when it had metastasized to the lungs. In the 1950s, the pathologist who probably knew most about this disease and the host of other tumors related to the chorion of pregnancy was Arthur Hertig of Harvard Medical School, a colleague of the gynecologist John Rock.

In the 1940s and '50s, Gertrude Elion and George Hitchings were working at the Burroughs Wellcome Company laboratories in the Research Triangle of Durham, Chapel Hill, and Raleigh in North Carolina. Elion and Hitchings had

2. B. A. Chabner and T. G. Roberts, "Chemotherapy and the War on Cancer," *Nature Reviews/Cancer* 5 (2005): 65–72.

3. M. C. Li, R. Hertz, and D. M. Bergenstal, "Therapy of Chorio-carcinoma and Related Trophoblastic Tumors with Folic Acid and Purine Antagonists," *New England J. Med.* 259 (1958): 66–74.

4. J. Laszlo, *The Cure of Childhood Leukemia. Into the Age of Miracles* (New Brunswick, NJ, 1995).

devised a series of nitrogen mustard gas-like compounds, which attacked several tumors of lymphatic tissues and a few other rapidly growing tumors. They worked at synthesizing antifolate and other compounds later found to be useful against certain cancers, and purine analogues such as 6-mercaptopurine.[2]

In 1954, Min Chiu Li, a naturalized American citizen, was working on cancer therapy at the Sloan Kettering Memorial Institute with the neurosurgeon Bronson Ray and the endocrinologist Rulon Rawson, who at that time were specializing in trying to cure or ameliorate cancers by ablating the pituitary, adrenals, ovaries, or any other area of the body. They had a patient they thought had metastatic melanoma, whom they were treating with methotrexate, which was apparently working dramatically. Being endocrinologists, they were collecting and measuring everything possible. Sometime in July 1955, Li moved to the NIH to serve his time in the service for the Korean Conflict (at the time, the fighting was not called a war). Imagine their surprise back at SKI when they found very high levels of HCG (human chorionic gonadotrophin, indistinguishable in their tests from the pituitary hormone FSH, follicle stimulating hormone). Upon reviewing the histology of the tumor, they concluded that it was not malignant melanoma, but a choriocarcinoma.

Roy Hertz's group at the NIH was in a perfect position to collect a good series of patients with metastatic choriocarcinoma, which might have otherwise been difficult to collect in one group, since they were not common. The NIH, with its new 500-bed Clinical Center—a public hospital devoted completely to clinical research—offered free care and treatment to patients with diseases of interest to the research doctors, many of whom, like Li, were serving military time in the Public Health Service. Hertz and Li were thus able to show that these agents could make the tumor masses literally fade away, so much so that there was a danger that a patient with extensive lung metastases might bleed dangerously from the lysing of the lesions. After the treatments, the lesions were often really gone, never to return.

They could cure this cancer![3]

TOWARD THE MIDDLE OF the century other advances were being made in chemotherapy, sometimes in connection with wartime studies in chemistry. Another area of success was childhood leukemia, uniformly fatal at the beginning of the 20th century when Tinsley first came on the scene. While the number of new cases rose as the population grew, the "deaths of children under the age of 15 with leukemia fell—the number of deaths changed from 2,140 in 1961 to 610 in 1991."[4]

As science and more careful clinical observations advanced with the 20th century, other successes in medicine occurred. Some beneficial treatments were devised for conditions that were not even recognized as diseases at the opening of the century. For example, once clinical workers could measure the arterial blood pressure in people, the *insurance companies* defined hypertensive diseases. Doctors realized that blood pressure could become chronically elevated in a number of abnormal states. In other words, there was no single cause of hypertension any more than there is one cause of cancer. Still, this chronic high blood pressure could be quite dangerous. Treatment could be beneficial.[5]

The patient seen by Dr. S. Richardson Hill in 1957 with hypertensive encephalopathy, complete with grand mal seizures, papilledema, a systolic pressure of more than 300 and diastolic to match, would surely have died had Dr. Hill not insisted that the surgeons remove the kidney which appeared abnormal on the intravenous pyelogram. With the kidney removed, the pressure returned to normal. The patient was discharged a healthy man. Around 1950, the only diuretic agents were the mercurials, Mercuhydrin and Mersalyl, which had to be given by injection, usually by a visiting nurse several times a week. The first orally effective antihypertensive agents began to appear in mid-century, such as hexamethonium in 1950, and the physiology of hypertensive disease and its effects became increasingly understood. By the end of the century almost half of all older Americans were taking antihypertensive drugs.

My original idea as a side story for this book was to trace the clinical appearance and understanding of each disease as it appeared in Chapter 1, the time of Tinsley's birth, to 1978 when he died. It is tempting for me to pursue the advances of each of the nearly 500 disease groups in the diagnosis related groups used for charging fees since 1983 even as new ailments are discovered—perhaps boring to some readers. For one who lived through most of the century close to the active spots of study and understanding, and who knew personally many of the participants, it is fascinating. There's much that is still not known. So many incredible thinkers, scholars, and doctors devoted their lives searching for understanding and cures. Nevertheless, it would require a multivolume encyclopedia by many, many authors to do a decent, thorough job. This isn't that book.

Some connections of Tinsley with the past are interesting. In this category was the occurrence of *worms* among many—not just a few, but many—of the adult patients in the VA Hospital in Birmingham as it opened in 1953. John Montgomery,

5. Postel-Vinay, Nicolas, ed., A *Century of Arterial Hypertension 1896–1996* (New York: John Wiley & Sons/Imhotep, 1996). The chronology on 192–95 gives a nice, if abbreviated, review of these advances. By 1994, according to Kaplan, 30 percent of all Americans from 55 to 64 years of age were taking an antihypertensive drug, and 40 percent of those from 65 to 74.

a medical student in the mid-1950s, was the champion worm finder in older rural veterans. As a third-year medical student in pursuit of a good grade he became a diligent worm hunter among the patients, usually older males from a rural setting. He found eggs, and sometimes adults, of hookworms, pinworms, strongyloides, ascaris, tapeworms, and others.

As time passed, many common problems disappeared. Gradually the black widow spider bites from outdoor privies disappeared (as did most but not all of the privies). The lead poisonings from bootleg whiskey made with automobile radiators also disappeared as more sophisticated methods of illicit distilling prevailed.

Tinsley had biases carried over from former times, such as one about initial treatment of late syphilis. He believed it should never be with penicillin alone. This belief was based on two patients he had had when penicillin first became available. Both had died, apparently of acute myocardial infarcts. He blamed these on the occurrence of Jarisch-Herxheimer reactions, the release of old antigens, swelling of the coronary ostia, and fatal heart attacks. A preliminary course of bismuth seemed preferable, as in the old days.

THE PROMOTION OF A useful clinical sign of disease, described by Tinsley's friend and co-editor of *PIM*, neurologist Raymond D. Adams of Harvard and the Massachusetts General Hospital, was one such clinical advance: the sign asterixis. This is the flapping tremor of the outstretched hands of a patient with impending hepatic coma, as described in a patient earlier in this text. Harrison saw such a patient on rounds just before he was to have a lung biopsy of a vascular malformation there. Tinsley saved the patient by recognizing the problem, by way of the flapping tremor, which had been missed by the other doctors.

Adams had recognized it in the early 1950s in an officer from the Charlestown Navy Yard across the Charles River from the MGH. Adams was able to do this because the officer had a particularly observant secretary who recognized that, when the officer's handwriting began to deteriorate, perhaps after an evening of heavy drinking with a large meal of beefsteak or other meat, he was headed for trouble and perhaps coma. He also had mild jaundice, so she sent him to Chester Jones, the liver specialist at the MGH. Jones noticed these jerking movements, and of course the patient was comatose, so he called Adams.

Adams suspected the underlying problem, essentially an Eck fistula, and wanted to confirm his suspicions, so he contacted Dr. Joseph Foley, another neurologist at the Boston City Hospital, where Adams had worked with Professor Derek Denny-Brown. The Boston City Hospital in those days had 2,800 beds, occupied largely by local derelicts, often winos who survived on a diet of cheap wine. These homeless drunks often sold blood for transfusions, thereby gaining $10 or $20, which they promptly spent on more wine. Hepatic cirrhosis was common in the BCH.

One weekend Adams and Foley spent Saturday afternoon making rounds on every patient they could find in the BCH, and asked each patient to hold out his hands for as long as he could keep his arms extended. They saw the flapping tremor in a substantial number of the patients; almost all had advanced liver disease. Foley had a friend who was a Catholic priest who knew Latin, and the priest suggested the term "asterixis" as appropriate for the clinical sign.[6] Thus, they had given clinical medicine a new clue of a serious underlying disease.

Or had they? In a wonderful article the hepatologist Adrian Reuben has described how asterixis or something like it was known to astute physicians from the time of Hippocrates or before, and how Shakespeare's Sir Andrew Aguecheek, "a minor player in *Twelfth Night* . . . [was] an alcoholic knight with chronic dementia and protein intolerance . . . a shallow fop, stupid, cowardly, and socially gauche, who exhibits fluctuating personality changes with occasional flashes of insight. 'Methinks sometimes I have no more wit than a Christian or an ordinary man. I am a great consumer of beef, and I believe that does harm to my wit.'"[7] Shakespeare and his contemporary physicians—remember, this was the time of Harvey and not long before Sydenham—must have been keen observers of clinical signs and symptoms, such as the irregular jerky movements of asterixis, and they recorded them. So Adams and Foley did indeed discover asterixis—it had just been discovered before. With no centralized system, the condition had been lost, forgotten, and then rediscovered and renamed. It is chilling to think that all of our medical knowledge and advances could be lost again.

TINSLEY WAS ABOVE ALL else a *teacher*. His most famous book was really only an extension of this. The book exemplifies the reasons why he was devoted to teaching.

Tinsley loved the subject and loved the students, the two essential criteria of being a good teacher. He was emphatic about this. Sometimes he took this beyond what most people would consider reason, as he promoted former students and fellows for faculty positions in another medical school or practice group, which he also did with great enthusiasm and energy.

6. R. D. Adams and J. M. Foley, "The Neurological Disorder Associated with Liver Disease," *Association for Research in Nervous and Mental Disease* 32 (1953): 198–237. See also M. Victor and R. D. Adams, "The Effect of Alcohol on the Nervous System," *Association for Research in Nervous and Mental Disease* 32 (1953): 526–73.

7. Adrian Reuben, "Landmarks in Hepatology: There is Nothin' Like a Dame," *Hepatology* 35 (2002): 983–85; William Shakespeare, *Twelfth Night*, Act I, Scene III.

8. On one occasion
McMannus had an
argument with a se-
nior resident about the
exact wording of Oc-
cam's Razor, an early
dictum important in
the development of
the scientific method.
McMannus proved
right.

Tinsley could take a lackadaisical, mediocre student and stimulate him to great accomplishments. Some of his students went on to become leaders in their fields and in other schools. Two were Dr. Joe Norman, who became chief of the pulmonary division of medicine at the University of Mississippi, and Dr. Sheldon Skinner, who became chairman of physiology at the Bowman Gray medical school in North Carolina. One former student, Dr. John T. Binion of Dallas, said Tinsley kept you believing you could do anything you want, and he stimulated you to want the very best. He would promote the careers of his students almost to the detriment of his own, and they would usually return the feeling and work ceaselessly to avoid disappointing him.

He knew his subject in great depth and breadth. He knew it cold. He knew not only the cardiology of the moment, but he knew the history of cardiology and had thought deeply about its probable future. He held tremendous knowledge of nearly every other topic in the modern medicine of his times, especially as he edited *PIM*. He was broadly knowledgeable in the humanities, especially English literature and European history, and he had a detailed knowledge of the history of medicine.

He had great natural histrionic abilities. In the 1950s, the chief of pathology, J. F. A. McMannus, originator of the Schiff-periodic acid stain and an excellent scholar well versed in Latin,[8] invited the well-known Canadian pathologist William Boyd to spend several of the coldest months of each year at the medical school in Birmingham, where he proved a popular teacher. Boyd occasionally poked fun at Tinsley in conferences for his "wonderful noises—you know, the swishes, whirrs, and whistles of cardiac murmurs, or the snores and groans of asthmatic wheezes one hears through a stethoscope, and so on." One former student said, "Harrison could make a great lecture out of a piece of old shoe leather!" Tinsley kept his audiences in rapt attention and got his points across in memorable style. He was always excited, enthusiastic, and fascinated by the subject as he explained it. He drew his audience in with him as participants in learning.

He was a master bedside teacher on rounds—in those days they really were rounds, in which several students and several residents would walk from patient to patient for several hours, usually during the morning. A student would present the history and physical findings, and sometimes the laboratory results. Then the teacher ("the attending physician" and the one with ultimate responsibility for the patient) would give his or her opinions and directions for further care of the patient. Attendings were all expected to write a note in the chart themselves, but otherwise they varied greatly in how they functioned. Some, such as the prominent gastroenterologist Chester Jones, of Harvard and the Mass General Hospital, would take the chart and write lengthy notes, then write orders in the chart themselves, sometimes without explaining much to the others. They were saved only by their recognized clinical excellence and abilities in treating patients. Others, such as Dr. Edward F. Bland, head of cardiology at the Mass General, always wrote just a two-word note: "I agree," after the notes by the student and the intern and resident, and signed it.

Tinsley did neither. He would listen only to the history, then he would examine the patient himself, often minutely, taking time to auscult the heart in particular with the patient in various positions. Then he would ask the presenter, the student or intern, what he/she had found. Next, they might discuss these findings. Then he would start with the person of lowest status in the group, perhaps a fourth- or even third-year student, and ask, "Well, Mr. Jones, what do you think is going on here?" Usually Jones wouldn't have a clue. So Tinsley would ask the intern; then the resident or fellow, then maybe even a faculty member on rounds that day. Tinsley might ask for the lab results at this point, but often not. After gathering all these opinions, Tinsley himself would deliver his opinions, always very clear, often with much historical background about the disease and patients like this one. He loved to predict lab results, such as the hematocrit or hemoglobin, and only then check his guess against the actual result. He was rarely far off the mark. (Tinsley's friend Raymond D. Adams, the prominent neurologist and co-editor of *PIM*, also frequently used this technique. John T. Binion, former Tinsley Texas student, said that "Harrison teaches medicine just like Adams teaches neurology.")

Tinsley was clever and opinionated and sometimes he disbelieved the lab. On one occasion he thought the blood urea nitrogen (BUN)[9] was erroneously high, so he had blood drawn on all those on rounds with him and sent the samples to the lab with phony names. In this case, he was right, but the lab was incensed. Tinsley had been in charge of the lab determinations at Hopkins as a house officer, later at the Brigham, and still later at Vanderbilt while on the faculty, so he knew about turning the urea into ammonia and CO_2 using urease, then determining the amount of ammonia formed spectrophotometrically. "You must know lots about the lab procedures," he often said. "You'll either be the slave of the lab or the master of the lab. You're bound to be one or the other, and you'll be a better doctor if you're the master!"

His bedside rounds weren't limited to teaching the facts and skills involved in

9. The BUN was determined in those days by converting it to ammonia and carbon dioxide by the action of urease. The ammonia formed in the enzymatic reaction was determined spectrophotometrically by the phenolhypochorite reaction of Berthelot using sodium nitroprusside as a catalyst.

examining a patient, making a diagnosis, and organizing a plan of management. The patient always came first, and he was at pains to make this clear to all present. He knew that the prognosis is important to the patient and that the spirit and outlook of the patient were important components of healing. He would sometimes sit on the bed and discuss these things with the patient, making the news as encouraging as possible without misleading the patient. When the patient was ready for discharge, Tinsley would dictate a letter into a dictaphone to the patient telling him or her about the situation, what must be done to care for it (by the patient), and what to look forward to. This was transcribed later by a secretary. Tinsley would then dictate a letter to the patient's local physician, usually also in the presence of the patients and other doctors. If it was a cancer patient or a patient with terminal heart disease, this doctor's letter would probably be dictated later in his office, but usually with the house officers and students present. They understood that care of the patient's spirit was as important to Tinsley as care of the body, and he did everything possible to emphasize that to them.

IN 1956 ON TEACHING rounds with the residents one morning, Tinsley was presented with a patient about 45 years old, a white man whose X-rays revealed multiple spider-like shadows throughout his lungs and abnormal liver functions. The patient was a goldmine of physical findings, including what appeared on X-ray to be small spider angiomata throughout the lungs. The possibility of a malignancy of the lungs could not be ruled out. On examination with his stethoscope, Tinsley found a loud hum over the liver. The students and residents wanted to biopsy both the lung—requiring surgery to open the thorax—and the liver, a simpler needle biopsy.

Tinsley spoke with the man. The patient seemed vague, unable to comprehend. He then asked the patient to hold his hands out straight in front of him, elbows straight, arms stiff. The patient did for a couple of seconds then relaxed his arms. "No. That's not it," Tinsley said. "Keep holding them out as long as you can or till I tell you to let them down." Out went the hands again and stayed extended. As the residents watched, the arms seemed to collapse momentarily then recover to the arms-out position. They would collapse for a second or less in a sort of flap. "See!" Harrison exclaimed. "I thought so! That's asterixis, the flapping tremor of impending hepatic coma! If we operate on him now or carry out any procedures, it may well kill him. He has the Cruveilhier-Baumgarten syndrome—cirrhosis and portal hypertension with some patent umbilical and paraumbilical veins, which account for the hum." He advised that a blood ammonia level be obtained, that neomycin given by mouth to cleanse the bowel, and that the patient be put on a strict low-protein diet. The blood ammonia level indeed was found to be markedly elevated; with the treatment prescribed the patient soon improved markedly and was later discharged. And the students were much the wiser!

In another situation about the same time, they presented a patient with malignant hypertension, the most severe and usually final clinical manifestation of essential hypertension. The patient had an extremely high blood pressure, papilledema (bulging of the optic disc on ophthalmoscopic examination), retinal hemorrhages and exudates. He had experienced several grand mal seizures. There was no effective antihypertensive treatment. He was clearly terminal. Tinsley asked to see the IVP (intravenous pyelogram, which outlined the kidneys and ureters on X-ray). Looking at the findings, Tinsley saw what he thought was an abnormal absence of part of one kidney. "This man probably has an infarction of the kidney and might be cured by nephrectomy!" he said. Some surgeons objected, but Tinsley had it done anyway. The blood pressure declined immediately, the patient improved so dramatically he resembled his premorbid normal condition, and walked out of the hospital feeling fine! The staff and students were impressed.

Sometimes when giving a clinic before a larger audience, as he did from 10 A.M. to noon on Thursdays for many years in a large conference room in the VA Hospital, there were 30 or 40 in the audience. On these occasions he would listen to the history only, then personally examine the patient in front of the group. Sometimes this would take 5 or 10 minutes, as he looked intensely, felt the abdomen and other areas including the precordial area (to determine the cardiac apex and for the presence of thrills or abnormal bulges), probed, poked, looked at the optic fundi with an ophthalmoscope, listened carefully to the heart after placing the patient in the appropriate positions, and so on. During this time the audience would be absolutely silent. (Tinsley was fond of saying, "The first duty of a cardiology consult is to get the patient into a quiet room.") Then he would deliver himself of his opinions, sometimes with the patient still present if he could be reassuring, or after sending the patient back to the room if the news was bad. He often predicted the results of yet incomplete laboratory findings.

In the 1950s, as older editions of the *Principles of Internal Medicine* were being reviewed and new editions being prepared, Tinsley seemed to know the whole book by heart. On rounds, he used the time during the fumblings of students, residents, and sometimes faculty members present, to organize his own thoughts about the problem at hand. Thus prepared, Tinsley would deliver a classic oration on the patient and the disease, often with references to history and non-medical literature.

Tularemia and brucellosis were often seen in Alabama in those days, as well as infestations with worms of various sorts, especially hookworms, ascaris, pinworms, and occasional tapeworms. Tinsley knew these in his usual great details, including the appearance of the eggs in stools, the complete life cycle, and the history of the disease. Sometimes he asked to examine the stools themselves, both grossly and under a microscope. He also knew the manifestations of late-stage syphilis, especially as it affects the heart. But his friend and colleague Ben Friedman (whom you recall ran the "L Clinic," for "lues," at Vanderbilt) could have known more in this area, and Tinsley chose him to write the chapter on syphilitic heart disease in the early editions of *Principles of Internal Medicine*.

Once a house officer who had been to Africa had brought back microscope slides of blood containing the microfilaria of the lymph-blocking worm *Wuchereria bancrofti*. In the VA Hospital at the time was a patient with massive edema of the legs and feet, unexplained despite intense and extensive investigation over several weeks. The patient was presented to Tinsley at a conference. He was puzzled as to the origin of the impressive edema. He could not explain it. The house officer thought he could trick Tinsley. So he pointed Tinsley to the microscope at the slide already set up on a nearby table. The tiny microfilariae were clearly visible in the sample, and Tinsley correctly identified them.

"I still don't understand," Tinsley said. "You said this man served in Europe during the war, but there are no such microfilariae there. The only veterans with this problem served in the South Pacific, or maybe in sub-Sarahan Africa, though I don't know that we had any troops there. Are you sure he didn't serve in the Pacific Theater?" He did not. "The only other possibility is that he lived near Charleston, South Carolina, since I've heard that there are some cases endemic there." He was from the Birmingham area. Finally Tinsley said, "Well, I just can't explain this man's edema. Maybe he has some odd abnormality of the lymph system." So the house officers had to explain the trick, much to the amusement of all. But again Tinsley had shown his extreme erudition in medicine and inspired the students.

The formal teaching sessions weren't the only venues for teaching. Since the Vanderbilt days Tinsley had the habit of inviting medical students and residents, and often a few faculty, to his own home for a medical evening. First, there would be drinks and perhaps some very light refreshments (such as cookies or cheese and crackers and peanuts). Second, there would be a light dinner. After dinner, a student would present a paper on some medical topic, usually a physiology or other research topic. In Birmingham one topic was the directions of the muscle fibers in the various parts of the heart and how this influenced the sequence and efficacy of the heartbeat. These were often substantial talks of a half-hour or longer. Then they would come to the main event of the evening: the discussion (although the informality did not entirely preclude questions and comments during the talk). Although he never overtly admitted it, in later years it seemed that Tinsley's secret agenda was to start a fight. If he could split the group into two or more segments disagreeing vigorously with each other, he knew that would motivate them. They would then rush to the library the next day and following weeks to study furiously for information to prove their opponents wrong and themselves right. The schools were small then, and he might have many of the same people at the next evening meeting a month later to continue the discussion and either settle it or provide a good question for further research.[10]

There was a large auditorium, holding 250 people, in a five-story building remaining from the old Birmingham Medical College, adjacent to the Old Hillman Hospital built in 1903 for charity patients.[11] During the mid- and late 1950s a weekly joint medical-surgical grand rounds was held here, and Tinsley and surgical chief Champ Lyons often held forth for more than an hour over some patient or clinical problem.

Lyons had been born to a physician family in central Pennsylvania. His parents divorced, and his mother returned to her native Mobile, there to marry into a family related to Luther Leonidas Hill, M.D., Senator Lister Hill, and other leaders in the state. Lyons had achieved a good academic record, making Phi Beta Kappa, then graduating cum laude and Alpha Omega Alpha from Harvard Medical School. He remained at the Massachusetts General Hospital under Chief of Surgery Edward D. Churchill from 1931 to '43, when he joined the U.S. Navy, returning to a position in the Ochsner Clinic and Tulane in New Orleans in 1945, leaving only to take the position in Birmingham as the first full-time chief of surgery.

In their grand rounds sparring, Tinsley often liked to needle Lyons about the intellectual superiority of internists over surgeons. On one occasion, he challenged Lyons about the blood supply of the thyroid gland. Lyons asked if Tinsley, a poor

10. Sometimes Tinsley had visiting scholars at these evenings. On one occasion his guest was Carl Moyer, whom he had recruited to Dallas to be professor of experimental surgery and who later became the dean and still later was professor of surgery at Washington University-Barnes Hospital, the chair formerly held by Evarts Graham, an originator of the standard test for gallstones as well as much of thoracic surgery. Most of that discussion concerned medical problems in surgery, but it drifted off into a contest as to which participants could speak the most languages—an unusual competition for Alabama, in those days.

11. H. L. Holley, *A History of Medicine in Alabama* (Birmingham: University of Alabama School of Medicine, 1982), 96–101. The Birmingham Medical College operated from 1894 through the graduation of 1915.

12. Harrison to Blalock, March 8, 1944.

internist who never got a chance to actually see inside a patient or deal with it, could know himself.

Tinsley answered, "It is the inferior thyroidal artery!—of course!"

Lyons just as promptly snapped back, "No! It's the subclavian artery! I knew no *internist* could be expected to know anatomy!"

To this Tinsley asked, "And what do you suppose the origin of the inferior thyroidal artery is? The subclavian, of course! But you could not expect a *surgeon* to know such details!"

Lyons was an excellent surgeon, and this was another occasion when the two were suspected of colluding for the sake of the show.

Another time Tinsley was asked how he would feel if he were presented with a patient at a rounds attended only by a dozen surgeons and no other doctors. He responded, "That would make it about equal intellectually."

On rounds one bright, sunny day Tinsley asked for an ophthalmoscope to examine the optic fundi of a patient. He requested that the lights in the room be turned down to better see the fundus and retina, whereupon a large dark cloud drifted across the sun, and the light outside became much dimmer and less bright. One student later wrote in a letter to Tinsley, "We practically worshiped you and were greatly impressed that the Deity himself would respond to your request so promptly and dramatically!"

He did indeed impress the students. Yet, as he had archly indicated to Al Blalock in 1944, despite his devotion to teaching, the students were not his main concern: ". . . You can be very sure that there is one thing above all else which will not be neglected—namely, contact with patients. I came into the medical picture originally as a doctor and expect to go out the same way . . . What feeble abilities I may possess are much greater in the care of the sick . . ."[12]

The Alabama Medical School

Birmingham, 1950–1958

Sometime in late 1949, several luncheon meetings were held at the home of Dr. Groce Harrison on Cliff Road in Birmingham, the same house he had built in 1906 when the family moved from Talladega. The luncheons were a gathering of storied medical professionals. The main participants were Drs. Groce Harrison and Seale Harris Sr., and on at least one occasion in 1950, Dr. John M. Gallalee, president of the University of Alabama, based in Tuscaloosa 60 miles to the southwest. Just when and where Seale met Groce is not known, but it must have been early in their careers, which had many parallels. Seale Harris's son Seale Jr. had been Tinsley's colleague on the Vanderbilt faculty of the 1930s and was now in practice with his father at the prominent Seale Harris Clinic in Birmingham. Also present at the foot of the table was a penurious young first-year medical student living at the Harrison home to earn some money assisting Tinsley's parents—Groce, 79, was by now almost blind. This medical student was Buris Raye Boshell, from Bear Creek in Winston County, in the hill country of northwest Alabama.[1] Boshell later took his last two years at Harvard Medical School then was on the house staff of the Brigham Hospital, where he was chief medical resident two successive years. He later returned to a faculty position at Birmingham, from which he rose to become a major figure in Alabama medicine. He remembered well the details of these conversations but was told not to repeat them. He kept this promise until the 1990s.

Seale Harris Sr. was one of the most prominent doctors in the city and in Alabama.[2] He was born in Georgia in 1870 to a prestigious family, his father, Charles Hooks Harris, having obtained an M.D. degree from New York University in 1857

1. The county is famously known as "the Free State of Winston" because it seceded from Alabama when Alabama seceded from the union to join the Confederacy.

2. James A. Pittman, *Seale Harris*, eds. J. A. Garraty and M. C. Carnes (New York: Oxford Univ. Press, 1999). E. B. Carmichael, "Seale Harris—Physician-Scientist-Author," *J. Med. Assn. State of Alabama* 33 (1954): 189–195.

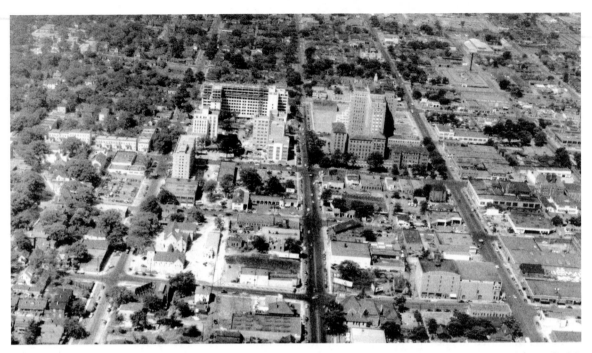

The UAB area of downtown Birmingham, looking west along Sixth Avenue South, about 1950.

and finished a year there teaching anatomy as an assistant to P. A. Aylett. C. H. Harris joined Robert E. Lee's army for the Civil War and afterwards served for 30 years as a horse and buggy doctor in rural Georgia. An older brother of Seale graduated from West Point and another was a U.S. senator from Georgia. Seale himself obtained his M.D. in 1894 from the University of Virginia (living in the room previously occupied by Edgar Allen Poe). He entered practice in Enterprise, a small town in southeastern Alabama. He quickly rose in rank in the county and state medical organizations. In 1906 he moved to Baltimore for a year's postgraduate study of medicine and gastrointestinal diseases, after which he studied in Vienna and elsewhere in Europe. He then moved to Mobile to become chairman of medicine at the Medical College of Alabama, the same post Groce had been offered earlier.

His life continued along interesting paths, including service as a lieutenant colonel under General William C. Gorgas and General Pershing, then later as a member of President Wilson's treaty party after the war ended. On the ship back to the U.S., he had several long conversations with Franklin D. Roosevelt, then assistant secretary of the Navy. He authored chapters on G.I. diseases in *The Medical History of the War* and several books on pellagra as well as biographies of Banting and J. Marion Sims.

Seale Sr. discovered and named "hyperinsulinism" while visiting and studying with Frederick Banting in Toronto immediately after the discovery of insulin. He created a major clinic and large hospital in Birmingham, but both were lost to the Great Depression of the 1930s. He recovered, re-establishing a medical clinic in Birmingham which continues as a leading practice of internists today. Seale Sr. was a major figure in Birmingham and Alabama medicine, known especially for his work in metabolism and pellagra. In 1949, he was awarded the Southern Medical Association's Research Medal—the same award Tinsley won in 1945. After Harris's death in 1957, that medal was renamed "The Seale Harris Medal" for "important research accomplishment in the broad field of metabolism, endocrinology, nutrition, or research which contributes to a better understanding of the chemical changes occurring in disease."

Another regular at the talks was James Somerville McLester, M.D. In accordance with the traditions of leading physicians of the area, he had graduated from the University of Virginia with an M.D. in 1899, then studied in Göttingen and Freiburg, Germany, returning to the Birmingham Medical College as professor of pathology in 1902. Later he became professor of medicine and active in the house staff training program. In 1907–08 he returned to Germany to study under the world-famous chemist Emil Fischer, who did seminal work on sugars, nucleoproteins, amino acids, and polypeptides and synthesized Veronal, popularly known as phenobarbital. Some of this work led to the discovery of vitamins and was closely related to nutrition. McLester had been a physician and lieutenant colonel in the American Expeditionary Force in World War I. He was the first physician in Birmingham to establish a clinical laboratory in his office, had been a member of the first board of regents of the American College of Physicians, and was president of the state medical association (1920) and of the American Medical Association (1935). He authored six editions of *Nutrition and Diet in Health and Disease*, and had been chairman of the Foods and Nutrition Council of the AMA, but he had also achieved in academe. He was a member of the top academic organization of internists in America, the Association of American Physicians, the Old Turks, and had written chapters for the standard American textbook of medicine, *The Cecil Textbook of Medicine* in the 1930–40s.

In 1920 McLester, while remaining in practice in Birmingham, was made chairman of medicine at the two-year medical school in Tuscaloosa and remained in that position until the late spring of 1949, when he retired at age 72 and the imminent

Capsule History of the Alabama Medical School

1859, Medical College of Alabama was in Mobile, a one-year program.

1920, moved to Tuscaloosa as a two-year program.

1944, moved to Birmingham as a four-year program.

November 1966, the Extension Center and the Medical Center merged to form the University of Alabama in Birmingham, a component of the University of Alabama.

1969, UAB became an independent institution within the University of Alabama System.

1984, name was changed to the University of Alabama at Birmingham. The medical school is now officially the UAB School of Medicine.

appointment of someone as "full-time" chairman of medicine. Thus, he was out of contention for that appointment, but he also had a son about Tinsley's age or somewhat younger, James B. McLester, M.D., who had graduated from Harvard Medical School and was prominent and eligible.

The senior McLester had played an important role in the development of the medical school since 1920 or '22 and must have been involved in discussions regarding the desirability of going to a full-time faculty system in the late 1940s. McLester and Seale Harris were vigorous competitors. Their competition was strong enough that some people thought they were enemies. Despite their antagonism, they were always cordial and sometimes generous towards each other in public. When Harris invited Banting to Birmingham to speak, he invited McLester to introduce Banting at that time. But they were often in professional opposition. All the chairs of the clinical departments were "McLester men." The "Seale Harris crowd" was simply out. One strike against the appointment of the younger McLester chair of medicine was presumably opposition from Harris. The younger McLester, in all fairness, was not of the stature of his father; he had a difficult personality, and was not popular among local physicians.

The main player in Alabama medicine was Roy Rachford Kracke, the Atlanta hematologist who had been appointed dean of medicine at the inception of the new four-year degree-granting school in Birmingham in 1944. Kracke was dedicated to the development of the school and was an excellent dean. In the late 1940s the medical school and its hospital ran out of money, like many other schools in the South, such as Southwestern and Vanderbilt. This was not a unique problem. Vanderbilt was so short of money that on January 7, 1949, Tinsley's friend and former colleague Dean of Medicine Ernest Goodpasture recommended to Chancellor Harvie Branscomb that the medical school be closed (at least the undergraduate portion leading to the M.D. degree; Goodpasture thought the research and residencies might be continued. This situation in Birmingham aggravated the already touchy relations between Dean Kracke and President Gallalee, and Gallalee had finally insisted that all requisitions be routed through his office, 60 miles away in Tuscaloosa, for approval before execution. Plans for moving to a full-time system were progressing nonetheless. Then Kracke died unexpectedly on June 27, 1950. It was in this atmosphere—a new school in extreme financial difficulties 60 miles distant from the university president and de facto administrator, and as of late June without a dean of medicine—that the conversations between Groce, Seale, and finally Gallalee took place.

We do not know the exact details of these conversations. They must have focused on problems facing Alabama medicine, the need to obtain the best, most outstanding chief of medicine possible and the likely difficulties of doing so in the current circumstances. The excellent record of Tinsley and his plans to leave Dallas were also discussed. The elders of Alabama medicine wanted Tinsley to come home and worked on a way to make this possible. No letters concerning this offer and acceptance have been found, but Tinsley himself has left a memoir which discusses these matters.[3]

"My impression [was] that Dr. Joseph Hirsch, a lifelong friend," Tinsley later wrote, "was the first to suggest to Dr. Gallalee that I be approached in regard to the Department of Medicine and that at about the same time Dr. Seale Harris Sr. suggested me for the position as Dean. When Dr. Gallalee discussed the situation with me, my reactions were mixed. I had no desire whatever to be a Dean again. Once had been enough! Indeed, too much! Furthermore, I knew that the Medical School was suffering from monetary undernutrition and that the Jefferson-Hillman Hospital, as it was then called, was in desperate financial straits. I did not then deem it likely that the Medical School would ever become first-class. . . . There were, however, certain favorable considerations. Dr. Gallalee impressed me as a forthright, outspoken individual with high ideals and strong personal integrity. All subsequent associations with him reinforced these initial opinions."[4]

Tinsley traveled to Birmingham and met the first full-time chief of surgery, Champ Lyons, and the dean of the new School of Dentistry, Joseph F. Volker, from Boston. He was impressed by both. In his memoir he wrote,

Insofar as academic and professional considerations were involved in the decision whether or not to become a part of the Medical School, the *pros* and the *cons* seemed to about balance each other. Actually the considerations that tipped the scales were not professional but personal. My parents had six children. By 1950, two were dead and a third hopelessly ill. Of the remaining three, none lived in Alabama. My parents were not only old and ill, they were lonely.

No children could have had a finer or happier home environment than we had during our formative years. Each of us had been generously provided with the quality and quantity of education he or she desired. Now my parents needed me. The need was not financial because although never wealthy, my frugal father, aided by my thrifty mother, had ample savings to meet their modest monetary wants.

3. T. R. Harrison, *The Medical School of the University of Alabama: Some Reminiscences,* manuscript, UAB Archives. Some of the other information about these times is also from this source.

4. Ibid., 18.

5. T. R. Harrison Jr.,
personal communica-
tion, 1993.
6. The best history
of its development is
given in *The His-
tory of Medicine in
Alabama*. There is
another account in
preparation as part of
a history of the overall
University of Alabama
at Birmingham by
Tennant McWilliams,
Ph.D., an excellent
historian nationally

Here was a chance to repay, at least in small measure, the treasures of guidance, education, happiness and wisdom that our parents had showered upon their children. This consideration seemed to outweigh such lesser matters as my own academic and professional future. My companion on life's journey supported me in that decision as she has in all others. Once again she said, "Whither thou goest."

Upon my telling Dr. Gallalee that I was deeply interested in the Professorship of Medicine but had no interest in the Deanship, he made an interesting comment. He said he deemed it improper for the President of a University to appoint a Departmental Chairman except upon the recommendation of a Dean. He therefore suggested that I accept the position as Dean and nominate myself for the Chairmanship. Perhaps I would then decide that I wished to retain both positions.

My reply was that I had previously been both Dean and Chairman of a Department of Medicine in Dallas and that I had been a failure as a Dean but perhaps a success as a Professor of Medicine. There was no chance that I would ever change my mind. My heart lay in teaching, research and patient care and most definitely not in administration. However, if he wished it, I would accept a position as Acting Dean for a few months in order to give him time to find a Dean, which I hoped he would do soon so that I could get on with the business of developing the Department.

The decision was made. The move would be to Birmingham. He would return to his homeland.

ANNOUNCEMENTS HAD ALREADY BEEN printed and the envelopes stamped to tell colleagues and friends that the now-reconciled Harrisons were moving to Nashville. The stamps were expensive: three cents each for a sealed envelope. So the envelopes were placed in a bathtub so the stamps could be soaked off for future use, and other announcements designating Birmingham were prepared and mailed.[5]

The house on Cliff Road was found to be in need of serious repair, and this could not be done while it was occupied, so in July 1950 Tinsley and Betty moved to an apartment in Birmingham. The family re-converged on Birmingham, Alabama's biggest city. Young John, having completed his fifth grade, came from Kennebunkport to Birmingham. Betsy started the senior year of high school at Brook Hill, an upscale private girls' prep school in town. Because Betty, Tinsley, and Betsy were living in an apartment, there was little or no room for John, who moved in with Randy and his new wife Evelyn and infant Laura (born March 2, 1950) in a spacious but spartan basement apartment; Randy had moved to Birmingham the year before and was working with Tinsley's nephew John Calvin Wilson in the construction business. Groce and Lula, with their live-in personal aide, the medical student "Bo" Boshell, now a sophomore, moved from Cliff Road up to the Altamont Apartments.

However, on March 5, 1951, Lula was found dead from a heart attack. She was 79 years old. Her death was a terrible shock for both Groce and Tinsley. Groce had lost his life mate, Tinsley his mother—she had been a constant in his life and always his most important supporter, an honest loving critic.

Boshell remembered walking with Groce a few days later from the Altamont to the Johns Ridout Funeral Parlor, a distance of about two miles. It was a very cold day for March, and they did not talk a great deal.

Soon thereafter, in the spring of 1951, the family—including John, Groce, and Boshell—moved into the refurbished house on Cliff Road, as Tinsley settled into his new job and new school. The family was reunited. Things were looking up.

TINSLEY'S NEW INSTITUTION, THE University of Alabama School of Medicine, had deep but tangled roots.[6] The school was started by an entrepreneurial surgeon, Josiah Nott,[7] in Mobile in 1859. The summer of 1858, Nott had toured Europe, purchasing anatomical models, specimens of various chemicals for demonstrations, pieces of equipment, and other items for use in the new school. He returned, and the new school opened in the fall of 1859. When the Civil War started in April 1861, the school closed as the students and faculty rushed off to support the Confederate army medical needs.[8] European-oriented physicians in Alabama had, for most of the 19th century, tried to bring order and science to local medicine.

In the 1950s, however, Tinsley was once again building a new school, his fourth. Tinsley's view always was that people count the most. Great facilities and lots of money help. But without excellent students, staff, faculty, and administrators, a school will not be a good school.

Tinsley had a wonderful secretary, Mrs. Katherine Morgan, whose husband worked for the Tennessee Coal and Iron Company, which was part of U.S. Steel. Kay was hired by Roy Kracke as the first employee for the new medical school. She knew all the local rumors and gossip. She also knew who could be trusted and who could not. She was discreet and loyal. She was the secretary for the first five deans of medicine and left that position only in 1968 when Dean Hill followed Joe Volker

recognized in his area of special interest (e.g., history of Hawaii), but his book on UAB does not focus on the medical school.

7. R. Horsman, "Josiah Clark Nott" in *American National Biography*, 538–539.

8. Some of the items purchased by Nott had not yet arrived and were on a ship bound for the Confederacy. The ship was captured by Union forces and brought to Massachusetts, through the port of Salem. A collection of chemicals and minerals in bottles somehow found its way into the *Collection of Historical Scientific Instruments* at the Cabot Science Center of Harvard University. Harvard retained these despite entreaties from the dean at University of Alabama School of Medicine to return them, including letters to Harvard President Derek Bok and Dr. Sara Schechner, curator of the instrument museum—despite the fact that the bottles are still labeled "Medical College of Alabama." M. Richardson, personal communication, September 22, 2003. James A. Pittman Jr., M.D. to S. Schechner, 2003.

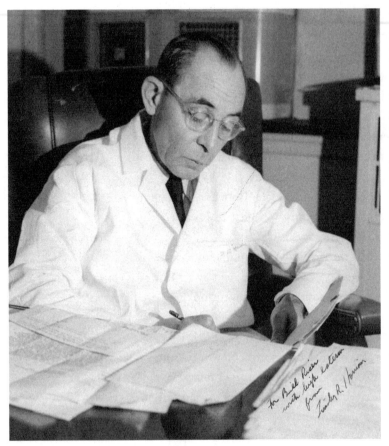

Tinsley Harrison at his desk in the Birmingham medical center, in the 1950s.

to become the second vice president for health affairs and took her with him to that new office.

A number of excellent physicians had already been practicing for years in Birmingham. Many had been teaching in the clinical portions of the medical school before Tinsley arrived in 1950. Tinsley knew, however, that in Birmingham, in the Deep South with no money, it would be difficult to attract the best medical scholars and clinicians from elsewhere. The South was a troubling place, no less so than 100 years earlier. Though the civil rights tensions had not yet openly flared enough to attract international attention, they and other aspects of the South—rumor, violence, racism—were bad enough to attract the scorn of academics everywhere and to generate songs like Tom Lehrer's "Dixie" parody, "Take Me Back to Alabammy," ridiculing the state.[9]

The South was poor but in other ways besides money. Educational achievements of the general public, statistical indicators of health, and prestige in the rest of the country and world—the South was viewed with pity and scorn. The South was the butt of jokes, was ridiculed, and derided in popular songs and films. True, Vanderbilt, Bowman Gray, and Southwestern were in Tennessee, North Carolina, and Texas, all also in the South. But there was a degree of difference, somehow, from Alabama. Birmingham had issues that Nashville, Winston-Salem, and Dallas did not, and though Tinsley could not know it yet, the degree of difference would only intensify in the coming two decades.

Isolated individual scholarship and academic excellence thrived in the Deep South as well as elsewhere, but it would be challenging to attract outstanding scholars and scientists from the world's leading institutions and build similarly excellent institutions of widespread renown.

Recruiting faculty and senior staff from centers in Boston or New York would be difficult if not impossible. Philadelphia and Chicago were remote possibilities, but smaller and not as promising. The west coast was out; medical schools there were either just starting or undergoing major upgrades. The medical schools of University of Washington in Seattle started only in 1945 and UCLA in 1951, and UCSF and Stanford were transforming themselves from sleepy schools in San Francisco for practitioners to biomedical dynamos. They were competing, and very successfully, for the scarce personnel needed for a new medical school. And of course there was little or no good hunting in the South. The University of Miami, with its more cosmopolitan ambiance, was about to open its medical school in 1952. The University of Florida in Gainesville would follow soon. If Tinsley wanted clinically active physicians also experienced and active in research, he would, with rare exceptions, have to bring them with him on the basis of his own personality and abilities or grow them *in situ*.

As for the students, though Alabama did not have laws which restricted acceptance of medical students to only residents of the state (as in the case of some state schools and soon in Texas as well), similar considerations applied to aspiring premedical students. The number of good applicants were adequate to bring together class after class of competent students who would become good and often outstanding doctors, but applicants often self-selected themselves geographically because of the cultural views in other parts of the country and because of their finances (as tuition in this new school was very low for state residents). Insularity of outlook and attitude with regard to place and time thus remained a major problem for the state (as it is everywhere).

TINSLEY'S COLLEAGUES AND STUDENTS were loyal to him, often fanatically so. He often exerted himself to promote their careers. His colleagues felt an obligation to him and admiration for him. He was fun to work with, an exhilarating presence. As had occurred in the moves from Vanderbilt to Bowman Gray and from there to Southwestern, he brought some of those he had worked with before, including Kathryn Willis, a research fellow who had work in progress in the summer of 1950. It was relatively simple clinical work which required modest financial support. Two of her papers were published in the journal *Circulation* in 1951, one on the

9. Sung in the 1950s by the talented Lehrer, a Harvard mathematician, to his own skillful piano accompaniment, and greatly cheered by sympathetic audiences at a Kenmore Square lounge near Boston University: "Won'tcha come with me to Alabammy, . . . / I wanna talk with Southern gentlemen / And put my white sheet on again, . . . / The land of the boll weevil, . . . / Where the laws are medieval, . . . / Be it ever so decadent, / There's no place like home." Tom Lehrer, "Take Me Back to Alabammy," *The Remains of Tom Lehrer*, CD (Los Angeles, CA: Warner Brothers Records, Inc. and Rhino Entertainment Co.).

10. W. N. Viar, B. B. Oliver, S. Eisenberg, T. A. Lombardo, K. Willis, and T. R. Harrison, "The Effect of Posture and of Compression of the Neck on the Excretion of Electrolytes and on Glomerular Filtration: Further Studies," *Circulation* 3 (1951): 105–115.

11. M. J. Greve, E. E. Eddleman Jr., K. Willis, S. Eisenberg and T. R. Harrison, "The Effect of Digitoxin on Sodium Excretion, Creatinine Clearance and Apparent Cardiac Output," *Circulation* 3 (1951): 405–512.

12. E. E. Eddleman Jr., K. Willis, T. J. Reeves, and T. R. Harrison, "The Kinetocardiogram. I. Method of Recording Precordial Movements," *Circulation* 8 (1953): 269–275.

13. T. R. Harrison, L. Christianson, E. E. Eddleman Jr, R. Pierce, R. Watkins and K. Willis, "Movements of Human Ventricles," *Trans. Assoc. Amer. Physi.* 66 (1953): 250–256.

14. E. Booth, K. Willis, T. J. Reeves and T. R. Harrison, "The Right Auricular Electrokymogram of Normal Subjects,"

effect of posture and compression of the neck on the excretion of electrolytes and on glomerular filtration rates in human subjects,[10] and the second on the effect of digitoxin on sodium excretion, creatinine clearance, and apparent cardiac output.[11] She had no publications in 1952 but three in 1953: on the kinetocardiogram as a method for recording precordial movements;[12] on movements of human ventricles;[13] and on the normal right auricular electrokymogram.[14]

The paper on ventricular movements was presented by Tinsley before the annual meeting of the AAP, the Old Turks. Like every other year, the annual meetings the first weekend in May at Atlantic City were immensely stimulating to young aspiring internists.[15] Tinsley was more famous than ever, with the publication and success of *Principles of Internal Medicine* only three years before.

The people mentioned in the following few pages are discussed in considerable detail. In the remaining 28 years of Tinsley's life, they played major roles, contributed much, and are interesting in themselves. Their lives also tell something of how medicine, especially academic medicine, and the world worked in those days.

A MAJOR EARLY FACULTY addition—an exception to recruiting difficulties Tinsley anticipated—was the fascinating Richard J. Bing. Born in Nurnberg, Bavaria, in 1909, he lived to age 101 and was one of the brightest stars to pass through 20th century medicine. A polymath and Renaissance man, Bing attended universities of Vienna, Munich, and Berlin, finally obtaining not one but two M.D. degrees from Munich (1934) and Bern (1935). He then took a fellowship at the Carlsberg Institute in Copenhagen, Denmark, in 1935–36. While there, he had a life-changing, and probably life-saving, encounter. This meeting is described in a biography of the American aviator, Charles A. Lindbergh, by A. Scott Berg, as well as in a profile of Bing by A. B. Weisse.[16] Lindbergh had just completed a tour of German air installations and factories at the request of the U.S. government and had managed to fly some of the Luftwaffe's superior new airplanes. He then went to Copenhagen to meet Alexis Carrel, with whom he had worked at the Rockefeller Institute on perfusion apparatuses for animal organs *in vitro*. While visiting the Carlsberg Biological Institute to demonstrate their perfusion pump, Lindbergh and Carrel met "a brilliant young doctor . . . Richard Bing, a half-Jewish German citizen . . . just [when Germany was] coming under 'the Jewish stigma.' Lindbergh and Carrel rushed to Bing's aid, helping him secure a grant from the Rockefeller Foundation, which enabled him to move to New York and become an American Citizen," as Bing was probably hoping to do.

Bing remained at the Rockefeller for the rest of 1936–37. He then took an internship and residency in surgery at Columbia's Presbyterian Hospital in New York. Although these were technically in surgery, they were really research positions. After serving as an instructor in physiology first at Columbia then New York University, Bing moved to Johns Hopkins in 1943 under Warfield T. Longcope, chairman of medicine. At Hopkins, Bing served as a resident and took part three of the National Board of Medical Examiners' tests so that he could obtain a license for clinical medicine. Thereupon he promptly entered the U.S. Army and was stationed at Edgewood Arsenal, about 40 miles from Baltimore. Alfred Blalock, desperate for help at the time, got Bing released to return to Hopkins, doubtless influenced by Bing's experience in departments of both medicine and surgery as well as his expertise in experimental physiology. (In addition, Bing had married the daughter of the famous Physicians and Surgeons-Columbia surgeon Allen O. Whipple, originator of the "Whipple procedure" for pancreatic cancer.)

Blalock wanted Bing to study the physiology of congenital heart diseases. To do this Bing returned several times to New York to learn cardiac catheterization in the laboratory of Andre Cournand, who in 1956 shared a Nobel Prize for his developing cardiac catheterization work. Bing was not 100 percent happy with his time at Hopkins; he later described his tenure there as being like "Daniel in the lions' den," the lions being Helen B. Taussig and Blalock. Still, he managed to publish 18 papers on congenital heart disease, one being the description of the Taussig-Bing complex. Only one of the papers was with Blalock, "The Surgical Treatment of Mitral Stenosis and its Physiological Consequence," presented at the Atlantic City meeting of the Old Turks and published in their 1951 *Transactions*.

During one catheterization, Bing's catheter slipped into the coronary sinus, considered very undesirable by Lewis Dexter, cardiologist at Harvard's Brigham Hospital. However, Bing was familiar with a 1914 paper by Evans and Matsuoka on cardiac metabolism and efficiency in mammalian heart-lung preparations, and saw this as an opportunity. He began to study this, his first paper appearing in 1947,[17] but the more his studies emphasized cardiac metabolism, the more unhappy Blalock became. He wanted *diagnostic* catheterizations done and congenital heart disease studied, not the general physiology of the heart.

Blalock's close friend and nearly constant correspondent Tinsley must have known about this. Once in Birmingham with the responsibility for the whole department of medicine to worry about, Tinsley, who had no personal experience

Circulation 7 (1953): 916–921.

15. Pittman and Miller, "Southern."

16. A. S. Berg, *Lindbergh* (New York: Berkley Books, 1998), 360–361;. A. B. Weisse, *Heart to Heart* (New Brunswick, NJ: Rutgers University Press, 2002).

17. R. J. Bing, L. D. Vandam, F. Gregoire, et al., "Catheterization of the Coronary Sinus and the Middle Cardiac Vein in Man," *Proc. Soc. Exper. Biol. & Med* 66 (1947): 239–240.

18. Longmire, *Alfred*, 283.

19. A. Cournand, Bing R. J., Dexter L., Detter C., Katz L. N., Warren J. V., and Wood E., "Report of the Committee on Cardiac Catheterizations and Angiocardiography," *Circulation* 7 (1953): 769-773.

with cardiac catheterization and always said he was clumsy with his hands, enticed Bing to Birmingham in 1951. This was a major recruitment. Tinsley had brought to his new department a world leader in the new technique of cardiac catheterization. Bing arrived that summer and did Alabama's first—probably the first in the South—cardiac catheterization in September 1951.

No discussion of Bing would be appropriate without mention of his musical activities, especially his compositions. Early in life he had to choose between music and medicine for a career, and unfortunately for music, he chose medicine. However, he played the piano and the harpsichord and composed more than 300 pieces, one of which, a mass for full orchestra, chorus, and soloists, was performed by the Vienna Orchestra. Some of his later publications related music to medicine, and were published in several languages. Some thought he was a brother or cousin of the musically famous Rudolph Bing of New York, but the two of them had gone over their ancestry together, and there was no close relation.

Bing must have had a major impact in forwarding Tinsley's agenda to build a sound base for medical research in Birmingham. His most recent bibliography includes 517 publications in four or more languages and a worldwide collection of co-authors famous in cardiology and medicine. Ten or more of these co-authors were on the medical school faculty in Birmingham, a large percentage of the tiny faculty at that time. Bing's prominence helped highlight Tinsley's new medical school nationally and internationally. Longmire writes, "The contributions of Bing and his associates did much to establish the value of cardiac catheterization as an essential component of diagnostic cardiology."[18] Bing was also involved in the development of angiocardiography and was a member of an American Heart Association committee chaired by Cournand to report on cardiac catheterizations and angiocardiography.[19]

OTHER NEW RECRUITS CAME from Dallas. One of the most important was T. Joseph Reeves, who had graduated from Baylor medical school in 1946. Reeves interned with Tinsley at Parkland Hospital in Dallas because of Tinsley's fame as a teacher of internal medicine, though this was a *rotating* internship complete with surgery, obstetrics, pediatrics, and so on, as required by the Army and Navy. In 1947, he was called to active duty in the Navy. After his tour of duty, Reeves returned to Dallas in 1949 for two more years of residency training in internal medicine. His plan was to qualify for board examinations in internal medicine; at that time the medical board required four years of hospital training plus two more years doing practice of internal medicine to qualify for the examination. Reeves interrupted his plan in 1951, following Tinsley to Birmingham for a year as a cardiology trainee supported by the new National Heart Institute. From 1952 to '54 Reeves operated a private practice in oil-rich Beaumont, Texas. But Tinsley induced Reeves to return to Birmingham's new school and a job as chief of medicine in the new Veterans Administration hospital.

Reeves replaced Walter Benedict Frommeyer, another interesting man. Born in Cincinnati, Ohio, in 1916, Frommeyer received his M.D. from Cincinnati in 1942. He interned at Cincinnati General, then entered the Army Medical Corps in 1943. Frommeyer was wounded in Europe, received a Purple Heart and Bronze Star Medal with Oak Leaf Cluster, and left the Army as a major in 1946. But before leaving for Europe, he got a three-day furlough in January 1944 to marry Elizabeth Ann Lee, a beautiful Southern belle from Birmingham; they had met while Frommeyer was in Birmingham for three months in the spring of 1943 to study nutritional deficiencies with Tom Spies, who was on the faculty of the University of Cincinnati College of Medicine but spent periods in Birmingham doing research. Spies apparently considered this missionary work in the destitute South. That Frommeyer was permitted this elective in the middle of the war—when medical school curricula were accelerated and internships were shortened—is remarkable. Spies must have liked Frommeyer, because he put his name as co-author on six papers between 1945 and '47. Spies resurfaces in Tinsley's story in the mid-1950s.

One example of Frommeyer's care for subordinates was his insistence on walking 100 miles in the desert with the troops among the scorpions and snakes, though as a medical officer he was entitled to ride in a vehicle. He did this, he explained, "so that he could know how the men he was caring for felt in such conditions."[20]

Out of the Army in 1946, Frommeyer took two years of residency training back at the Cincinnati General Hospital at $15 a month. He followed this with a research fellowship at Harvard's Thorndike Memorial Laboratory with William B. Castle. Here he worked chiefly on blood coagulation and clotting defects, achieving three papers in that one year, one in *Blood*, one in the *Journal of Laboratory & Clinical Medicine*, and one in the *New England Journal of Medicine*. Castle wanted him to stay, but he had promised Betty they would return to Birmingham. They returned in 1949 to the Deep South, where he entered private practice with Dr. Keehn Berry.

Soon he began to work with hematologist Dr. William Riser in the blood bank of the university hospital, then still called "Jefferson-Hillman." In 1950 he became

20. Mrs. Walter B. Frommeyer, interview, November 15, 2003.

21. E. E. Eddleman, telephone interview, November 17, 2003.

director of the University of Alabama Tumor Clinic, and in 1951 director of the blood bank. In 1953, the brand new Birmingham Veterans Administration Hospital opened, and he became its first chief of medicine. He started as an instructor in medicine at the medical school, then was promoted to assistant professor by Tinsley in 1951, and with the appointment as VA chief of medicine was promoted to associate professor. This was a full-time job, which he appreciated. Frommeyer never really liked private practice and always admired and enjoyed academic medicine. He remained at the VA for a year, then from 1954 to '57 served full-time at the medical school as associate dean. Like others on the medical faculty, Frommeyer provided major help in building the department and benefited from Tinsley's international visibility and prominence.

ANOTHER EARLY ARRIVAL WAS Elvia E. "Eddie" Eddleman Jr., originally from Birmingham but a graduate of Emory medical school in Atlanta. He had interned at Emory's main teaching hospital, Atlanta's Grady Memorial Hospital for the indigent, where the medical service and department of medicine were chaired by Paul B. Beeson, a good friend of Tinsley's and co-founder of the Southern Society for Clinical Investigation. Upon nearing completion of his internship, Eddleman talked with Beeson about the best place for a residency. Beeson suggested Dallas, and when Eddleman was positive, he called Tinsley, and it was arranged. Eddleman moved to Dallas in 1949 and was just finishing his first year of residency in June 1950 when East Germany claimed sovereignty over the Sudeten residents, the North Korean army crossed the 38th Parallel, and Chiang Kai-shek ordered a halt to attacks on the Chinese mainland from Taiwan. Eddleman entered the U.S. Navy.

In the summer of 1952 Eddleman mustered out of the Navy and followed Tinsley to Birmingham. He served as a research fellow in cardiology, funded by "money Tinsley had from somewhere."[21] In 1953, he entered private practice for several months, but he was recruited back to the new VA hospital where there was a salary for a staff physician in medicine. It was a joint appointment with the medical school, which also paid him a small amount for teaching activities and gave him an academic appointment. Eddleman rose rapidly, supported by the VA salary for clinical care of patients and research money from the VA and other sources (the NIH, and the American Heart Association, among others). Soon Eddleman was appointed associate chief of staff for research and education. Shortly thereafter he became chief of medicine. After a few more years, he resigned as chief of medicine and concentrated on the research, remaining ACOS for research and education for some years. As he got older he developed severe diabetes with neuropathy, which so incapacitated him that he retired. By the time of his retirement he had published extensively, risen to professor of medicine, and was an important figure.

THERE WERE OTHERS ALREADY in Birmingham working for the medical school as clinical teachers. These were town practitioners who used multiple hospitals in the area and who taught without financial compensation. Among these were Keehn Berry, Joseph Welden, Joseph Hirsch, Samuel Cohn, soon Stanley Kahn, and many others. One who was already actually at the medical school was Howard L. Holley. These were all excellent doctors.

Holley had been born in Alabama but received his college and medical school educations in South Carolina before taking a 1941–42 internship at the U.S. Marine Hospital in Norfolk, Virginia, and serving 1942–45 in the U.S. Public Health Service, Holley came to Birmingham for a residency in internal medicine under McLester. He then joined the faculty as an instructor in medicine. Years later he founded the Division of Rheumatology and Immunology at UAB, was awarded an endowed chair, and became a major player in building Tinsley's medical school.

As Tinsley shed his acting deanship of the whole medical school in 1951 and could concentrate on the department of medicine and his own teaching, research, and patient care, his prominence in teaching and cardiovascular research drew others, mainly from the Southeast. Lloyd L. Hefner from Vanderbilt and William Bailey Jones from Duke joined the staff, Jones arriving in 1952 for his internship and residency under Tinsley and Hefner in 1953. Previously, Hefner had interned at Vanderbilt and served two years in the Army Medical Corps. In 1955, both began cardiovascular fellowships with Tinsley and later became important factors in building the medical school.

ONE OTHER PHYSICIAN CRITICALLY important in Tinsley's life arrived in December 1954: Samuel Richardson "Dick" Hill Jr. Born in North Carolina in 1923, Hill obtained his B.S. from Duke and began medical school at Bowman Gray in 1943 while Tinsley was chief of medicine. Hill developed hepatitis during medical school and was Dr. Harrison's patient as well as his pupil. With the accelerated program, Hill graduated from medical school in December 1946. He was awarded a Rockefeller Traveling Fellowship "to inspect and evaluate the medical schools of recently

22. S. Richardson
Hill Jr., interview, July
2002, UAB Archives.

devastated Europe." This tour occupied the six months before he began his internship at Harvard's Brigham Hospital in July 1947. In addition to examining the schools and writing his report, he gained invaluable experience and insight into what it took to make a medical school one of the best in the world.

Having done exceptionally well in medical school, Hill obtained his competitive internship and two-year residency in internal medicine at the Peter Bent Brigham Hospital with George W. Thorn, the leading endocrinologist and expert on steroid hormones. Hill then began a chief residency back at Bowman Gray. After two years as chief of medicine at Lackland Air Force Base, he returned to Boston and Thorn as an assistant in medicine for Harvard Medical School. During this time he co-authored two chapters—on the thyroid and testes—for the second edition of Tinsley's *Principles of Internal Medicine.*

In 1954 Hill received a telephone call from Joe Reeves, just back with Tinsley from his two years of practice. Reeves had never met Hill, but at Tinsley's suggestion he invited Hill to come to Birmingham to look at the possibility of joining his old Bowman Gray professor and personal physician in the newly developing department of medicine as a full-time faculty member with excellent laboratory facilities and secretarial and technical support.

Hill took the job for $10,000 a year. His wife, the former Janet Redman from Andover, Massachusetts, and a graduate of the prestigious Smith College, had never been to Alabama. From Smith she went to the Brigham, where she worked in Dr. Thorn's laboratory. When they arrived and Hill showed her their modest dwelling in a long row of rather industrial-looking apartments, she burst into tears. Her family soon visited, and said, "There's no way you can live in this god-forsaken place!"[22] The Massachusetts view of Alabama was clear. They nevertheless stuck it out, and things over the next half century worked out well. Hill became a major factor in building Tinsley's new medical school, as well as the new university: UAB.

HOW DID TINSLEY AND his deputy, Joe Reeves, manage to make such an offer to Hill in the midst of a poverty-stricken medical school? The U.S. Veterans Administration was the answer.

The meager financial resources in Birmingham resulted from low annual appropriations from the state legislature for the new school, but especially from the hemorrhaging of funds and low revenues at the associated Jefferson-Hillman University Hospital. The problems were probably similar to those at Vanderbilt and

Southwestern. Jefferson-Hillman was so poor that vendors would not even leave milk or produce at the hospital loading dock unless a recipient was there to pay with cash. Checks weren't accepted.

However, Roy R. Kracke, the first dean of the four-year medical school in Birmingham, was a visionary. He saw that after World War II the Veterans Administration would play an important role in medical care in the United States. The VA would also, in Kracke's eyes, prove critical in the development of what would later be called an "academic medical center"—a collection of institutions including at least one medical school and one university hospital.

Kracke was a member of SMAG, the VA's Special Medical Advisory Group, and this probably helped shape his ideas. SMAG was established during World War II and made up of fewer than a dozen leading physicians from around the country drawn from organized medicine (the AMA), medical schools, practicing physicians from the community of labor, private practice, and other sectors. It met several times a year in Washington where it advised on policy matters regarding the VA's medical care system. The meetings were always attended by the VA's chief medical director (now the undersecretary for health affairs), and often the VA administrator (now called secretary of the VA and a member of the president's cabinet on the same level as secretaries of State, Defense, and so on).

The history of the U.S. Veterans Administration is too long and complex to be detailed here, but a brief review is necessary to understand the VA's important role in Tinsley's life.

It is impossible today to recapture the feeling of gratitude to its soldiers that pervaded the U.S. population during and after World War II. Despite the usual congressional wrangling, the GI Bill was signed by President Roosevelt on June 22, 1944,[23] paving the way for some 16 million veterans to gain an education and a better life. As the end of the war grew even nearer, popular concerns mounted over the postwar medical care for veterans. There was also worry about the supply of well-trained physicians for the U.S. populace as a whole. Most of the thousands of doctors in the armed forces were young men who had been rushed through medical schools on accelerated three-year schedules followed by quick nine-month internships before entering the war for their first actual practice of medicine. Almost all of the medical specialties of the time had been established in the 1930s, and sustained economic depression had restrained their growth. It was correctly anticipated that as they were discharged these young physicians with field experience in medical

23. M. J. Bennett, *When Dreams Came True. The GI Bill and the Making of Modern America.* (Washington: Brassey's, 1996), 192.

24. R. Adkins, *To Care for Him Who Shall Have Borne the Battle* (Washington, DC: House Committee on Veterans Affairs, U.S. Gov. Printing Office, 1967).

25. Benjamin Lewis, *VA Medical Program in Relation to Medical Schools* (Washington, D.C.: Committee on Veterans Affairs, U.S. Gov. Printing Office, 1970), 11, 45.

26. A. Deutsch, "Veterans Hospitals Called Back Waters of Medicine," *PM* [New York], January 9, 1945, Complete Edition, 20.

27. Benjamin Lewis, *VA Medical Program in Relation to Medical Schools* (Washington, D.C.: Committee on Veterans Affairs, U.S. Gov. Printing Office, 1970), 105.

28. Ibid., 107.

29. As we saw in Chapter 9, Southwest Medical School signed up for the VA plan while Tinsley was there. By the time the plan was detailed and discussed in the December 15, 1945, issue of the *Journal of the American Medical Association*, 27 of the country's 77 approved medical schools had signed on. *By the end*

practice would want to specialize in surgery, medicine, psychiatry, and so on, which were becoming popular with the public. The VA medical system could participate in this training while also improving the care for veterans.

The VA had long had a program of hospital care for veterans,[24] but most knowledgeable medical people believed the medical care provided by the existing VA professionals, facilities, and arrangements was far inferior to that available to the general public in the private sector. The belief was pervasive, justified or not,[25] as indicated in a January 1945 newspaper article which referred to VA hospitals as "medical monasteries . . . because of their physical and scientific isolation," and because of this they were "backwaters of medicine" and providers of inferior care.[26]

General Omar N. Bradley, a leader in the European Theater, expected that after Germany fell he would go to the Pacific to help conclude the fighting against Japan, but General George Marshall wanted him to take over the dispirited Veterans Administration as the top boss reporting directly to the president—responsible for veterans' benefits as well as the medical program. Bradley assumed the position of VA administrator on Wednesday, August 15, 1945. The next day he received a letter from presidential adviser Bernard M. Baruch recommending "establishment of 'effective VA ties with centers of medical education and skill.'"[27]

In Chicago, Paul G. Magnuson was thinking along these same lines. Magnuson, professor of orthopedics and chairman of the Department of Bone and Joint Surgery at Northwestern Medical School, contacted three medical school deans in Chicago and Minnesota to ask if they would affiliate with a local VA hospital for residency training of returning doctors, which he believed would also upgrade the medical care at the VA hospitals. All three agreed. Soon Magnuson was talking with his friend Major General Paul R. Hawley, just back from his post as chief surgeon of the European Theater, who had been recruited by Bradley to run the VA's medical programs. Magnuson left his job and moved to Washington as a full-time VA employee, taking an income reduction of about 90 percent. His "first accomplishment . . . was the writing of a detailed 'statement of what I believe General Hawley has in mind for the immediate future for the staffing of veterans hospitals and for cooperation with teaching institutions.'"[28] Hawley made some minor modifications, and the plan was begun in November 1945 as the "Hawley-Magnuson Plan."[29] Letters regarding this cooperation were sent to the medical school deans, and their essentially uniformly positive responses were then sent to the VA hospitals for implementation.

William S. Middleton, dean of the University of Wisconsin medical school wrote, "Splendid! I am indeed sorry to hear that the American Board of Surgery beat the American Board of Internal Medicine to the gun, but I have no doubt that the several boards will fall into line."[30] Even as dean, Middleton was a clinically active physician in half-time practice and a real soldier, who later served two terms as chief medical director for the VA. He was, like his colleagues Magnuson, Hawley, and Tinsley, first and foremost a physician. They got along well.

The affiliation between a VA hospital and a medical school was remarkably informal—just a few letters signed by people with no apparent legal authority to make such extensive commitments and accomplished mainly on the basis of personal contacts and mutual trust. The real fight came at the end of 1945 and first few days of 1946. To make this plan work well and over a long term, the Bradley-Hawley-Magnuson team needed more legal underpinning. They found a potent enemy in the U.S. Civil Service, which correctly saw itself as losing control. The accounts of Lewis and Magnuson[31] detail the dramatic bureaucratic battles of those days, culminating in Truman's signing on January 3, 1946, of Public Law 293.[32] The law created the Department of Medicine and Surgery in the VA and established Title 38 of the U.S. Code, removing VA physicians, nurses, and dentists from the Civil Service and placing them in this special VA professional category, which was run by the real professionals in medical care, not the bureaucrats looking in some direction other than directly at the individual veteran patient. The Veterans Administration central office was and remains an 11-story building directly across Lafayette Square from the White House.

Public Law 293 led to the issuance of the VA's Policy Memorandum Number 2, written in Hawley's warm and personal style, detailing the obligations and responsibilities of the VA on one side (care of patients) and the medical schools on the other (maintenance and promotion of high standards and training of resident physicians).[33]

By 1951 a special subcommittee of the U.S. Senate Committee on Labor and Public Welfare—chaired by Alabama's Lister Hill—had investigated VA policies on hospital administration. In its report of August 2 that year, the subcommittee opened with the following statements:

> The medical care program of the Veterans' Administration is one of the largest in the world . . . Obviously, a program of this magnitude is one of considerable and continuing interest to the Congress and the people of the United States. . . .

of 1946, 63 of the 77 were on board.

30. Lewis, *VA*, 109.

31. Lewis, *VA*; P. G. Magnuson, *Ring the Night Bell: The Autobiography of a Surgeon* (Boston: Little, Brown & Co., 1960). Reprinted by UAB, Birmingham, AL, 1986.

32. H.R. 4717, Public Law 293, 79th Congress, 1st Session.

33. U.S. Veterans Administration, policy memorandum No. 2. "Policy in Association of Veterans' Hospitals With Medical Schools," January 30, 1946, Washington DC. This is reprinted in its entirety in Lewis's book, 123–25.

34. Quoted in Adkins, *To Care*, 1, with original reference. Italics in Adkins's original.

35. The historic U.S. Supreme Court decision in *Brown v. Board of Education*, reversing the 1896 "separate but equal" doctrine of *Plessy v. Ferguson*, was still a year away. During Birmingham's increased racial strife soon to come, the VA often served as a haven for beleaguered souls and bodies.

That interest is considerably heightened by the fact that during the last few years the quality of the medical care available to the beneficiaries of the Veterans' Administration has been raised to a point where it unquestionably represents the best medical care available anywhere in the world at any time in the world's history.

When one realizes that this program also represents an attempt on the part of the congress to *partially discharge our obligation to the men and women who have offered their lives in defense of our country*, it is obvious that anything materially affecting that program should be of immediate concern to the Congress.[34]

SENATOR LISTER HILL MUST have known Kracke; perhaps he played a role in Kracke's appointment to SMAG. In any case, Kracke was able to secure a city block of land across from the existing university hospital (the Jefferson-Hillman complex) for construction of one of the new VA hospitals. Birmingham's was a solidly built 479-bed facility, one of the biggest hospitals in the state. Its equipment was the newest and best available. Salaries for the nurses and other personnel were higher than those across the street in the university hospital, perhaps the highest in the state. It was racially integrated from the day it opened in 1953, when all other similar facilities in the state were strictly segregated by race, including the university hospital across the street.[35] The VA hospital in Birmingham was clearly a federal institution; local police and state troopers were required to leave their sidearms outside or with the guards when entering the facilities.

The VA's important role in development of what became the UAB Medical Center in Birmingham was first apparent in its provision of money and space for the recruitment of physicians for the faculty, just as Paul Magnuson had hoped and planned.

It was into this facility, with its money and new and empty space, that Tinsley was able to recruit Walter B. Frommeyer as its first chief of the medical service and an assistant professor of medicine in the school. And a year later, when Frommeyer was named assistant dean of the school, the chief of medical service position became vacant and Tinsley recruited Joe Reeves, his former resident and fellow from Texas, where Reeves was just finishing his second year of private practice in mid-1954.

Reeves then recruited S. Richardson Hill from his position with Harvard's George Thorn at the Brigham; Hill became an assistant professor of medicine and full-time member of the medical staff of the new VA Hospital in late 1954. This may not seem such a remarkable recruitment in the 21st century, when the little medical school has become the University of Alabama at Birmingham with its UAB Medical Center—by many measures one of the most prominent and excellent in the nation and world—but in the early 1950s, bringing Hill from Boston was a major coup.[36]

By the end of 1954, Tinsley, no doubt with the aid of Champ Lyons and Joe Volker, had recruited Frommeyer, Reeves, and Hill to his department of medicine. The three were important to him for the rest of his life and they played crucial roles in building his new medical school. All three began their new academic careers with the school in the VA, so they had intimate knowledge of its philosophy and workings. In his *Reminiscenses,* Tinsley's Chapter 10 on the VA was titled "The VA to the Rescue," and he concluded, "There can be little doubt that without the University Medical Center affiliation, the standard of care in the Birmingham Veterans Administration Hospital would have been low. But it is equally true that without the Veterans Administration hospital affiliation, the Medical School would have remained second class. Each institution has been essential to the other in their joint escape from mediocrity."

TINSLEY ACCEPTED THE POSITION of dean of medicine only after University of Alabama President John Gallalee suggested that if he really preferred the chief of medicine position, he could as dean appoint himself to the latter position then later decide which he would prefer to keep. Tinsley had no doubt about this, having served in both positions in Texas, but Gallalee said that his decision could be made within a few months, so Tinsley accepted both positions. He later felt that he had ameliorated some political conflicts among the physicians and had avoided a potentially damaging fight over space occupied by a non-teaching, non-cooperative squatter consuming much valuable space needed by the faculty, especially if the school was to profit from the oncoming flood of federal and private research dollars, which Tinsley correctly saw coming in the near future.

That fight was with Tom Spies, the Harvard-degreed nutritionist from Ohio who was interested in proving that pellagra was caused by dietary niacin deficiency rather than an infectious agent. Spies had been invited to Birmingham by James S. McLester and had come in 1938 because of the large numbers of patients there with pellagra. McLester, whose major accomplishments and writings were in nutrition, thought there might be an infectious component to the full-blown clinical picture of pellagra. Spies was building on the shoulders of the earlier studies of Dr. Joseph Goldberger of the U.S. Public Health Service. Goldberger had sought the "P-P

36. UAB's reputation exists, despite the lingering impression among some academics in New England, New York, and elsewhere that Alabama is culturally, economically, and educationally the least desirable place to live.

37. A good brief account of Goldberger and his studies on pellagra is in the *American National Biography*, vol. 9, 180–181.

38. Partly at the urging of Groce Harrison Sr., but mainly at the urging of Dr. Flexner.

39. J. D. L. Holmes, *A History of the University of Alabama Hospitals* (Birmingham: University of Alabama in Birmingham Print Shop, 1974), 73–. Although Volker was appointed dean on June 9, 1948, he had forewarned the administration that he was committed to traveling in Europe (especially Czechoslovakia) as part of a rehabilitation/reconstruction effort and would not be available until the end of the summer. It was a hectic time, arranging for space and money, selecting and recruiting the first faculty and getting them in place, arranging with the medical faculty to teach both medical and dental students, to arrange curricula, to admit the first students, etc., all of which he accomplished in 45 days. Fifty-two students started October 18th the same year!

Factor"—pellagra prevention factor—in various foods but died in 1929 before the vitamin niacin was discovered in 1937.[37] In 1937 or '38, Spies and McLester had a discussion at a meeting where McLester challenged Spies's idea that pellagra was caused *solely* by a deficiency of nicotinic acid. At this meeting McLester invited Spies to Birmingham to do a clinical trial, since patients with pellagra were common there but rare in Ohio. Spies had accepted and opened offices, laboratories, and a large clinic in a building of the medical school complex, part of the old Birmingham Medical College closed in 1915. Now, as the war ended and the issue of pellagra pathogenesis settled, McLester as chairman of medicine for the new four-year medical school and physician-in-chief of the hospital, and all his staff, expected Spies and his group to return to Ohio. But Spies refused to leave.

To UNDERSTAND THE GENESIS of the Spies-Medical College fight one needs to know the physical structure of the medical school-hospital complex as it was then. The old Hillman Hospital had opened as a private charity hospital in 1903 and had expanded over the next three decades, culminating in the Jefferson Hospital, a 17-story structure built mainly with federal funds under a Roosevelt New Deal program. It opened in January 1941. The much smaller Hillman Hospital was being transformed into an office building for clinical faculty. Just behind the old original Hillman Building was the building which had housed the defunct Birmingham Medical College, closed in 1915.[38] This building was a substantial five-story structure currently used for outpatient clinics. It was in this building that Spies had set up the "Spies Clinic" in 1938 and which he now refused to vacate despite the needs of the new four-year medical school.

As the school moved its two-year program, with faculty, staff, and equipment, from Tuscaloosa to Birmingham in the summer of 1945, no facilities had been constructed to house the new four-year school, which now occupied the 17th floor of the already filled Jefferson Hospital. To aggravate the space problem, a totally new School of Dentistry had been started in 1948 by President Gallalee and Joseph F. Volker. When Volker opened the dental school in October 1948, having become dean of dentistry that June,[39] there was no additional space, so he crowded in with the medical school. He reasoned that for the first two years the dental students would be occupied mainly with the basic sciences anyhow. Thus, 52 dental students were squeezed in with the 130 medical students who transferred from Tuscaloosa rather than moving to schools in other states after the second year as had been the procedure since 1920 when the Mobile school closed.[40] Both the medical and the

40. Ibid., 57, 73.

dental schools were in desperate need of space as well as money.

Spies had raised considerable money for his quarters, which were lavish in comparison to the facilities of the medical and dental schools. This money had come chiefly from the socio-political powers of the city—the iron, steel, and coal barons. They were grateful for the success he and others had gained in controlling pellagra and other debilitating diseases affecting their non-affluent labor force, and they were attracted to his suave, sophisticated, entrepreneurial style. In *Reminiscences*, Tinsley said of Spies that he was a "natural born fundraiser." Nonetheless, Spies's occupation of a majority of the space in the old Birmingham Medical College was damaging the medical school by preventing its use by the full-time faculty who were desperate for space and squeezed into the already filled Jefferson Hospital.

Kracke, the former dean—with the full support of his faculty, the approximately 30 full-time basic science group as well as the 75 volunteer clinical teachers from Birmingham's practicing community—had previously attempted to extrude Spies. Spies's powerful friends were extremely influential in the state legislature, and they vigorously rejected the idea. They also threatened President Gallalee that if Spies were expelled, the budget and support for not only the new medical school in Birmingham, but also for the entire University of Alabama would be severely cut. Coming so soon after the decision to place the school in Birmingham, such a fight with the state legislature might reopen the wounds of prior fights between Mobile, Tuscaloosa, and Birmingham and conceivably result in moving the school out of Birmingham. Gallalee sympathized with and agreed with the goal of McLester and his faculty, but he felt that the Spies problem would sooner or later resolve itself; simple procrastination was the best course.

This was devastating for Kracke and the faculty but undoubtedly was the right decision at the time, according to Tinsley's reminiscences. Tinsley knew the details of this fight and knew the people involved, having grown up with the McLester children. He admired Galallee and considered his avoidance of this statewide fight one of his accomplishments as dean of medicine. Spies departed later in the 1950s, as Gallalee had predicted, and his space reverted to the hospital and medical school.

IN THE MEANTIME TINSLEY wanted to fulfill his wish to be just chief of medicine (with designations as both chairman of the Department of Medicine and chief of the medical service in the University Hospital) and definitely not dean of medicine.

Small and primitive as it was, Tinsley had the embryo of his cardiology program up and running. It was the research, writing, and teaching he really wanted to devote the remainder of his life to, not sitting in committee meetings and trying to allocate the scarce resources or referee power struggles. He was already prominent and distinguished in medical circles, with his service as president of the American Heart Association and membership on the first Council of the new National Heart Institute, for which he received a commendation from the U.S. Public Health Service on April 29, 1952, as well as a Distinguished Service Award and Silver Medallion from the American Heart Association in October of that year. But the main reason for his prominence, of course, was the appearance in 1950 of the first edition of *Principles of Internal Medicine*, which had taken the country by storm—and won him the Marchman Award for Oustanding Contributions to Medical Education from the Dallas Southern Clinical Society—and would continue to occupy Tinsley's energy into the 1970s. Meanwhile, as Tinsley went about building the new school in the early 1950s, the second edition of *PIM* was in preparation and needed much attention. As it was coming out in 1954, Tinsley was presented the Modern Medicine Award for Distinguished Achievement from the *Journal of Modern Medicine*.

When he accepted the position of dean of medicine, Tinsley promised that he and Chief of Surgery Champ Lyons would form a search committee of two and help Gallalee recruit a new dean. They launched into this immediately, identified seven leading physicians from elsewhere, and attempted to recruit each to the deanship. In each case the position was refused. Tinsley felt the reasons were based less on emotional impressions of potential candidates about the South and more on money and space. He further felt that this was aggravated by similar views of the local citizens themselves. He said:

> For eighty years the people of the state had slumbered, dreaming of past glories (many of which had never existed) rather than facing present realities and preparing for future challenges. Like most other areas in the deep South, Alabama suffered from an inferiority complex and from self-pity. The lament: "We lost the War between the States; we were persecuted during the Reconstruction period; we are poor; we cannot afford to pay for first-class education"; was firmly planted in the minds of many political, business and professional leaders. The young Moses who was eventually to lead the people of the state out of their self-imposed bondage and

point them towards the Promised Land of educational excellence . . . had not yet appeared on the scene. Despite a few exceptions, the public schools were, by and large, mediocre and distinctly inferior to those in most other states.[41]

The candidate who eventually surfaced for the deanship was James J. Durrett, a 1914 graduate of Harvard Medical School who also held a pharmacy degree from Mobile. A native of Tuscaloosa, Durrett had served as the first county health officer in Tuscaloosa, then in Memphis, where he also taught 1920–28 at the University of Tennessee medical school as professor of public health. He next worked as chief of drug control for the U.S. Food and Drug Administration (FDA), then as director of the medical bureau of the Federal Trade Commission.[42] He had a good academic background, a familiarity with medical administration, and the search committee felt he was probably favorably disposed toward Alabama. Durrett accepted the position of dean of medicine and assumed his duties in September 1951. Unfortunately, he was a poor choice and turned out to be a poor leader. His years in bureaucracies had trained him more about bureaucracies than about medicine or the teaching of medicine. He was a piddler and procrastinator. "Decisions were again and again postponed."[43] He lacked a vision for the school.

A new Basic Science Building across the street from the Jefferson Hospital was completed in 1951, and a dental clinic was added. Durrett, however, allocated none of the space vacated in the Jefferson Hospital to the surgery department. Lyons had complained bitterly about the lack of surgical beds for charity patients and teaching, and Tinsley, after some agonizing, yielded two medical service beds to Lyons, rationalizing that many students can be taught on a single medical patient, but fewer on surgical patients (who usually have only one operation). "Durrett, whose main concern was to avoid rocking the boat, decided that Champ [Lyons] was Public Enemy Number One. He was to hold this opinion for two years and then change it. During this period he continually frustrated Champ by delaying, time and again, action on the urgent requests from his department."[44] The result of Durrett's chronic procrastinations and bureaucratic personality was loss of confidence in him by the faculty and chiefs of service. He held endless meetings which accomplished no decisions or actions. "The net result," Tinsley said, "seemed to be perpetual motionlessness."

Durrett was more intent on avoiding bad decisions than making good decisions. The result was stagnation. One decision he did make proved to be a major blunder.

41. Harrison, *Reminiscences*, 1.

42. V. E. Fisher, *Building on a Vision: A Fifty-Year Retrospective of UAB's Academic Health Center* (Birmingham: University of Alabama at Birmingham, 1995), 180.

43. Harrison, *Reminiscences*, 2.

44. Ibid., 3.

45. Zachary, *Endless*.
46. Harrison, *Reminiscences*, chapter 6.
By the first decades
of the 21st century
SRI had become an
official and legal af-
filiate of UAB. Many
of the two faculties
and staffs held joint
appointments, and
there was considerable
joint research done on
NIH and other grants
and contracts. The
model which SRI and
similar organizations
attempted to emulate
was the Batelle Insti-
tute in Ohio.

At the end of the war, Thomas Martin, a much admired president of the Alabama Power Company and a wealthy and influential citizen, helped found the Southern Research Institute, a private institution dedicated to continuing and advancing the spectacular research led by the charismatic Vannevar Bush under the wartime Office of Scientific Research and Development.[45] The directors of the SRI were the most prominent, wealthy, and influential citizens of the area and beyond, and Durrett tried to divert their support to the medical school. The result was a rift between these individuals and SRI versus the medical school, which lost support rather than gaining support. This rift was still a concern in 1969 when Tinsley wrote his reminiscences.[46]

Finally Frommeyer, having served a year as chief of medicine in the new VA Hospital, was convinced to give that position up and become associate dean. In Tinsley's view, Frommeyer saved the dean's office from total collapse during Durrett's tenure, which ended in 1955 with his retirement.

One catastrophe which occurred despite Frommeyer's influence was the appointment of Elmer Caveny as chief of psychiatry, a department which had been founded by Dr. Frank Kay years before. Kay resigned to devote more time to practice, and Durrett asked Tinsley to chair a committee to recommend a successor to be appointed on a full-time basis. A new building for psychiatry was being planned, and it was important to obtain a good leader.

Tinsley describes the situation well:

At the first meeting of the committee, Dr. Durrett urged the appointment of Dr. E. L. Caveny, who was retiring from the Navy. The Dean saw no need to go through the usual procedure of instituting a nationwide search. When questioned, the Dean admitted that his candidate had had little experience with teaching and that he, himself, had not read Dr. Caveney's publications. Nevertheless he had talked with the candidate and was convinced that he was just the right man for the position. These arguments were decidedly unconvincing to Dr. Lyons, Dr. Frommeyer, and myself. It seemed to us that our committee had been summoned to rubber stamp the Dean's choice. A departmental chairman has a minimum of three responsibilities, i.e., for leadership, teaching, and research. In the case of a clinical department, there is a fourth, that of patient care. The Dean's nominee had ample experience in the latter function and was presumably entirely competent therein. But we had been offered no evidence concerning his achievements as a teacher or an investigator, or his potential for leadership. Upon this somewhat stormy note the first meeting ended.

During the next several days I read all of Dr. Caveny's publications. They were few in number and mundane in quality. I saw no evidence of originality, imagination, deep insight, or an aim at new concepts. This opinion was presented to the committee when it next met. Champ Lyons strongly supported my view that we should not act in haste but should institute a broad search for the best possible man.

Durrett now became adamant. He saw no need in wasting more time. The committee should forthwith recommend his nominee. Champ and I declined to yield. We both now began to suspect that the Dean had actually offered the position to Dr. Caveny even before appointing our committee. The Dean was asked why he had appointed our committee if he had already made his decision. The reply was of the usual diversionary irrelevant variety.

Champ and I now elaborated on the extreme importance of departmental chairmen. There would be only a few such appointments in the near future. The caliber of these men would presumably set standards for a score or more years. They should be imaginative, energetic and critical investigators. They should be stimulating teachers and inspiring leaders. Preferably they should already have achieved a national reputation in order that they could attract brilliant young teachers to their departments. Again we urged delay during which the views in the field could be obtained, not only concerning the Dean's nominee but about other possible candidates.

During most of these discussions, Walter Frommeyer had maintained the judicious discretion that was appropriate to his difficult position. The Associate Dean would ordinarily be expected to support his superior. But Wally is made of tougher material. He saw that now the chips were truly down. Tactfully but firmly he expressed concurrence with our views. Despite this the committee, with the Dean and the Associate Dean abstaining, voted three to two in favor of the Dean's nominee.

There had been nothing personal in this disagreement. The department of medicine was in no way directly involved. But a vital principle, that of a deep obligation to search for the best possible man for any faculty appointment and most especially so in the case of a departmental chairmanship, had been at stake. From that time forward every glimpse of Durrett brought to mind the line from Canterbury Tales: "The gretteste clerkes been noght the wysest men."

The Department of Surgery did reap one indirect dividend from this episode. After the battle concerning psychiatry, Champ Lyons was no longer Public Enemy Number One. Henceforth, I would be so regarded. . . . The Medical College floundered because the helmsman neither knew where he wanted to go nor how to get there even had he known.

During five decades in academic life, one observes many errors. Probably the most frequent serious mistake involves the appointment of mediocre persons to faculty positions. In most instances this stems from the recommendations of insecure individuals who occupy positions of leadership for which they are unfit. Men with second-rate minds appear to have a subconscious fear of those with first-rate minds.

One occasionally observes a superior leader who misjudges a person and makes a weak appointment. The reverse situation, a strong appointment by a weak leader, is much rarer. As a rule the outstanding leader selects outstanding followers while mediocrity perpetuates mediocrity. The failure of department heads, deans and presidents to make an intensive, almost agonizing, search for men with brilliant minds and future potential leadership is probably the single greatest defect in our system of higher education. Too often there is only a half-hearted search for an outstanding individual. In many instances there is a preference for an agreeable personality rather than for a superior intellect. Thus Portia's assessment—'God made him and therefore let him pass for a man' describes many appointees."

In his *Reminiscences*, Tinsley does evince some sympathy for the problems facing Durrett, such as serious inadequacies in some professional areas, weak teaching, and a near total lack of research in most departments, grossly inadequate physical space, a weak hospital administration, and a terrible if improving fiscal situation. Tinsley continued to push everybody to be active in research, and the new NIH began providing increasing amounts of money, as did the VA in smaller but still significant quantities.

In 1953, Gallalee was replaced as president of the University of Alabama. He had been a patient of Tinsley's and died after a mercifully brief cardiac illness. The replacement was O. C. (Oliver Cromwell) Carmichael, a native of rural, Protestant Alabama, who had a remarkable career in teaching and education administration. Trained in Romance languages in local colleges, he won a Rhodes Scholarship and studied at Wadham College, Oxford University, earning a B.S. in anthropology. During the war, Carmichael also worked in Belgium, befriended Herbert Hoover, joined the Y.M.C.A. (Young Men's Christian Association), and worked in East Africa where he learned Urdu and Swahili, took a fellowship in languages at Princeton, became head of foreign languages at a Birmingham public high school, then served as principal of several grammar schools and high schools in the Birmingham area. After serving in administration at Alabama State College for Women in Montevallo, he took administrative positions in Tennessee, finally becoming chancellor of Vanderbilt University, then president of the Carnegie Foundation for the advancement of teaching. At age 62, Carmichael returned to Alabama to finish his career in what he expected to be a relatively tranquil period as president of the University of Alabama. His background and native intelligence seemed to put him in a good position to understand and lead the state's major old university.[47]

When Tinsley was a youthful medical student, his father entertained Carmichael and other Birmingham school officials at home. Young Tinsley came to know and admire them. When Carmichael moved to Vanderbilt in 1935, Tinsley was the family's internist. Tinsley reports that his reaction to Carmichael's return as university president and overall leader for the medical school was "more than pleasurable; it was joyful." Here was a man who could surely help the school move rapidly forward to new heights. The year was 1953. The school was stagnating for a variety of reasons, and Durrett was one of them. Yet Tinsley later wrote that, contrary to local gossip, he never "politicked President Carmichael on the Durrett problem."

THOUGH TINSLEY MET CARMICHAEL at several large university functions over the following months, and had seen him as a patient for several check-ups during that time, they had not discussed the situation of the medical school. One day Carmichael telephoned and asked for a meeting in the president's office in Tuscaloosa but did not state the reason or agenda. Tinsley guessed. During the 60-mile drive he worried about how to tell the truth without seeming malicious and destructive. He need not have worried, for the wise and experienced Carmichael simply told him that he believed the medical school had great potential and that they should obtain the best possible "advice from an external, unbiased and therefore objective group concerning future plans. . . . [And he] asked [Harrison] to suggest the name of the best possible person to be chairman of such a committee." Tinsley explained the situation further:

When I proposed Dr. Duckett Jones, the president asked about our previous

47. M. G. Synnott, "Oliver Cromwell Carmichael" in *American National Biography*, 404–406.

48. Jones was prominent in medicine as the one who established the "Jones Criteria" for the diagnosis of rheumatic fever, which has no pathognomonic finding. T. D. Jones, "The Diagnosis of Rheumatic Fever," *J. of the Amer. Med. Assn. 126 (1944)*: 481–484. The "Jones Criteria" were prominent in medicine late in World War II and into the 1950s, when rheumatic fever had a brief resurgence. They underwent two modifications later and were being further modified by Bauer, et al., during Jones's visits to Birmingham. P. C. English, *Rheumatic Fever in America and Britain* (New Brunswick: NJ, Rutgers University Press, 1999).

associations. I explained that Duckett had been one of the pioneers in the study of rheumatic fever and was currently the Chief Executive Officer of the Helen Hay Whitney Foundation.[48] We had worked together for about eight years on various Boards and Councils, and I had served under him, the Chairman, as a member of the Health Subcommittee of the Study Committee for the Ford Foundation. I assured him that with the possible exception of Dr. Alan Gregg of the Rockefeller Foundation, there was no man in the medical field whose judgment, integrity and courage I had more confidence than in Duckett Jones.

Dr. Carmichael asked me to telephone Dr. Jones. Fortunately the call immediately found him in his office. After the introduction, Dr. Carmichael was handed the phone. When it was clear from Dr. Carmichael's words that Dr. Jones was about to decline the request, I asked for the telephone. Duckett Jones was reminded that more than five years previously I had been "too busy" because of responsibilities and problems in Dallas, the Presidency of the American Heart Association, and membership in the Heart Council of the NIH, to accept his offered position on the Health Study Committee for the Ford Foundation. But when he had put the matter on a personal basis and had said that I *had* to accept because of friendship for him, I yielded. Now the situation was reversed and I expected to "cash the check" of personal obligation. He *had* to accept because of personal friendship for me. Duckett then agreed. Dr. Carmichael asked him to select whichever two other persons he desired for his committee. Those selected were Max Lapham, then Dean at Tulane, and Jack Mazur, who was Director of the Clinical Center of the National Institutes of Health.

Aside from several joint visits by the entire committee, each of the three members made separate visits to us. Duckett Jones came repeatedly [and made a thorough investigation]. . . .

After some months of interviews, the report of the Jones Committee was made to the President in August 1954. This report marks a landmark in the history of the medical college. The most important of its many findings was the conclusion that the Medical College was suffering from "weak leadership." Dr. Carmichael subsequently initiated the necessary remedial measures. . . . The period of stagnation was thereby ended.

The story has a tragic sequel. Duckett Jones had, at my urging, agreed reluctantly to Dr. Carmichael's request that he serve as Chairman of the External (Jones) Committee. . . . Neither then nor later did he mention to me that [his] initial reluctance [to accept the chairmanship] had stemmed from the headaches he was having as a consequence of increasingly severe hypertension [for which there was no effective treatment then].

A few months after the Jones report had been submitted, Duckett's secretary called and told me that he had been hospitalized and was well nigh moribund. When I mentioned that I would like to fly to his bedside and see him, not as a physician but as a friend, she told me that he was no longer conscious. Within a few days he expired.

Tinsley had the highest regard for Jones, "a kindly man . . . forced by his conscience to offer unkind and critical comments" which would hurt some decent people. "We can only revere the name of a noble character and honor the memory of a wise and strong man" whose perceptiveness, insights, energy, and articulateness had led to the report. Tinsley later felt that the Jones Report probably hastened Jones's death—that the stresses of multiple hasty trips, too frequent heavy meals in tense situations, the self-imposed deadlines for writing reports, and the heavy impact of the report itself had shortened the days of Jones's life. He felt that he personally had contributed to this. Many times in subsequent years Tinsley commented that he felt sad that Jones's crucially important report for the school had come at such a price.[49]

The Jones Report also stimulated the medical school by observing that the other major school in the medical center, the School of Dentistry, was making strong progress and had already come to be recognized as "among the leading such institutions in the country," with high morale, good teaching and well-supported research, and "young dentists from other nations . . . beginning to choose Birmingham for advanced training." It also stated, "The University of Alabama School of Dentistry is at present the best functioning unit of the Medical Center." "The spirit of inquiry was leading to productive research."[50]

The most important recommendations of the Jones Report were:

1. A Vice President of the University in Charge of Health Affairs should be appointed (to separate the hospital from the responsibilities of the Dean of Medicine).

2. The Dean of Medicine should be qualified by experience for leadership.

3. The name of the largest unit, the hospital, should be changed from the Jefferson-Hillman Hospital to the University Hospital and Hillman Clinic.

4. A well qualified administrator with experience in university hospital work

49. Harrison, *Reminiscences*, chapter 6, 13–chapter 7, 2.
50. Ibid., chapter 7, 1.

51. Ibid., chapter 7, 3; John E. Dietrick and Robert C. Berson, *Medical Schools in the United States at Mid-Century* (New York: McGraw-Hill, 1953), which "comprises the formal report of the Survey of Medical Education."

52. Harrison, *Reminiscences*, chapter 7, 3.

53. Despite the lack of an earned doctorate, Carmichael had many honorary doctorates.

54. Ibid., chapter 7, 4.

55. Durrett, however, cast a long, uncomfortable shadow. Elmer Caveny was appointed chief of psychiatry by Durrett on January 1, 1955. He retired from that position in April 1959, but Carmichael kept him on as a special adviser to the president until 1969, which calmed Caveny's anger, humiliation, and resentment and also helped with his retirement (though he already had retirement incomes from the Navy and U.S. government). In accordance with Tinsley's predictions, he had accomplished little other than to occasionally make other faculty members angry, especially Lyons.

should be appointed as the chief executive of the hospital.

5. Several smaller clinical departments should be incorporated into the departments of medicine or surgery.

6. An independent department of psychiatry should be established.

7. The Executive Committee of the faculty should be reactivated.

8. Regular meetings of the Medical College should be resumed.

9. The School of Nursing should be moved from Tuscaloosa to Birmingham.

President Carmichael began implementing Jones's recommendations by identifying and recruiting Robert Berson as vice president and dean of medicine. Berson had been a student of Tinsley's at Vanderbilt, where he had the unusual distinction of making excellent grades while playing first-string tackle on the football team. Tinsley and Lyons were invited with spouses to dine with the Bersons at the Frommeyers' home and urged Berson to accept Carmichael's offer, which he did.

Berson was well-suited for the job, having served as associate dean at both Illinois and Vanderbilt and having co-authored a well-received book on medical schools and medical education in America, "the first comprehensive study of this subject since the Flexner report four decades previously."[51]

Subsequently, Carmichael drove himself and Tinsley to Talladega for the funeral of one of the university trustees. Tinsley claims[52] that on this trip he had his one and only conversation with Carmichael about Durrett: "I congratulated Dr. Carmichael[53] upon the appointment of Dr. Berson and told him that the change in leadership of the Medical College had been absolutely necessary to prevent chaos and to insure progress. Despite our physician-patient relationship and our personal friendship, this was the only time we ever discussed Dr. Durrett."[54] Tinsley believed that Carmichael had handled this situation with wisdom and effectiveness. Durrett soon retired to Florida where he died in 1968.[55]

The next item in the Jones Report was recruitment of an able administrator for the hospital. This time a good man was close at hand: Mathew Francis McNulty, the first administrator of the new Birmingham VA Hospital. He had arrived with his wife, a native of Montgomery, Alabama, whom he had met while serving there in the U.S. Army Air Corps in 1943–44. McNulty, like Frommeyer, was thus a staunch Roman Catholic from the North who had married a girl from the South. He had studied and done hospital administration for years. Some indication of his abilities was his 1941–46 rise from private to lieutenant colonel. The VA had

moved him from an administration position in its Washington, D.C., hospital to
Birmingham when the VA hospital opened there in 1953. It was necessary only
to move McNulty across the street to the newly renamed University Hospital and
Hillman Clinic in 1954, and the next major change recommended by the Jones
Report was accomplished. McNulty was effective and popular and held many
positions in the medical center over the subsequent 15 years. The hospital began
to regain solvency and improve the laboratories and radiology facilities. Finally,
things were moving ahead.

IN 1957 TINSLEY ANNOUNCED that he was retiring from his role as chairman of
the department of medicine. Walter B. Frommeyer was selected to succeed him.
Frommeyer was less bound by his own biases and more future-oriented, and he
immediately established administrative divisions in his department. This was the
sort of sub-specialization that Tinsley despised. He continued to rail against "the
'ologists, who know all about one organ but nothing about a whole patient."
He compromised, however, accepting appointment as chief of the division of
cardiology. He recognized that if the school was to prosper in the years ahead it

*Department of
Medicine faculty
and house staff
on the steps of
University Hospital,
1957–58. The
front row includes
(from left):
Tinsley Harrison
(third), Walter
B. Frommeyer
(fifth), James A.
Pittman Jr. (sixth),
S. Richardson Hill
Jr. (seventh), and
Howard L. Holley
(eighth).*

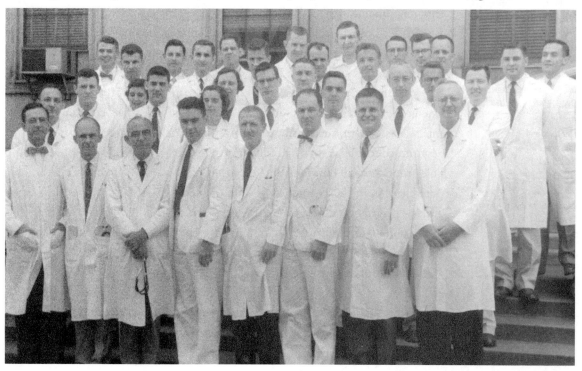

56. As discussed in Chapter 8, Williams, a Tennessee native, took year of medical school at Vanderbilt then the last three years at Hopkins, as Harrison had. He interned and took a residency year at Vanderbilt from 1935 to 1937, then a year back at Hopkins with Longcope, and in 1938–39 he was chief medical resident at Vanderbilt. After working with J. H. Means at the thyroid unit of Mass General Hospital, he spent several years at Harvard's Thorndike Memorial Laboratory at the Boston City Hospital. In 1949 he became the University of Washington's first chairman of medicine in Seattle, where he is given much credit for making that one of the world's leading medical schools. He was still chair of medicine in 1957–58. Maxwell Finland, *The Harvard Medical Unit at the Boston City Hospital* (1983), 708. "The Thorndike," now moved to Harvard's Boston Beth Israel Hospital, was a center for excellent medical research and productive conduit for leaders in academic medicine for the latter half of

would have to create specialty or subspecialty administrative units within its larger departments. And despite his loud protests to the contrary, he was first of all a superb cardiologist. Thus, he began the retirement from administrative medicine. He was 57 years old.

Some internists do not begin a career as a departmental chair until their mid-fifties. Tinsley talked much about staying too long and cited his old Brigham chief Henry Christian as an example. He believed that a chief who stayed too long did not help, but rather impeded, the progress of his department. Probably his experiences as the chief at Bowman Gray and Southwestern, and the problems he had in later years there, also influenced him as he tried to help his newest school get on its feet and move ahead. He now had a substantial faculty and solid house staff, as the applicants for residency positions became more abundant. It seemed time to move on.

Secretly, a friend in Seattle was plotting. The famous endocrinologist Robert H. Williams, who had been a student and resident under Tinsley at Vanderbilt in the 1930s, was planning a going-away present for his old mentor and close medical friend. Maxwell Finland says in his book on the Harvard Medical Unit at the Boston City Hospital (BCH), which included the famous research unit, the Thorndike Memorial Laboratory, ". . .Williams has been one of the most dynamic and creative architects of scientific and academic medicine in the third quarter of the 20th century."[56] He was the right man for this commemorative job. It was to be a grand party and banquet at the 1958 Atlantic City meetings of the Old Turks, the AAP.

It was indeed a grand occasion. Tinsley had announced his retirement as chair of medicine effective as of October 1957, and Frommeyer had taken over in September. Tinsley continued his non-administrative activities outside cardiology, but he continued to attend many administrative meetings, since by later standards the whole group was still quite small. He continued private and clinic practice, taught, worked hard in the lab, wrote, worked on the new editions of *Principles of Internal Medicine*, played a bit more golf at the Mountain Brook Club with old friends (often wealthy donors to the medical school), and spent more weekends at his cabin on Lake Martin, 90 miles south of Birmingham.

The Old Turks' annual meetings were held the first weekend in May 1958. They were a great illustration of how medical and other sciences progressed in the 20th century: observations, collections of data, presentation at meetings of others with similar interests, arguments about the data and interpretations and sometimes the underlying postulates, and after the meeting publication in some journal. All papers given at the Old Turks meetings were published in a thick hardbound book, *Transactions of the Association of American Physicians*, automatically sent annually to all living members. The center of activities was the Chalfonte-Haddon Hall Hotels, the Haddon Hall complex at the middle of the Atlantic City boardwalk. Those meetings were concurrent with (but certainly not mixed with!) those of the nation's other two leading clinical/medical research societies: the American Society for Clinical Investigation and Henry Christian's American Federation for Clinical Research.[57] The grandeur of the hotels, especially the great Traymore south of Haddon Hall, which had glorious huge fireplaces a tall man could stand in, surrounded by figures of nude women supporting the mantel, the great history of the meetings attended by many old Nobel laureates and nearly all the chairs of departments of medicine in the country, as well as chairs of some other departments (especially pediatrics), and herds of their followers and aspiring academicians, from other countries as well as America, made this the perfect place for the surprise about to be unveiled.[58]

President W. S. Tillett called the meeting to order. Vice President Walter Bauer, Tinsley's old Michigan Navy colleague and now chief of medicine at Mass General, was present. Secretary Paul Beeson, chief of medicine at Emory, Yale, then Oxford, and A. McGehee Harvey, who had replaced Tinsley at Vanderbilt in 1941 and later moved to Baltimore to become chief of medicine at Hopkins, were there, as well as other famous friends. The proceedings were duly listed in Harvey's history of the association published by the AAP (the Old Turks) in 1986, the 100th anniversary of its founding.[59] It was a remarkable gathering of physicians who were themselves largely responsible for the advances in the scientific aspects of clinical medicine in the preceding century—the most spectacular advances in the entire history of medicine.

As usual, the meetings themselves were held in the large auditorium on the Steel Pier, which jutted out into the waves of the Atlantic. There was a rope or ribbon across the first few rows of seats, which were reserved for the members only. After a paper was given, 15 minutes long, there was the usual discussion, all recorded for later publication. Non-members sat to the rear of the auditorium and could not speak or ask questions unless introduced by a member. On Monday, the business meeting was held and newly elected members for the year were announced. Each volume of the *Transactions* recorded the whole meeting, including the list of members—*all* the members, living and deceased, including the original founding members from 1886: William Osler, J. M. DaCosta, William Draper, Reginald H. Fitz (who described acute appendicitis), R. Palmer Howard of Montreal, S. Weir

the 20th century. Williams was brought to the Thorndike by Nobel laureate George Minot in 1940 and remained till 1948. Others who passed through the Thorndike and were known to Williliams included Eugene Stead (later Duke), Soma Weiss (Brigham), Herrmann Blumgart (Harvard/Beth Israel), Charles Rammelkamp (Cleveland), T. Hale Ham and Joseph T. Wearn (Case Western Reserve), Harry Dowling (Univ. of Illinois), John T. Lawrence and Joe Ross (UCLA), Jack D. Myers and Jessica Lewis (Pittsburgh), Monto Ho (Taipei, Taiwan), Glen Leymaster (Philadelphia), Chester Keefer, Tinsley's old friend (Boston U.), Franz Ingelfinger (BU and the *New England J. Medicine*), Manson Meads (Bowman Gray), Charles Burnett and Reece Berryhill (UNC/Chapel Hill), Thomas Mou (Syracuse), Cheves Smythe (MUSC, South Carolina), others from Britain and other countries, and many more. Obviously, the gregarious Bob Williams knew everybody in academic medicine,

Head table guests (and opposite page) at the Atlantic City party, May 1958. From left: Hugh Morgan, Sidney Burwell, Al Blalock, Betty Harrison, and William Dock.

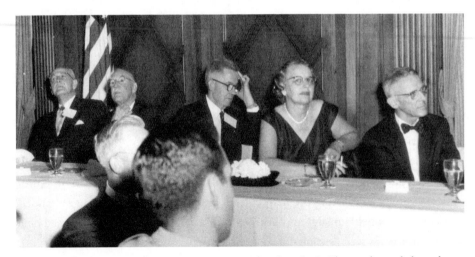

not only in North America but around the world.

57. Later the American Federation for Medical Research, the youngest and least prestigious but most numerous of the three, sometimes called the Young Squirts.

58. Pittman and Miller, "Southern." Discusses the origins of these societies.

59. A. M. Harvey, *The Association of American Physicians 1886–1986: A Century of Progress in Medical Science* (Baltimore: Waverley Press, Inc., 1986).

60. Some of the memorable honorary members included George M. Sternberg, Alfred Stillé, William H. Welch, T. Mitchell Prudden, Francis

Mitchell, William Pepper, James J. Putnam, Frederick C. Shattuck, and the others, as well as honorary[60] and emeritus members, living and dead. All past winners of the Kober Medal were also listed, a number of Nobel laureates among them.

On Monday evening, while others were talking about the formulas of some new or especially interesting molecule or some physiological regulatory system at the Brighton Punch Bowl near Haddon Hall or eating a lobster dinner at Hackneys to the north along the boardwalk, Bob Williams took his old friend Tinsley to a "private dinner to discuss things" at Haddon Hall. Both were active in these societies, especially the Old Turks, and both would later be awarded the AAP's Kober Medal, the highest honor which could be bestowed on an academic internist.

As the two of them walked through the door into the dining room, they were greeted by a huge crowd of the world's leading internists. It was a complete surprise—Tinsley knew nothing about it.

I was present at the festivities. As they came in, I was standing at the door beside Miss Minnie Mae Tims, his technician, secretary, administrator, and academic caretaker since the early Vanderbilt years in the 1920s. (She is now buried with the Harrison family in Birmingham.) Tinsley was very happy. I asked him if he would like a drink, and of course he said, "Yes," so I handed him the bourbon and water I already had in my hand beside my drink. At this he kissed Miss Tims. She was always called "Miss Tims," never, "Minnie" or "Minnie Mae." Upon receiving the kiss, she cried, "I've been waiting 30 years for that!"

After cocktails, the group of more than 200 people, possibly more than 300, were seated for dinner at round tables of eight. There was a long podium with an elevated

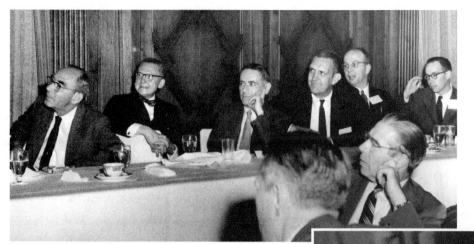

From left, Tinsley Harrison, Chester Keefer, William Resnick, Robert Berson, Joseph Crampton, and Louis Tobian. Below, a cake for the occasion, decorated to look like PIM.

head table on the south side of the somewhat gaudy high-ceilinged hall. Thirteen people were at the head table, which prompted one wag to comment, "Well, there they are, the Deity and the 12 disciples." At the center, near the microphone, sat Robert H. Williams, organizer and master of ceremony. At his right sat Tinsley, and next to him Bill Dock, then Betty Harrison, Al Blalock, C. Sidney Burwell, and Hugh Morgan at the right end of the table. To the left of Williams, in order, were Sam Levine, Chester Keefer, Bill Resnick, Bob Berson, Joe Crampton, and Louis Tobian. The audience was a worldwide image of internal medicine nearing its zenith in 20th century America. It included most leading figures of internal medicine throughout the world, including hypertension expert George Pickering (Sir George Osler's successor as Nuffield Professor and chief of medicine at Oxford); Paul Dudley White (the Boston cardiologist, originator of the Lee-White bleeding time test for clotting disorders and co-discoverer of the Wolf-Parkinson-White syndrome of accelerated conduction in the heart, a long-time friend of Harrison, also famous as the cardiologist called to care for President Eisenhower during the heart attack of September 1955; George W. Thorn, Hersey Professor of the Theory and Practice of Physic at Harvard and the Brigham; and others included in the *PIM* book as "really part of internal medicine," most notably Raymond D. Adams, M.D., Bullard Professor of Neuropathology and professor of neurology at Mass General, one of the editors of *PIM*. A notable absence was Paul B. Beeson, one of the original editors of *PIM* and a good friend. He was probably residing at Yale or Oxford at the time. But he was there in spirit. There were hordes of current and former residents and fellows of Tinsley's, as well as colleagues and friends from his six medical schools: Michigan, Hopkins, Vanderbilt, Wake Forest/Bowman Gray, Dallas Southwestern, and Birmingham.

Williams ran the affair as only he could, calling first on Sam Levine, Tinsley's first serious mentor, dedicated to Tinsley from the beginning. Tinsley had helped Sam form and create Sam's life in cardiology and medicine, and Sam had helped form Tinsley's future successes. It was Levine who identified the empty laboratory of Dr. Grant, recently departed from the Brigham, and engineered its assignment to Tinsley for the real beginning of his serious physiological research, and who published with Tinsley on rheumatic fever in the South, and who had nurtured him in academic medicine over the years. When Levine died years later, Tinsley published an obituary, even though one had already been published.

That evening in their beloved old Atlantic City, as everybody realized their permanent departures were approaching and their treasured competitive collegiality was gradually coming to a close, Sam spoke of what a great student and fast learner Tinsley was—a quick study of whatever he tried to understand. And how productive he had been during his Brigham years, despite a load of clinical care. And, of course, he spoke of a patient, one which resulted in the bet which Tinsley lost, when he failed to identify a myocardial infarct in a patient but called it pericarditis instead, probably never having recognized an MI in a living patient before that. Things had changed in the years between 1922 and the spring of 1958.

One by one, the others at the head table took the podium to speak. Betty did not comment. She sat silent and attentive, smoking cigarette after cigarette. Bill Dock reminisced about their early years together. Blalock spoke briefly and seriously, but with some needling of Tinsley about the superiority of surgery over internal medicine as a medical career. Burwell and Hugh Morgan talked of "the great days at Vanderbilt Medical School in the 1920s and '30s," when people worked so hard and the department of medicine led the school in productivity and publications, thanks mainly to their "human dynamo," Tinsley.

Chester Keefer spoke of how his work with penicillin at the end of the war prevented him from participating in the historical publication of the first edition of Harrison's *Principles of Internal Medicine*, and Resnick of his enjoyment at participating as "the only real doctor here." Bob Berson, dean of medicine in Birmingham at the time, told of the tribulations and triumphs of having Harrison as the chief of medicine. The testimonials were completed by two former fellows with Tinsley, Joe Crampton now at the Virginia Mason Clinic in Seattle, and Louis Tobian on the faculty of the University of Minnesota.

Tinsley was the final speaker. He thanked everyone—all his friends for so many years—and spoke of "the traditional three-legged stool of academic medicine." He said it was difficult to say which had been the most significant and important for his life in medicine—essentially the whole of his existence: "The tear in the eye of a grateful patient, the joy of a student suddenly comprehending a point in medicine, or the thrill of himself understanding a concept in research." He concluded that the last was probably most significant to him personally, and probably his most lasting contribution.

Many years later, people would still discuss this question, and opinions would be divided into the three camps. The care he gave patients was invaluable to those patients and their families, and it was the basis of all else. But once he passed from the scene, that care itself would be gone. Likewise, the book, much as it was and remains admired, was destined ultimately to the dust heap. The research findings alone, he believed, would advance medicine and be more permanent and a greater contribution to medicine. A half-century later, it appears Tinsley had got it right that evening.

Before the event closed. Williams announced that a group of Tinsley's friends had started an endowment at Birmingham (at what is now UAB) to fund an annual Tinsley Harrison Lecture, and additional contributions would be welcome. Second, he announced that they were working on a festschrift of Tinsley's friends to be published in a major medical journal. Thoughts turned to the *Annals of Internal Medicine*, the *Archives of Internal Medicine*, of some national or international cardiology journal. Unfortunately the festschrift was never published, but the lecture series did become a reality in 1958,[61] the same year Tinsley was inducted as a Fellow into the American Academy of Arts and Sciences.

Minot, William Councilman, Francis Delafield, Henry Bowditch, and John S. Billings. There were many others.

61. By the fall of 1958 there was sufficient money in the Tinsley Harrison Annual Lecture Fund to invite the first speaker. Tinsley wanted to invite his old cardiologist friend and fellow intern, Bill Dock, because Bill had mild angina pectoris and might not live many more years. The iconoclastic Dock's talk rambled but was interesting. Then he did live for many more years in Paris with a French wife, until moving to the Caribbean island of Guadeloupe where he died at age 91.

12

Back Down the Academic Ladder

1958–1978

The 1958 tribute dinner in Atlantic City, where so often Tinsley had actively participated in the reports and discussions of the Young Turks and the Old Turks and in their political machinations, seemed a fitting conclusion to Tinsley's life in academic medicine. But this was not so. Several years later he was scheduled, according to tradition, to move up the hierarchy in which he had been active for so long to become president of the Association of American Physicians, the Old Turks and the oldest American association or society of physicians devoted to medical research. This was recognized at the time as the peak of academic medicine. However, he declined to be promoted and deferred to George Thorn, who thereby became president a year earlier than scheduled.[1] Whether Tinsley declined because he was somewhat depressed or just tired or concerned about his new medical school and wanted to spend more time there and work harder on the immediate problems is not known. He did not relate well to the unfolding cultural changes of the late 1950s and '60s.

As Tinsley remarked on several occasions, "It may be more difficult to climb down the academic ladder than to climb up."

We must believe his repeated complaints that he really did not like administrative work and did not believe he was good at it. He was a great recruiter, but he disliked the distance from actual patients. He was also chronically disorganized, erratic in his scheduling, and often distracted in the application of his office.[2] He longed to return to his first loves of patient care, research, and teaching.

As mentioned earlier, his successor as chairman, Walter Frommeyer, presented

1. G. W. Thorn, personal conversation, HHMI office, Boston, March 1993. This hierarchical succession of AAP presidents can also be confirmed by the records published in the annual *Transactions of the Association of American Physicians*.

2. Harrison, *Reminiscences*, chapter 6, 9. "The failure of department heads, Deans and Presidents to make an intensive, almost agonizing, search for men with brilliant minds and future potential leadership is probably the single greatest defect in our system of higher education."

Tinsley with a new challenge. Tinsley had always preached against the growing specialization of the times and "splitting up the patient into ever smaller organs and minute parts, with little regard for the whole patient" and had steadfastly refused to divide his department into divisions devoted primarily to hematology, endocrinology, gastroenterology, cardiology, and so on. Frommeyer had done that and offered him the position of director of the Division of Cardiology in the Department of Medicine. Tinsley accepted. He had already taken a more drastic concrete step as chairman of medicine when he led the effort to abolish rotating internships in the hospital. He had contended that a single year of very brief exposures to multiple areas of practice would not make a new graduate competent in any of the fields but would be only a quick repeat of the fourth year of medical school. Further, it would interfere with his or her developing internal medicine residency, since that would be the area he or she would most need in general practice.

IT WAS STILL DIFFICULT to attract house staff from elsewhere in the country, despite Tinsley's prominence as *Principles of Internal Medicine* became ever more popular and used throughout the nation and world. In 1956–57 there was one resident from Yale, two from Harvard, one from Puerto Rico, two from New York, one from St. Louis, and one from Germany. The rest were from the South, mostly University of Alabama graduates.

Tinsley's oft-expressed view was that the best way for medical students to learn about clinical medicine was to have some personal responsibility for patients and to do clinical medicine under the supervision of experienced physicians. He pursued this as a goal anywhere he taught and could influence the curriculum, at all his prior medical schools as well as in Birmingham.

There was also a pragmatic side which probably influenced him. Paid hospital help, both house staff and nurses, were in short supply. Nurses were scarce because of lack of money and competition from other hospitals, and because there simply were few registered nurses or licensed practical nurses around. House staff were scarce because of both lack of money to pay them and lack of applicants, many new local graduates going to other Birmingham hospitals.

Patients were separated not only by race, but also by economics. The charity patients, called ward patients because they were usually hospitalized in large rooms of about 20 poorly separated beds, were primarily the day-to-day responsibility of the interns and residents, and in the early days even senior or junior medical students.

The students often carried out nursing duties, including administering medications, moving patients in the bed, escorting them to X-ray or other areas, starting IVs, even charting TPR (temperature, pulse, respiration). The private patients were primarily the responsibility of their private doctors practicing from their individual offices around town, or more rarely, groups of doctors in a single office building.

For the residents, the patient load was large, some 30 or 40 patients for a single intern and one student, sometimes the student alone. Regular nursing was grossly inadequate on many wards. On one occasion a resident was told by an elderly nurse that an IV had infiltrated into the arm of a post-operative patient but not to worry. "I've got it restarted and put up a new bottle of D&W," she said.

"Dextrose and water? Are you sure that's what it is?" he asked.

She reassured him that this was correct.

"Don't you put another drop into that patient!" he said. "I'll be right over to check." He found that it was indeed D&W rather than dextrose and saline. Dextrose and water could lyse the red blood cells, block the kidneys, and kill the patient. The elderly nurse caring for this private patient apparently had forgotten the difference. A brief discussion of the differences followed, and the resident vowed to himself to check the patient more often.

On another occasion a resident complained to the head nurse about lack of attention to a particularly sick elderly black man, and the nurse, a middle-aged white RN (at the time all the nurses were female), replied, "Do you know it is actually illegal for me to be caring for a black man?" Jim Crow Alabama law forbade that sort of interracial care. Nevertheless, in this instance the nurse provided it.

Some of the most egregious medical results, for the residents but mainly for the patients, were the results of the segregated emergency rooms—one white and one black. Technically the separation was not the result of racial segregation but of a division of the private ER from the public ER. As the 1950s progressed, the private white ER began to take a few of the more affluent black patients. The public ER had always had a few serious emergency patients who were white, but the separation was a legacy of many earlier years.

As good as things were in the medicine world, as many advancements as had taken place, things were still rough. We lost patients due to mistakes, miscommunication, faulty equipment, all the time.

Late one afternoon as I was headed for supper and passed the hallway door into the private ER, I was surprised to see a well-dressed and neat young black man about 30 in a wheelchair. He was gasping for breath as pink frothy foam came from his mouth. It was clearly acute pulmonary edema and the patient was in extremis. I rushed into the small neat ER and asked the nurse (again a very elderly white lady) where the doctor was.

"At home, but I've called him, and he's coming in," she said.

"If he doesn't get here in the next five minutes, this man is a goner," I said. I then learned that the doctor was William Hawley who had trained at Harvard's Brigham Hospital, an excellent town doctor and a friend. So I telephoned him at home and learned the patient had mitral stenosis but had not yet even received digitalis. No diuretic drugs were available other than two mercurial preparations which had to be injected, Mercuhydrin and Mersalyl. Hawley gave me permission to treat the patient—apply tourniquets to the arms and legs, inject Mercuhydrin, give morphine and oxygen, and so on. But when I turned around in the small ER, the patient was gone.

"I sent him up for a chest X-ray," the nurse explained.

The X-ray department was on the seventh floor, and the ancient elevators were slow and crowded at that time of day. Finally I arrived at the seventh floor only to find the orderly in the empty hall curiously leaning over the patient, slumped down in the wheelchair. "I think he's gone, Doc," the orderly said. And indeed he was. At that moment, a senior surgical resident passed, noticed the situation, and we opened the chest for cardiac massage—closed chest cardiac massage and resuscitation had not yet come into use. Under our hands, the heart restarted and it appeared the patient might revive. Then a mistake was made. This surgeon said, "We're in here, we might as well try to fracture that tight mitral valve." We did. The heart stopped. This time the patient was dead and stayed dead. Had appropriate treatment been given immediately on the young mans arrival, he probably could have been saved, been given chronic treatment, and lived for some months or years—perhaps long enough for helpful cardiac surgery.

Another case was that of a white infant with extreme diarrhea brought to the private ER by his mother. The child was wrinkled and somewhat listless, but no doctor was immediately available, as usual. The nurse had called, but the town pediatricians were overwhelmed. She responded simply that he would "get there as soon as he could." Several hours passed. As the child grew obviously weaker, the nurse finally recommended that the mother take him around the corner to the other

ER, which she did. It was too late; the little patient did not make it in time. He died about the time of arrival at the other ER. He could—should—have been saved.

Tinsley was told of these patients and the belief that they might have been saved had they been taken immediately to the public ER. It was primitive and so crowded that the residents called it "the Hole," but it was staffed by interns and residents at all hours. The separation and the inadequate staffing in the private ER was bad medicine, the one thing Tinsley would not tolerate. The immediate response was that this had been discussed with the hospital authorities, who had explained that they had promised the city fathers they would continue to maintain separately a private ER and a general ER. However, several weeks later the private ER was abolished, and all emergency patients black or white were taken to the general public ER.

The town doctors used several hospitals around town, traveling from one to another every day to visit their patients or carry out procedures. Pediatricians especially covered multiple hospitals to see newborns, since obstetrics was included in nearly all the hospitals. Most patients thus already patronized the private hospitals in town.

The charity ward patients were poor, plentiful, often neglected, and fascinating, frequently presenting with advanced manifestations of serious disease. In 1956 one elderly black man said he was 106 years old. I asked if he had been a slave, and he answered, "Yassuh. I shore was."

When asked if he remembered much about the time before the War Between the States, he answered that he remembered his childhood well.

"How was life then?" I asked.

"Not bad. We had plenty of food, and a warm cabin in winter; and we played a lot in the summer with all the other children, black and white," he said. He was suffering from advanced congestive heart failure; he was in no condition for a prolonged conversation. He died a few days later.

This was life as a doctor.

There were patients to see and medical students and residents to teach as well as conferences and clinics for other physicians, and Tinsley was, as always, enthusiastic about these things. He also was still involved in various aspects of organized medicine both locally and nationally.

PROBABLY THE EASIEST WAY to visualize the routine teaching activities is to look at the weekly schedule.

Mondays were consumed with trying to dig out from the mass of uncompleted work which had accumulated over the weekend—reviewing findings and progress of new as well as old patients, looking for unattended details, and of course handling the new patients and new work always pouring in. There were occasional special meetings and the usual daily routine.

The house officers and fourth-year students would rise about 6 or 6:30 in the morning (surgical house staff perhaps an hour earlier), have breakfast, then get the morning's lab work done—CBCs, urines, stool guaiacs, urinalyses, perhaps a few other simple lab tests. Blood was drawn from of the patients with reusable needles and syringes, placed in small glass vials, and sent to the hospital laboratory. Work rounds began no later than 8 A.M.

Work rounds consisted of the group's walking from patient to patient throughout the ward and into the semi-private or private rooms of the sickest, seeing each patient, reviewing the chart. Did the temperature subside during the night? Has he or she become more conscious of the surroundings? Less pale than yesterday after the transfusions last night? What is the hematocrit this morning? What do the blood chemistries show?

Next, there would be a visit to the cafeteria for a quick cup of coffee and perhaps a doughnut, followed by a group visit to the X-ray department where the films would be reviewed with the radiologist, usually a faculty member or senior resident. By then it would be nearly 10 A.M., and they would hasten back to the patients.

There, on the ward, they would be met by the attending physician or Visitor who would make teaching rounds with the group. Ideally, these were usually senior faculty with years of experience, charged with teaching as well as ultimate care of the patient. Attendings were legally responsible for the care of the patient. In postwar Alabama and most of the South, staffing was thin. The lack of faculty often dictated that the attending was a new practitioner or even a senior house officer.

The attending would see each new patient admitted in the past 24 hours and be briefed on any patient who had been admitted and died overnight. Each patient would be presented in detail, and the attending would question the members of the group closely about the course of the patient's illness, each physical finding, the results of the last and previous laboratory findings, and other details. And woe to the house officer who did not know the correct answers! The only thing worse was to confabulate, to make up an answer when you didn't know. When the resident or student had been busy all night caring for new patients and very sick established patients, running to the emergency room, wheeling patients around the hospital, starting IVs, and writing notes, with only an hour or so of sleep, there seemed no time at all to study. Of course, the residents and students on a ward were expected to be up to date on *all* their patients with current observations, lab results, and so on. Any especially difficult patient or problem was also presented to the attending. In the established hospitals of the Northeast, the attending also signed off on each patient about to be discharged. But there was usually no time for that in Alabama. There weren't enough beds.

Somewhere around 12:30 or 1 in the afternoon, attending rounds would finish and the group would adjourn to the dining room for lunch. Some attendings would join in the lunch group, but most would not, preferring to go to a separate table with fellow attendings their own age or to go care for their private patients elsewhere.

The residents' and students' afternoons would be taken up with ward duties, reviewing the sickest patients, visiting new patients in the ER, and working up newly hospitalized patients (often up to a dozen or more). There would be afternoon work rounds, supper, then continued coverage through the night for half the residents, who were given every other night and every other weekend for rest. This was the schedule most frequent through the U.S. hospitals around 1950.

Some programs and hospitals demanded more. For years, if you were lucky enough to intern and take residency training at Hopkins, you knew you would be on duty 24 hours a day, seven days a week, all year. Cornell-New York Hospital had a similar schedule of duty, as did other major hospitals in the buyers' market for residents. Beginning in the 1960s, there was a gathering of some of those on duty in the cafeteria around 10 each night. Before this, some would visit a local diner, especially if they had missed supper.

In the late 20th century, amid concerns about sleep deprivation and its deleterious effects on the professional abilities of physicians such as overworked house officers, laws were passed to limit the hours to not more than 80 hours per week. Older physicians remembered how, even in the best hospitals, they would go on duty, for example in the emergency department, on Friday morning, work through Friday night, all day Saturday and that night, then the same for Sunday and all day Monday, going off duty at 7 P.M.—a total of 60 hours from Friday morning to Monday evening—then into the next week with its night duties before collapsing the following weekend. It was usually possible to squeeze in at least a few hours of sleep when things were quiet, but not always and not many hours. One exhausted house officer was shaken awake by an elderly man whose heart he had been ausculting with the admonition, "Young man! You need rest!"

The Libby Zion case at Cornell's New York Hospital (a young woman died, apparently due to an unknown conflict between two drugs; but her family sued, attributing the cause to overworked interns and lack of supervision) was important in drawing attention to this situation,[3] but no easy answer was available. How was a house officer to follow correction of severe diabetic ketoacidosis back to recovery if he could not follow that particular patient, essentially at the patient's bedside monitoring progress, for more than 24 hours?

In Tinsley's new medical school in the South, there really were no concerns about overworking the house staff. There were sick patients to care for. Nor were long work hours restricted to students, interns, and residents. At this time, Alabama had fewer physicians per capita than any other state save one. In the late 1950s, the chief medical resident would often receive calls from harried solo physicians in rural Alabama, such as one from Carbon Hill, a small Appalachian coal mining community about an hour north of Birmingham. He said, "Doc, can't you find some intern who wants to make a little extra money moonlighting? I've been two months without a single night off, often having to take a really sick patient into Jasper [a larger nearby town] where there's a hospital. I'm just not getting any sleep at all! I need somebody to spell me for just 24 hours so I can rest. I'll pay $100." Occasionally somebody could be found.

There was also clinical teaching on private patients of both faculty members and town doctors with offices elsewhere in Birmingham. For medicine, most of this teaching was on the 14th floor of the University Hospital. These rounds were more complicated for two reasons: First, there was no question about who had the responsibility—the private physician. Usually these doctors required that any order other than the simplest routines be personally signed by them. And they had to later countersign even these routine orders written by the resident. Second, since these practitioners had patients in other hospitals, they arrived at different times each day.

The unmarried house officers—the majority in those days—lived on the 16th and 17 floors; women on the 16th and men on the 17th. As the years passed, the HOs were increasingly married and usually lived in small houses near the hospital.

HOUSE STAFF ALSO ATTENDED weekly conferences including medical grand rounds (a comparable surgical grand rounds was held for the surgeons), the clinical-pathological conference, death conference, Tinsley's "Chief's rounds" for the third-year

3. Natalie Robins, *The Girl Who Died Twice: Every Patient's Nightmare—The Libby Zion Case and the Hidden Hazards of Hospitals* (New York: Delacorte Press, 1995).

4. In the last years of Tinsley's life—the mid to late 1970s—there were competing noon conferences of various sorts, and on days other than the Wednesdays when medical grand rounds were held, the various subspecialties had noon conferences in nephrology, neurology, GI, etc. Box lunches were provided for the audience. Sometimes one would hear discussions among residents or students as to which conference served the best lunch—food for the tongue and stomach, not the brain and medical soul.

students, and during some years Saturday morning joint medical-surgical rounds. Individual live patients were almost always presented, and the discussion centered on clinical care, the traditional diagnosis, treatment, and prognosis. There was also almost always a discussion of recent advances and research on the disease involved and related matters.

Medical grand rounds were from 12 to 1 one day a week on Saturday mornings, later changed to Wednesdays at noon. Attendance increased accordingly, often swelled by numerous Ph.D. and postdoctoral students and technicians, some of whom sat in the back of the auditorium and left after a few minutes.[4]

In the 1950s and '60s, the VA Hospital and the University Hospital were more or less equal partners, so medical grand rounds were held on alternate weeks on one or the other side of the street. The patient was usually present for the presentation and occasionally for the discussion, depending on the gravity, sensitivity, or privacy of the situation.

The weekly CPCs (clinical-pathologic conferences) were also well attended, and these were real tests of a clinician's diagnostic skills. The patients discussed had either died in the hospital and been autopsied or, in a few cases, had some tissue biopsied to provide the pathology portion of the conference. The presentation was written up ahead of time and read by the discusser, who might make a few comments as he or she stood before the audience and read it. Some write-ups were used for a discussion with junior and senior medical students prior to the conference, who would vote on the diagnosis.

One conference important for both learning and patient care was the weekly death conference, usually late on a Thursday or Wednesday afternoon. At these the cases of every patient who had died in the hospital (except those few reserved for a later CPC) were presented to the other residents by the resident who had been responsible for the patient at the time of death. The resident would present the case and discuss the reasons for failure to prevent death. Then the autopsy findings would be presented by the pathology department. If there were no autopsy, unusual in those days, an explanation had to be given why the autopsy had been missed. Some residents were better than others in obtaining autopsies, probably the result of better rapport with the family. Poor families, in Alabama at that time often uneducated blacks, were superstitious about the body and often denied autopsy requests. There are rumors about a "gold ball" story being told to ignorant people, in which a therapeutic ball of solid gold had supposedly been placed in the abdomen of a sick patient as part of the treatment effort. "If we are not able to recover that gold ball, we'll have to charge you over $5,000 before we can release the body for burial," the family would be told. This was always, according to these stories, sufficient to convince the family to sign permission for an autopsy. Otherwise, the response was often, "No 'topsy! No 'topsy!"

The death conferences were valuable both for learning about the course of a fatal disease as well as a way of exposing deficiencies in care. All the various public airings during conferences were important in elevating and maintaining standards of care in medical schools and large hospitals, advantages sometimes difficult to come by in smaller hospitals or rural settings.

PERHAPS THE MOST INSTRUCTIVE weekly conference for the students was Harrison's clinic every Thursday from 10 to noon in the second-floor conference room of the VA Hospital. Tinsley's clinics were attended mainly by third-year students. Two patients in succession would be brought in wheelchairs or beds and presented by students. After the presentation, Tinsley would query the patient about various details, some perhaps omitted or misinterpreted by the presenter, then he would examine the patient in detail. This might consume fully five minutes or more, while the audience sat in rapt attention (or asleep, if they had been up all night). He might have the patient assume various positions on the bed as he listened carefully for an obscure murmur or bruit or felt for a thrill. Though he liked to see patients with cardiac problems, his appetite was universal. One could almost see him flipping though the pages of *PIM* in his head as he gave beautiful discourses on tularemia, brucellosis, syphilis in all its stages, typhoid, typhus, malaria, lead poisoning, and many other medical topics. At some point, usually immediately after Tinsley's physical examination, the student would give the physical findings and conclusions according to the ward team. There would be more discussion, and they would move on to the next patient or the end of the conference. Tinsley was rarely wrong, though he might miss a very high-pitched or very soft cardiac murmur, which he attributed to his failing hearing. He always said that one of the most important contributions a consulting cardiologist can make is to take the patient into an isolated, very quiet room for examination.

In the early days Tinsley also used these conferences for more general instruction, especially in spoken English. He felt students from Alabama were basically as smart as anybody else, but that they lacked a basic education. At times he would interrupt

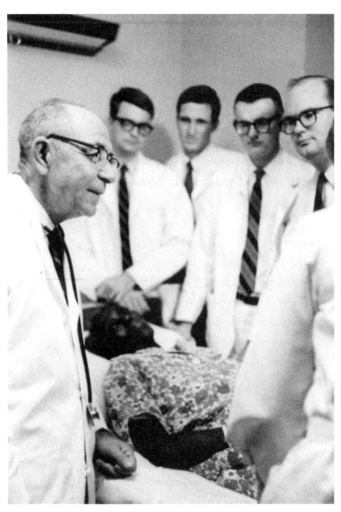

Tinsley Harrison with house staff and students, circa 1960s.

a student's presentation with a question such as, "What color were the feathers?" The student, confused at this point, might ask, "What was the question, Dr. Harrison?" at which Tinsley would repeat it. If the confused student still did not catch on, Tinsley would say, "Well, you said the patient was laying there, so I assumed the patient was a chicken laying eggs." There would also be occasional questions of basic grammar— "Conjugate the verb 'to do'"—on the long written test all third-year students were required to take.

ON SATURDAY MORNINGS AT 8, joint medical-surgical grand rounds were held in the huge Old Hillman Auditorium, a remnant of the former Birmingham Medical College. A patient would be presented, often in a wheelchair even if ambulatory in other circumstances. The usual presentation would be by a student, intern, or resident, who would review the history and physical findings in some detail, and the laboratory findings if available. The X-rays would be presented at some point, usually with discussion by a radiologist. Then there would be joint discussions between Champ Lyons and Tinsley, and these would be especially enjoyable to the audience. When doctors disagree, thing can get heated, as the disagreement often lies at the cross-section of ego, knowledge, and life and death.

Lyons could be quite explosive, to the amusement but also to the awe of the students. All doctors have stories. One of mine involved a conference when Tinsley was absent. A patient with hyperthyroidism was presented to Lyons. This patient, a young woman of about 20, would not take her antithyroid medication as directed but instead took the pills for a short time then discontinued them and became thyrotoxic again. The only solution seemed to be to keep her in the hospital with her medications monitored until she was euthyroid and suitable for surgical thyroidecomy. At that time radioiodine thyroidecomy was considered too hazardous over the long term to be used in patients under 40. Finally after several weeks, she was clearly euthyroid clinically and by lab tests, mainly a BMR (basal metabolic rate) and a PBI (protein-bound iodine level in the blood). There were very few charity beds, and there was no reason to delay operation. However, surgery disagreed, because she had been on this course of medications only three weeks. Lyons had detailed, inflexible rules for every surgical situation, and one was that a thyrotoxic patient must have six weeks of pre-op medication to make her sufficiently euthyroid for surgery. The argument had raged between the surgical and medical residents for several days, so it was finally decided to present her to Dr. Lyons at the Saturday conference. I was present.

The presentation went as usual, by a medical resident who pointed out that her hands were cool, without a tremor, and the lab results confirmed that she was euthyroid. Lyons stepped up and had her hold out her hands. "Look at those hands! They're shaking and trembling. And they're hot as a stove. And she's sweating!" (Perhaps it was because of the looming presence of Lyons and the drama of the occasion.) I was a member of the new division of endocrinology directed by S. Richardson Hill, so I said, "Dr. Lyons, I'm sure she's euthyroid and ready for the Lugol's and operation."

He replied, "No, she's not! I just demonstrated that!"

The chief medical resident responded, "Dr. Lyons, medicine has only 13 white female beds, and we really do need an empty bed for other patients. If surgery wants to treat her medically for another three or six weeks, let them do it on their wards."

Lyons insisted that it was for the surgeons, not the internists, to decide when to operate, and they would accept her on surgery when only she was ready, as determined by them, not the internists.

"Dr. Hill also says she's euthyroid," I added.

He exploded, "I don't care if Jesus Christ says she's euthyroid! She's hyperthyroid! And she's going to get the proper surgical preparation! Then and only then will surgery take her on our wards!" With that the surgical chief resident hurried Lyons out of the room, and medicine kept her for another three weeks.

TINSLEY HAD HIS OWN method of R&R for the interns and residents: water skiing. He owned a lake cabin about 90 miles south of Birmingham on Lake Martin, the largest of Alabama's several man-made lakes created by damming rivers to generate electricity. If Tinsley felt one or two residents were showing the strains of long tours of duty with little rest, he would offer them a weekend at his cabin.

Tinsley had owned this lake house for many years. It was a fairly large frame cabin with several bedrooms, large dining and sitting rooms, kitchen, several baths with modern flush toilets, and a large screened porch reaching around most of the house, all surrounded by the woods. The cottage was on a hill and the screened porch faced southwest, so family, friends, and guests often sat in the twilight having a drink and watching the sunset over the tranquil lake. The cabin was a bit rough, but it was usable any time of the year. This is where Tinsley and his family retreated to escape the pressures of Birmingham. He loved to water ski or pull children or guests skiing behind his motorboat.

On one occasion he suddenly called two senior residents to his office by having them paged over the hospital's loudspeaker system. On their way to Tinsley's office on the fifth floor of the Old Hillman Building, now with a new but noisy air conditioner cooling his office via a ragged hole in the ceiling, they wondered why they were being summoned. Probably it was to obtain some documentation to help get a particular old physician, Dr. L., kicked off the hospital staff. Tinsley considered him incompetent, and the night before Dr. L. had admitted a patient with congestive failure and acute pulmonary edema but had treated him intravenously only with quinidine. The house staff, unbeknownst to Dr. L., had administered the accepted treatment—morphine, oxygen, tourniquets, Mercuhydrin, and so on, and the patient was much better the next morning. Tinsley objected not only to Dr. L.'s failure to use the accepted best therapy, but also to the use of intravenous quinidine, which he considered absolutely contraindicated.

When the residents arrived in Harrison's modest office, he threw two keys on his desk and said, "You guys have been working hard and need a rest. Take these keys and go down to my cabin on Lake Martin for a couple of days and take it easy. Take your wives. One of these keys is for the house, and the other is for the boat. There are water skis in the boathouse. I'll see you Monday."

This was one example of Tinsley's desultory mode of day-to-day management. The exchange with the residents occurred on a Wednesday, but he had not discussed it with the chief resident, and no arrangements had been made to cover the scheduled duties of the about-to-be absent residents. Nonetheless, things were muddled through, and one of the residents was sufficiently impressed to remain another year.

IN THE LATE 1950S, NIH funding began growing in earnest, and Tinsley was goad-
ing his faculty to apply for it. One successful staff member was Howard L. Holley,[5]
a rheumatologist whose patients in the VA Hospital shared a 20-bed wing with the
endocrine patients of Dick Hill. Holley, for his part, tried to stimulate research by
sponsoring the John R. Irby Research Conferences each summer. These were held
at the Ann Jordan Farm, a 5,000-acre former hunting preserve and lodge about an
hour's drive from Birmingham. The preserve had been donated to the University of
Alabama years before and had a rustic but comfortable main building suitable for
such a meeting in a quiet environment, with quarters for perhaps 30 participants.
The meetings began Friday afternoon or evening with presentation of several papers
by research fellows, students, residents, or faculty followed by drinks and informal
discussions. Saturday morning was the same format. Saturday afternoon was free
for hunting, hiking, or other activities. Tinsley also offered accommodations and
water skiing to the participants at his Lake Martin cabin, 30 minutes away.

Holley, desiring better connections with the National Institute of Arthritis and
Metabolic Diseases of the NIH, invited its director of extramural research, Ralph
Knutti, to attend the conference in July 1957. Dr. Knutti accepted, and the first
portions of the meeting went well. He seemed impressed with the presentations,
asked many questions during the formal discussion period after each paper, and
seemed to enjoy mixing with participants at other times.

On Saturday afternoon he accepted Tinsley's hospitality at the cabin. This consisted mainly of Tinsley in his boat dragging Knutti around on water skis in multiple
attempts to get the director up and sliding smoothly over the water. These were
mostly not very successful and resulted in almost drowning the important visitor.

On the drive back to the lodge, the car carrying Dr. Knutti was slowed to a snail's
pace by an old sedan with a large wooden cross attached to its roof; the cross was
outlined by electric light bulbs. The three cars of Tinsley's safari managed to pass the
religious-looking car, the occupants of which were dressed in white—perhaps some
sort of religious group. Farther down the road, we were surprised to see two men of
about 25 or 30 standing at the turnoff to the lodge. They wore conical white hats
and were clad in clean white robes clearly marked KKK. Dr. Knutti, a California
native and Yale medical graduate, made no comments of record.

I was driving the lead car, so I stopped and asked, "What's the occasion?"

"We're having a parade," the Kluxers answered. "Go on down the road. You can
join. You'd be welcome."

5. Holley, *History.*
Holley was also author
of the classic—and
exhaustive—history of
medicine in Alabama.

6. The slogan was
removed in 1966.

This was the direction we were going anyway, so we proceeded. A short way farther there was a large group of perhaps 50 or more white people, some in white robes and regalia, several with crosses. They were of all ages—little children to old men and women, some with bare feet and clad in overalls or bedraggled dresses. The children were nearly all barefooted. We stopped again, and I asked one fellow who seemed in charge, "What's the occasion?"

He answered, "We're having a parade. Go on down a little more and you can get in."

"But what's the event?" I asked.

At this point he understood that we weren't part of their group. "It's my birthday, Buddy!" he said. In the back seat of our car was a Viennese psychiatrist who had escaped Austria just ahead of the Nazis. He pleaded, "Move on! Move on! I have a wife and child at home!" Indeed we did, having made some sort of impression on Dr. Knutti—maybe that we had potential but needed lots of help, including that from NIAMD.

That encounter on the road should not have surprised the local attendees and probably did not except for the unexpected embarrassment from it. After all, it was not rare in those days to see posters advertising KKK picnics, or signs on chain link fences as one entered a rural town advertising civic meetings, with the KKK logo— "Meets Thursday Noon at Joe's Diner"—mixed in amongst those for the Rotary, Kiwanis, Lions, etc. Since 1904, electoral ballots in Alabama had carried the slogan "White Supremacy for the Right" above the party symbol for the Democrats.[6]

This was the climate in the late 1950s and early 1960s in which Tinsley was trying to build a modern medical school. The only large sources for potential re-cruiting of young academic physicians were in the Northeast—Boston, New York, and to some extent Philadelphia, and new schools were starting in Connecticut (1961), New Jersey (1956 and 1966), and elsewhere—and Chicago. The University of California San Francisco was getting started, as was Stanford. The University of Washington in Seattle had started in 1949 with Tinsley's former resident and friend Robert H. Williams, and it too was in a recruiting and building mode. UCLA had started its school in 1951, UC Irvine and UC San Diego in 1962, UC Davis in 1963, and so on. Even in the South Tinsley had to compete with other new medi-cal schools: Florida in 1952 and 1956, Louisiana in 1966. Further, like Alabama, some of the older schools had only had two-year basic science schools—Mississippi and North Carolina—and these were upgrading to four-year schools. Some older schools elsewhere were excellent (Washington University in St. Louis for example), and a very few clinical faculty were recruited from them.[7] All these other schools were competitors for academic workforce, not sources or helpers. If Tinsley could not recruit from the big pools in the Northeast, he simply could not recruit. The situation would grow only worse over the next decade.

Why did this situation occur? Probably it was the concurrence of an increasing demand for medical care (soon to be transformed into "health care," then "healthcare") and the rapid evolution of biomedical research and financial support in the 1950s, especially from the NIH and NSF. To these would be added the tremendous impetus of Medicare/Medicaid in 1965, together with a frequent attitude of disdain and revulsion in the North toward the South and its multifaceted poverty in that period, to which was soon added a missionary fervor—but not enough for people to actually move and live there.

Sometimes Tinsley thought of the offer he had declined years ago to join the Harvard unit at the Boston City Hospital as a very junior person, perhaps a sort of instructor. He had declined Boston to stay at Vanderbilt and had cast his lot with the South. He did not regret that; he had done well. But nevertheless, during some times of special stress, his mind wandered back to Boston to wonder what might have been. Suppose he had married his early girlfriend then at Wellesley, Virginia Foster of Union Springs and Birmingham.[8] How might have things gone over the years? But he was where he was, and things were as they were. He carried on.

A YOUNG PHYSICIAN FROM Santiago, Chile, H. Cecil Coghlan, son of a prominent physician there, arrived for a cardiology fellowship with Tinsley in 1957. One day Coghlan was called for a surgical consult. A patient in the immediate post-op period had gone into shock, and no explanation could be found—no indication of internal or external hemorrhage, no other serious trauma anywhere, no problems with the heart, nothing—just no blood pressure. This was duly reported to the Chief. Tinsley came to examine the patient himself and explained, "Why, this man has had a heart attack, a myocardial infarct."

Coghlan and the residents protested that all tests of the heart were normal, including the EKG, which was entirely normal. "Just wait a few hours," Tinsley said. "The EKG will turn abnormal and you'll see the elevated ST segments, inverted T-waves, and the rest. Just wait, and in the meantime give supportive treatment."

How did Tinsley know this? He showed them the physical finding: a prominent

7. Some additional details of the establishment of medical schools, their size, etc., can be found in the "Annual Medical Education Number" of the *JAMA* 290 (2003): 1119–1268.

8. Virginia Foster Durr's rich life is not easily summarized in a footnote. Sister-in-law of Hugo Black, close friend of Eleanor Roosevelt and Rosa Parks, Henry Wallace ally, U.S. Senate candidate, anti-poll tax activist, founding member of the Southern Conference for Human Welfare (SCHW) are just a few of the phrases which can be attached to her name. See Virginia Foster Durr, *Outside the Magic Circle: The Autobiography of Virginia Foster Durr*, ed. Hollinger F. Barnard (Tuscaloosa: University of Alabama Press, 1990).

9. Eddleman "Ki-netocardiogram." Harrison later published a number of other papers on the KCG and gave reports of results with it at several large national/international medical meetings.

10. T. R. Harrison and L. Hughes, "Precordial Systolic Bulges During Anginal Attacks," *Trans. Assoc. Amer. Phys.* 71 (1958): 174–185. N. S. Skinner Jr., R. S. Liebeskind, H. L. Phillips and T. R. Harrison, "The Effect of Exertion and of Nitrites on the Precordial Movements of Patients with Angina Pectoris," *Amer. Heart J.* 61 (1961): 250–258.

bulge of the chest wall over the infarcted area. Missed by the other doctors, Tinsley's experienced hand caught the growth. Many years later this episode stood out brightly in the memory of Coghlan, by then a distinguished cardiologist himself.

Tinsley had long been interested in the movements of the heart during the cardiac cycle, and when he came to Birmingham, faced with no substantial laboratory facilities or financial support, he turned to cheaper methods of investigation, such as the ballistocardiogram and the kinetocardiogram. The ballistocardiogram was a platform hung like a swing from the ceiling on which the patient would lie quietly. A stylus recorded the swinging of the apparatus as it was moved by each stroke of the heart, the same mechanism as that which produces movements and sometimes sounds in one's bed as he or she lies quietly at night. The ballistocardiogram was popularized by Dr. Albert Starr of Oregon.

Tinsley's group built a ballistocardiograph machine, a BCG, with the aid of local engineers William Bancroft and Andrew Spear, to study cardiac outputs and other aspects of cardiac function in patients. It consisted of a very light aluminum bed suspended from the ceiling with electronic recording apparatus attached at one end. It had to be carefully calibrated with a small motor swinging a weight back and forth and other measures. Late one afternoon as the group of five or six cardiologists were standing in the BCG room discussing results, one by one they sat down on unoccupied chairs or benches. Tinsley's main protege, Joe Reeves—standing about 6 feet 4 inches and weighing 240 pounds—finally sat down also, on the BCG bed! And that was the end of that particular BCG apparatus.

The kinetocardiogram KCG was Tinsley's own invention.[9] It consisted of a blunt probe attached to a small bellows, which was in turn attached to a recording device. The whole apparatus was rigidly suspended to a frame over the subject and the probe placed against the various areas of interest of the precordium. This allowed the in-and-out movements of the chest wall to be recorded graphically. Tinsley and colleagues showed that even during an anginal attack, while the myocardium was weakened in the affected area, a distinct bulge could be demonstrated in a large percentage of patients.[10] Tinsley published at least 19 papers on this topic of precordial movements between 1953 and 1967, usually with his cardiology fellows as first or co-authors. Some were published in prominent places, such as an address to the prestigious and well-attended annual May meeting of the Old Turks in 1958. As Tinlsey aged and his writings became less concerned with new data and more with medical and educational philosophy, and as more dramatic and quantitative

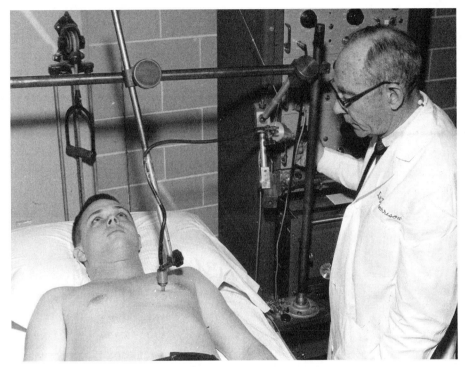

Tinsley Harrison demonstrating the kinetocardiogram on a medical student at the University of Alabama School of Medicine, about 1965.

studies became prominent with newer technologies—like cardiac catheterization, angiography, rapid biplane X-rays of cardiac chamber sizes and changes, and others—kinetocardiography faded from memory and from use.

There were interesting patients those days, patients with classic manifestations of advanced disease—hyperthyroidism so severe that the patient had congestive heart failure and jaundice, all resolved when the hyperthyroidism was controlled. Or male patients in their 20s but so poor or ignorant that they allowed their gynecomastia to become massive, coming to a doctor only after being taunted by associates for having "better breasts than any woman in town." Only then would they come for examination and have the adrenal, ovarian, or other tumor discovered and removed, with regression of the gynecomastia (but remnants needing attention). Some middle-aged female patients with similar disorders, some with striking advanced male pattern baldness and beards, seemed more common than in more developed parts of the country, perhaps because in rural, poverty-stricken Alabama such illness was permitted to reach advanced stages before medical help was sought. Even more common were patients dying of almost completely untreated advanced rheumatic valvular heart disease. Tularemia, brucellosis, and other infectious diseases were routinely part of the differential diagnosis. Occasionally trichinosis appeared. One striking group of diseases was the *worms*—ascariasis, strongyloidiasis, pinworms (in adults), or hookworms. Interestingly, some of these patients were on medicine and in the VA Hospital, yet they had these diseases of the past.

The percentage of families without indoor plumbing was high, and sometimes the outdoor privy was located uphill from the well. This led to contamination of the drinking water with whatever might drain downhill from the privy, such as hepatitis virus or some infectious bacterium like salmonella or shigella. This was worse in the poorest counties, like Lowndes County to the southwest of Montgomery on the way to Selma, about 85 percent black and said to be the poorest county in the U.S. Even the genius of Harrison's friend J. J. Kirschenfeld, educated at New York University medical school and a solo practitioner in the county from 1946 to 1960, could not correct all these problems.

The terminology of the patients was sometimes quaint and picturesque. Many of the patients older than 40 or 50, when asked if they had experienced fevers in the past would respond, "Oh, yes. I had typhoid-malaria," as though that were one disease, and sometimes the doctors told them that was the diagnosis. Occasionally they would say, "He died of Smilin'-Mighty-Jesus," which meant spinal meningitis.

In 1958 while making rounds in the VA Hospital, Tinsley was shown a patient who had very high blood pressure with papilledema and had experienced a grand mal seizure. It was assumed that he had "malignant hypertension," that there was nothing to be done about it, and that the patient would soon die. As always, Tinsley examined the near-comatose patient. "Did you see these lines in the mouth? The nearly black lines on the edge of the gums?" The residents had noticed them but assumed they were due to poor dental hygiene, as this was a white man and not a blue-gummed black man.

"Can you get me some fresh urine from him?"

"Yes, but his kidneys are failing, too."

Tinsley, with residents watching, obtained some acetic acid and ether, added these to the urine in a test tube, and shook it vigorously. He then took a Wood's lamp (UV) into the lab and placed the test tube under it in the darkened room. "I thought so!" he exclaimed. "Lead poisoning! Start an infusion of Versene immediately."[11] Tinsley saved this man's life.

In the 1950s adult patients sometimes were admitted because of plumbism—lead poisoning. The lead often came from bootlegging. During World War II, it had been impossible to obtain copper tubing needed for the moonshine stills which were tucked away in the mountains and hollows of Alabama. Lacking the proper materials for condensers, and usually not knowing any better, the whiskey-makers used automobile radiators, which contained lead solder. The bootleggers usually partook liberally of their own products and the victims entered with various symptoms, sometimes saturnine gout, or just severe abdominal pains and constipation.

One patient was treated and at discharge much improved. The problem with using car radiators instead of copper coils was explained, and the danger of lead from the soldered joints explained as well. The patient said he understood, but a few months later he returned with a full blown encephalopathy, and was again treated. When he had recovered he had explained to the puzzled doctors that he had understood the dangers, but "it just didn't taste right, so I added just a little of that lead [acetate]," which apparently tasted sweet. He got another explanation and stronger warning.

In the hot August that summer, another patient with severe pains in the abdomen was seen, with cramps and pains in the arms and legs. After examining the man, Tinsley asked, "Were you bitten by a spider?"

"Maybe so," the middle-aged black man answered. "I was usin' the privy, and just after I sat down I felt this stingin' on my pecker. I got up and looked around, but there was nothin' there, so I sat down again, and it happened again, but I was able to finish. Then in a few minutes I started gettin' sick."

Though the patient had not seen the spider, Tinsley was fairly certain from the familiar history as well as the physical findings that this was another case of black widow spider bite. After treatment, the patient recovered.

Patients in the hospital or outpatients at the clinics were not the only clinical material that provided opportunities to teach and to learn. Sometimes Tinsley would be called by local physicians to consult at the homes of patients at home perhaps too infirm to come to the doctors' offices. He would sometimes drive his own car for such house calls, but increasingly he asked one or two residents to join him and drive his car. These visits were usually in the evening after the regular day's work, and they were among the most valuable teaching exercises for the residents, allowing Tinsley to discuss various medical and nonmedical topics with the residents in another less-formal setting.

IN 1957 THE U.S.S.R. launched Sputnik, the first artificial satellite. (It was said that

12. As a member of
the U.S. Congress,
Carl Elliot also wrote
and introduced the
original bill for the
creation of the Bir-
mingham VA Hospital
in the late 1940s.

Russia got into space first because it had first choice of the German rocket scientists. But America got Werner von Braun, who came to Huntsville, Alabama, and some of his German associates came to Birmingham for medical care.) In 1958, amid the subsequent near-hysteria in the U.S. over the Russian advantage, two Alabama politicians, U.S. Senator Lister Hill and Congressman Carl Elliott,[12] persuaded Congress to enact the National Defense Education Act. Medical Education for National Defense, or MEND, soon followed, and Tinsley's medical school benefited. The very conservative people of Alabama have never seemed to understand the degree to which the economy of their state has been underwritten by the federal government they love to criticize, not only through health-related allocations, but also from military expenditures and the major space industry along the Tennessee River valley.

In the fall of 1958 when the radiologist Lawrence Reynolds donated his library of old medical books to the University of Alabama medical school, Tinsley was asked to write the dedication plaque. Like Tinsley, Reynolds was a graduate of the Johns Hopkins medical school. After being the first radiology resident at Hopkins, then serving in France in World War I, Reynolds joined the radiology staff at the Peter Bent Brigham Hospital just across Shattuck Street from Harvard Medical School's administration building for three years. He then moved to Detroit, where he practiced radiology for many years and was said to have eventually acquired personal ownership of four radiology departments. He never married, but he did have one passion: antiquarian medical books. Armed with plenty of money, especially after both World Wars, and a personal friend of one of the best booksellers and collectors in the country, Mr. Henry Schuman, Reynolds assembled a remarkable collection. The collection was so interesting that Yale, as well as several less libidinous suitors, was determined to get it. The collection contains more than 13,000 rare books (including 30 incunabula), first printings of William Harvey's *De Motu Cordis* of 1628 and Andreas Vesalius's *De Humani Corporis Fabrica* (1543), a collection of letters of the likes of Louis Pasteur, Florence Nightingale, O. W. Holmes, and William Osler, some medieval manuscripts, and a large collection on Civil War medicine. Reynolds had been born in Ozark, Alabama, and his physician family had been educated in the old Medical College of Alabama in Mobile. His physician father had loved books but had been blind, so young Lawrence read to him from Osler and other classics, especially on long buggy rides in the country as the blind father made house calls. Four of the medical books given him by his father are still in the collection. The collection finally went to Birmingham with the conditions that the school build an adequate structure to house it and that this structure have an efficiency apartment for Dr. Reynolds to use when in town. These conditions were met; the collection came to a small building near the southeastern corner of the University Hospital. In 1958 the Reynolds Historical Library was dedicated, and Tinsley's dedication on the bronze plaque reads [with added punctuation]:

> Here are housed the books collected and loved by Lawrence Reynolds, physician, scholar, and philanthropist. The official dedication ceremony of the Reynolds Library was held on February 2, 1958. But the more meaningful dedication will come from you who read these books. Each time one of you reaps from the great minds of the past the desire for finer achievement in your profession and nobler development of your own character, the Reynolds library will have been rededicated.[13]

Heavily influenced by his father, Groce Sr., who lectured on the history of medicine during Tinsley's years at Vanderbilt, Tinsley loved the subject and continued to study it. His Reynolds dedication obviously reflects both this love and his own values.

THINGS AT THE MEDICAL school were getting better, there was more money, and competition among applicants for residencies was growing. Freed from administrative details after he retired from his last chairmanship, Tinsley was able to concentrate more on his own interests. However, the culture was overtaking him. The continuous changes in the culture and environment around him, eddies in the overpowering but usually unnoticed current of history, grew into two large and pervasive waves: the overall alterations in society often referred to as the sixties; and the related activities and changes in race relations and civil rights. Both cultural movements are far too complex for treatment in a biography of a 20th-century physician, but Tinsley did live through them, and they affected him.

There is a saying in China: "Revolutions begin in the South." Some argue that the American cultural revolution of the sixties began in the South. Much of the spirit of the sixties was captured in music which had origins in the South, especially jazz, the blues, country and western, rock and roll, and later hip-hop.

The sixties were about more than a rejection of conventional social and political values. The various movements were about more than just teenage rebellion. Widespread changes were taking place amid shifting concepts of equality, sexuality, expanding social consciousness, and ideas of community. The very definitions

13. H. L. Holley, "Highlights in the History of Medicine in Alabama (fourth Reynolds Historical Lecture)" in *The Reynolds Historical Lectures 1980–1991*, ed. Marion G. McGuinn (Birmingham: UAB, 1993), 66–99.

14. Carl Djerassi, *The Pill, Pygmy Chimps, and Degas' Horse* (New York: Basic Books, 1992); A. O. Maisel, *The Hormone Quest: The Story of the Century's Most Exciting Advance in Health and Human Welfare* (New York: Random House, 1965). Djerassi is not only a superb synthetic organic chemist, but also a polymath—artist, creator of movie films and plays, etc. He shows, with references to specific patents, how his work in the 1940s and '50s originated nor-ethynodrel, the active component of Enovid, and how his patents antedated those of Colson's by several years (56–63). Colson was employed by the Searle Co., which was more totally committed to the market and making money than were Parke-Davis or Pfizer, which were constrained by societal and religious concerns. Pfizer, in fact, would not touch anything that might have to do with birth control, since its president was a staunch Roman Catholic. Maisel's book, which I reviewed in the *Archives of Int. Med.*, is a nice popular story

of society, of voting, of participatory democracy, of government, were all being challenged and redrawn. Many of the ideas that were radical at the time are now considered mainstream to U.S. society. No one went through the sixties unchanged.

Before the sixties, many beginning medical students in America had probably never even heard of marijuana, magic mushrooms, Quaaludes, LSD, or other drugs. In the sixties' new youth culture, these drugs became pervasive.

The drug with the most long-term social effect, however, was "the Pill," introduced as Enovid in 1960 by the American pharmaceutical company G. D. Searle.[14] With the Pill came sexual liberation and feminism. Then there was the coming out of homosexuals, who had by now co-opted the word "gay." The British author Arthur Marwick, in *The Sixties: Cultural Revolution in Britain, France, Italy, and the United States,* argued that America's sexual liberation, with the other changes, made permissiveness and promiscuity practically mandatory.[15]

The transformation was dramatic and, for many older adults, accustomed to what they viewed as more refined decorum and intelligent manners, the changes were abrupt, wrenching, and painful. Prior to 1965 it was illegal in Connecticut for a physician or pharmacist to provide contraceptives (including condoms or diaphragms) to anyone, even a married woman or couple. In the 1940s and '50s, laws in other states, especially those with large Catholic populations like Massachusetts, were usually similar. The U.S. Supreme Court case that changed this was *Griswold v. Connecticut*, decided June 7, 1965, which found that "though the Constitution does not explicitly protect a general right to privacy, the various guarantees within the Bill of Rights create penumbras . . . that establish a right to privacy.[16]

The sixties movement reached extremes. "Hippies" was a term that was popularized in 1967 with the publication of "The Social History of Hippies" in *Ramparts,* "the intellectual, left-leaning, even crusading magazine."[17] Hippies were largely full-time derelicts—layabouts and beatniks—often children of affluent parents. Their headquarters were in three places: Berkeley, the Haight-Ashbury in San Francisco, and Greenwich Village in New York City. By 1970 there was a Haight-Ashbury Free Clinic run by David Smith, M.D. I worked there one night. It was a haunting, sobering experience. Patients there included many single mothers now in their thirties with genital problems and infections, even though their syphilis and gonorrhea had been treated with penicillin. They often had several children, but most of the fathers had long since disappeared.

The old attitudes and values were not safe anywhere in America, not even in the hyperconservative South. The erstwhile Harvard faculty member and apostle of LSD as the route to true understanding, Timothy Leary, lived in Birmingham for a time. He coined a catch phrase that helped define the era: "Turn on. Tune in. Drop out!" Many young people followed, even in Birmingham.

Even among physicians, the use of illegal drugs became alarmingly frequent. This included medical students at Tinsley's school. A survey done by the medical students themselves found that 50 percent had used marijuana during the past 4 weeks, and 8 percent had used drugs such as cocaine.[18] An article published about the same time in the *New England J. Medicine* showed similar results for physicians and pharmacists in Massachusetts.[19]

To the generation being left behind, it was all connected. Raw sexuality, rampant drug use, riots—society seemed to be unraveling. Even the general language of physicians and patients changed. Before the war years of 1937–45, most physicians had at least attempted to avoiding vulgarisms and obscenities, even mild words like "damn" or "hell," substituting "darn" or "dern" or "heck." Coarse language had always been around, but beginning in the sixties, language seemed to the elders to undergo an immense degradation, not only in the words chosen but in grammar and logic, perhaps partly the result of large increases of population, urbanization, and television. When one father observed to his son that an ass is just a donkey, the son replied, "No, Dad. That guy is an "ass-*hole*!" So *asshole* was more definitive, as was *shit-ass*, a term sometimes used by Governor George Wallace of Barbour County in rural south Alabama. Even that most forbidden word in earlier years, *fuck*,[20] became increasingly common in motion pictures and on TV as the 20th century rolled on. It was no longer surprising that movie and TV stars like Eddie Murphy and Jerry Seinfeld used the word for its shock value, but in 2004 U.S. Vice President Dick Cheney, a leader for family values and fundamentalist Christianity, told an obnoxious reporter to, "Fuck off!"

These words, phrases, and usages were more than mere solecisms and were now being used publicly. Tinsley, like many of his generation, regretted these changes in the language in which the communicative value (and thus the transfer of understanding) of words, phrases, and constructions had been degraded by casual overuse of cursing and inappropriate vulgarisms. Tinsley was more concerned with the changes he saw in the fabric of society itself.

These changes tried Tinsley's patience, especially with the students and house officers he dealt with. The interaction was often unfavorable. Though Tinsley loved

of endocrine research, but mostly devoted to Enovid, called by that name after the first few mentions of the compound, which it praises highly as a major contribution to humanity. I was later told by another ghostwriter that Maisel was under contract with Searle and that the manuscript was typed in Searle's corporate offices.

15. A. Marwick, *The Sixties: Cultural Revolution in Britain, France, Italy, and the United States, c.1958–c.1974* (Oxford-New York: Oxford University Press, 1998).

16. *Oyez. U.S. Supreme Court Multimedia, ThisNation.com.* American Government & Politics Online, October 4, 2005. The actual decision, written by Justice William O. Douglas, concludes as follows: "We deal with a right of privacy older than the Bill of Rights—older than our political parties, older than our school system. Marriage is a coming together for better or worse, hopefully enduring, and intimate to the degree of being sacred. It is an association that promotes a way of life,

not causes; a harmony in living, not political faiths, a bilateral loyalty, not commercial or social projects. Yet it is an association for as noble a purpose as any involved in our prior decisions." (*This-Nation.com.* American Government & Politics Online. Accessed October 4, 2005). Hence, the laws banning contraceptives were overturned.

17. Marwick, *Sixties*, 482.

18. Med students at UAB—survey published in *Alabama J. of Med. Sciences*, 1975.

19. *New England J. Med.* Article on drug use by MDs and pharmacists in Mass.

20. J. Scheidlower, *The F Word* (New York: Random House, 1999).

21. T. R. Harrison, with various co-authors, often as first authors: "Kinetocardiogram"; "Movements"; "Movements and Forces of the Human Heart," *Arch. Int. Med.* 99 (1957): 401–410; "Movements and Forces of the Human Heart: Precordial Movements in Relation to Ejection and Filling of the Ventricles," *Arch. Int. Med.* 101 (1958):

his students and believed that genuine affection between student and teacher is as important to learning as the intellectual exchange, he refused to tolerate students who were unkempt, discourteous, used filthy speech, or didn't care about their patients or the preferences of those patients, especially older patients. On one occasion in 1968 he expelled two hippieish students from his rounds; he later regretted how he had handled the incident and felt depressed about it.

Tinsley's ire was not entirely unfounded. His mental and emotional environment was from earlier in the century, when youngsters treated their elders with respect, even when they disagreed. On one occasion Tinsley asked a resident to name one *physical* finding which might be a clue to the patient's having a silent myocardial infarction or a severe anginal attack with atypical symptoms. The resident, unfamiliar with Tinsley, answered, "Where have you been, Gramps? Everybody knows that there are no *physical* findings in an anginal attack, only *subjective symptoms*, unless you want to count sweating or anxiety." The resident was not only grossly disrespectful and ignorant of Tinsley's status in medicine, but also ignorant about clinical medicine itself. Beginning in 1953, Tinsley had published a whole series of papers in prominent places about precordial movements as affected by changes in coronary blood flow[21] and had regularly demonstrated to cardiology fellows such bulges in patients.[22]

(Many years later, after Tinsley had died, an article appeared in the *Journal of the American Medical Association*, perhaps the most prestigious journal concerned with clinical medicine in the entire world. The article was titled "Does This Man Have a Myocardial Infarction?" It discussed the symptoms of angina pectoris and myocardial infarcts, pointing out along the way that these patients have no actual physical signs, other than profuse sweating, indications of the anxiety of *angor animimi*, and alterations in the blood pressure. There was no mention of precordial bulges or their use in the quick, cheap assessment of the patient's problem. The closest the authors of the article came was a recommendation for a search for changes in the volumes of the heart using echocardiograms that would be obtained by a technician for the clinician.)

At one supper in the hospital in 1968 I asked a student wearing torn blue jeans, a plaid open-collar shirt with no tie, tennis shoes, and a Pittsburgh Pirates baseball cap if anybody ever complained about his dress. He replied, "Only once," and related that as he was making late rounds one evening at the VA Hospital an older gentleman, in a sparkling long white physician's coat, white shirt, and tie, had approached him and asked his name, which he told. The older man thanked him and they went their separate ways. The next day Chief of Medicine Joe Reeves showed the student a letter. It was from the new chief of surgery from the Mayo Clinic, John W. Kirklin. "If this man were on my service," the letter said, "he would be expelled immediately and permanently!"[23] But the resident was not on surgery, Reeves had many other very pressing problems, and the resident was not expelled.

The sixties were a polarizing time. The schism involved behavior, religion, language, art, politics, music, fashion, and economics. The generation gap was never more defined. The youth felt the older generation had messed things up; the older generation saw their progeny heading for a hedonistic disaster. The events of the sixties formed the ground on which Tinsley's later years stood.

NOWHERE WAS THE SECOND aspect of cultural change, the changes in race relations, more vivid than in Birmingham, the point of the wedge pushing civil rights forward in the United States. Governor George C. Wallace led Alabama's quixotic resistance to the inevitable future. Wallace came to symbolize the violent 1960s resistance to change with his 1963 inaugural cry, "Segregation today! Segregation tomorrow! And segregation forever!" This was followed six months later by his orchestrated, and toothless, "stand in the schoolhouse door" at the University of Alabama. He encouraged resistance rather than quiet discussion in attempts to work out the problems.

The people of industrial Birmingham, and especially the largely Northern-populated medical center faculty, did not support Wallace. He returned the favor, calling people like them "pointy-headed pseudo-intellectuals who can't even park their bicycles straight." He pronounced "pseudo-intellectuals" as "swaydo-." And though he had plenty of federal funds for highway construction, the new interstates were completed everywhere in the state except around Birmingham.

At that time state law prohibited successive terms for governors. Wallace failed to persuade the legislature to change the law, so he ran his wife, Lurleen B. Wallace, who became the state's first woman governor.[24] While George worked from his office in the capitol across from Governor Lurleen's office, mainly as a lobbyist in the legislature and on plans for another run at the U.S. presidency, Lurleen quietly did her best to implement George's policies, though she genuinely preferred being a wife and mother to their four children. She was popular and loved the outdoors, especially fishing quietly in the country. She occasionally hunted turkeys with the boys. But five months after her inauguration in January 1967 she was found to

582–591; "Movements and Forces of the Human Heart V: Precordial Movements in Relation to Atrial Contraction," *Circulation* 18 (1958): 82–91; "Problems in Evaluation of Pain in the Chest," *Modern Concepts of Cardiovascular Dis.* 27 (1958): 461–466; "Precordial Systolic"; "Effect of Exertion." And at least half a dozen more during this period and later relating to precordial bulges related to diminished coronary artery flow.

22. H. C. Coghlin, personal communication. See also video recording of "Centenary Anniversary of Harrison's Birth," 2000, UAB Archives.

23. Weisse recounts an interesting story in his interview with Kirklin (*Heart To Heart*). While Kirklin was a freshman medical student at Harvard, one Saturday morning he was in a lecture by Robert E. Gross on wound healing. Kirklin asks Weisse, "Did you ever see him in person? Well, he walked in, the very image of a surgeon: probably five foot eight or nine, with his hair in perfect order, immaculately

dressed in a beautiful blue suit and red tie. He gave a lecture that was not particularly inspiring, but he was clearly Robert Gross, and he was the world's opinion of a surgeon in appearance. And all those medical students were going to be heart surgeons at the conclusion of that lecture because it was only a few weeks before that he had successfully closed a patent ductus." (107).

24. Sledge, J. L. "Lurleen Burns Wallace" in *American National Biography*, vol. 22, 540–541.

25. Anita Smith, *The Intimate Story of Lurleen Wallace, Her Crusade of Courage* (Montgomery: Communications Unlimited Inc., 1969). Sledge, *"Lurleen."*

26. Holley, *History*, 159–161. Hill had studied suturing the heart, had found 17 known cases, two of which he had witnessed and had published a review of these in 1900. In 1902 he sutured the heart of a young black man who had been stabbed in a dramatic tale recorded and documented by Holley.

27. Virginia Hill to

have a recurrence of her uterine cancer, for which she had had surgery two months before the election. The rest of her term was marked mainly by her fight against the relentless disease, well-described by her friend the popular Birmingham reporter and historian, Anita Smith.[25]

As THE SIXTIES UNFOLDED, life for Tinsley and his academic medical center continued much as before despite the social problems. Toward the end of 1959 the "Hill Heart Center" was dedicated and named after Dr. Luther Leonidas Hill of Montgomery, "first American surgeon to suture the human heart."[26] Dr. Hill was also the father of U.S. Senator Lister Hill, powerhouse for health legislation in the Congress.[27] This heart center, a newly built operating room complex in the hospital, recognized the attempts of the Hill family's relative, Chief of Surgery Champ Lyons, to establish a strong program for cardiovascular surgery in Birmingham in an attempt to catch up with other medical centers. To that end Lyons had recruited an engineer, Leland C. Clark Jr. from Cincinnati, to build a heart-lung machine comparable to that developed in the early 1950s at the Mayo Clinic, which enabled operating *inside* the heart.[28] (The many coronary bypass operations of later years were not open-heart surgery.) In addition, W. Sterling Edwards, M.D., a Birmingham native, had recently returned from a surgical residency at Harvard's Massachusetts General Hospital and was eager to move forward with CV surgery. Local lore holds that Edwards, working with the Chemstrand Corporation of Alabama, developed and used special Dacron aortic grafts long before anybody in Texas, such as Michael Debakey. Lyons and his team performed some cardiac surgery, such as repair of the Tetralogy of Fallot in several patients. These early efforts were crucial to the later course of things, as we shall see.

The dedication address was given by Luther Leonidas Terry, M.D., from Red Level, Alabama, assistant director of the National Heart Institute and namesake of Dr. L. L. Hill.[29] Terry later served as U.S. surgeon general from 1961 to 1965 and was the first major government official to condemn smoking as an important health hazard with the Surgeon General's Report of 1964.

In 1962, Tinsley's former Bowman Gray student, S. R. "Dick" Hill, was made dean of medicine. I was named chief of endocrinology to succeed Hill. One story may illustrate some of the difficulties in recruiting excellent, well-trained faculty:

Carl Bentzel was a promising young physician working in the Harvard laboratory of the biophysicist A. K. Solomon. Bentzel was born and educated through

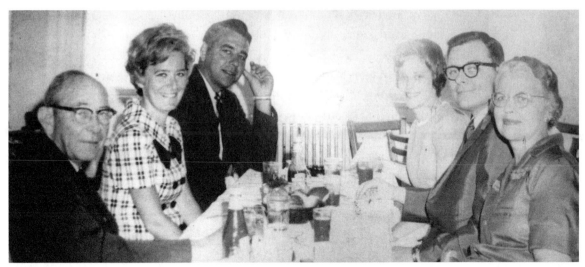

college and medical school in Alabama, then he interned at Columbia's Presbyterian Hospital in New York. After that he went to the NIH for a stint working on calcium metabolism, thence to Harvard. When I offered him more space and base money than he would ever find in the Northeast, plus an assistant professorship with great likelihood of making tenured associate professor within five years, he said, "No, I couldn't possibly live in Alabama." I was amazed and pointed out that he had attended college and medical school in Alabama, had been the recipient of a scholarship which required that he practice in a rural community for a year, which he did in Dadeville[30] some 90 miles southeast of Birmingham, and that his background fit him for a successful career in academic medicine. He said that he knew all that but that his wife was from Brooklyn, New York, and that their year in Dadeville had been the most miserable of his life.

He had been there just a short time, working in a new Hill-Burton hospital, when a nurse approached him and said some of the locals were complaining about his handling of obstetrics. He had delivered a baby and placed it in the new nursery, then delivered a second baby and done the same. The problem was that the first baby was white and the second black. They solved the issue by tying a string across the room and putting the black babies on one side and the white babies on the other. But Bentzel wanted no more of that, and his wife certainly wanted to get out of that atmosphere, so he refused the job I offered him. He later became a professor of medicine specializing in nephrology, but in a school further north.

Tinsley Harrison with his wife, Betty, sons, and daughters-in-law: left, Joan and Randy Harrison, and right, Janice and John Harrison, 1968.

J. A. Pittman, 1999. Senator Lister Hill's full name was Joseph Lister Hill, after the famous Scottish surgeon who introduced antisepsis and corresponded with Pasteur. His father had studied with Joseph Lister in Britain and hoped his son would become a famous surgeon. However, when he took the son into the OR at

the age of 9, the son
had fainted and lost
interest in practicing
medicine, except from
the U.S. Senate.

28. Fisher, *Building*,
46, 99.

29. Virginia Van Der
Veer Hamilton, *Lister
Hill: Statesman from
the South* (Chapel Hill:
University of North
Carolina Press, 1987),
239.

30. Dadeville, a lovely
town near Tinsley's
beloved Lake Martin,
claims to have been
the site of the first
medical school in
Alabama in 1852
(actually it was the
second).

31. His life and much
of his work is recorded
in a fascinating auto-
biography, *No Greater
Privilege* (Montgom-
ery: Black Belt Press,
1992), a title taken
from Tinsley's intro-
duction in the first
edition of *Principles of
Internal Medicine*.

ONE STALWART WHO WAS a remarkably excellent physician and practically a genius at keeping on despite all sorts of difficulties was Tinsley's good friend and colleague Jack J. Kirschenfeld, who practiced in Fort Deposit in Lowndes County near Montgomery for 14 years before moving to Montgomery in 1960.[31] Jack, a tall dignified physician, had graduated from the New York University medical school in 1943. He was born into a conservative orthodox Jewish family in the Austro-Hungarian Empire in 1919, and his father brought the family to New York in 1923. For such an impecunious Jew, getting into a northeastern medical school in the 1930s was no easy matter, but Jack was extraordinarily bright and resourceful.

He was drafted into the Army Air Corps and soon married a Methodist nurse at Bellevue from upstate New York. After the war they bought a very used car and planned to move to California and enter private practice there. But first they visited friends at the Maxwell Air Force Base in Montgomery, Alabama, where Jack had served. They were introduced to an elderly pharmacist from nearby Fort Deposit in adjacent Lowndes County. The pharmacist implored them to live there for "just a few weeks, until we can find a doctor to replace the one who just died." Jack had almost no money, internal medicine residencies throughout the U.S. were overfilled, nothing attractive or workable was available in New York, and California was an unknown, so he agreed; he and Mrs. Kirschenfeld remained in Fort Deposit nearly 16 years.

Kirschenfeld had a practice perhaps unique in American medicine—a Jewish doctor from New York practicing in a Deep South rural area in Alabama. He made many friends, had unusual medical experiences, and witnessed a rapidly disappearing culture, already past in most of America. Some of these he captured in his excellent autobiography, such as the fact that during his practice he encountered a number of white men living with black wives and families, but that after the desegregation orders of the 1960s, such partnerships disappeared—either went underground or actually stopped, at least temporarily.

Fort Deposit had no paved streets. The county had no hospital. The county population of 18,000 was 80 percent black. The area was desperately poor with almost no indoor plumbing or clean water in many of the shacks that served as housing. He saw many patients in his office in the back rooms of the pharmacy. He made house calls on horseback and did surgery and delivered babies in the backs of horse-drawn wagons as he tried to get the patient to his car at Fort Deposit then to the hospital in Montgomery.

Meanwhile he subscribed to medical journals and read them thoroughly. He even published a few papers, such as one describing a blood disorder seen in black women, probably with a pica, who ate moist clay and developed a peculiar anemia. After 1950 he traveled frequently to the new medical school in Birmingham and befriended Tinsley, who, always eager to associate with highly intelligent physicians, was drawn to Jack's experiences, so often reminiscent of his own father's a half-century earlier. Soon Jack began making rounds with the residents and students at the new medical school, often quizzing them (and sometimes the accompanying faculty members) about recent articles and advances and finding them less informed than he.

LOWNDES WAS ONE OF the poorest counties in the U.S., with a per capita income of less than $200 *annually* even in the late 1930s. (A few other Alabama counties had annual incomes as low as $156 per capita in 1935.[32]) Prior to 1965, everything remotely public was strictly segregated, and there were no registered black voters. The vast majority of blacks were tenant farmers chronically in debt to the white land owners. In 1861, probably nearly 100 percent of the white population favored secession.[33] In 1946, slavery was long gone, but rich planters and industrialists remained in control, and much of the population lived just above the subsistence level. As hard as times were during the Great Depression, for the majority of Lowndes County people circumstances had worsened during World War II as the county began losing population—especially young males—to urban areas, a shift that did not begin to change until after 1970.[34] Medical care was nearly nonexistent for much of the Lowndes County population; there just were not enough doctors.

About 1964, several of us were summoned to the office of Dean S. Richardson Hill to meet with Dr. John Chennault, a power in the state medical association. He had received a call from officials in Washington with word that something had to be done to improve the situation in Lowndes County. A meeting was arranged for a Sunday morning in Joe Volker's office, a rather small room on the ground floor of the new Lyons-Harrison Research Building. No Lowndes County doctors were available to attend (Jack Kirschenfeld had by then moved to Montgomery), but about seven general practitioners from adjacent Wilcox and Dallas counties were present. They were interesting physicians, wearing jeans and plaid shirts, and several had on broad-brimmed straw cowboy hats. One was chewing on a long straw, and another a plug of tobacco. The Feds were late. So we sat and chatted a bit about what we could do to keep the Feds happy, or at least satisfied. The atmosphere grew

32. Wayne Flynt, *Poor But Proud: Alabama's Poor Whites* (Tuscaloosa: The University of Alabama Press, 1989), 71.

33. Ibid., 37–38.

34. N. G. Lineback, ed., *Atlas of Alabama* (Tuscaloosa: The University of Alabama Press, 1973), 32.

35. Accreditation of medical schools was done by the LCME (Liaison Committee for Medical Education), and the residencies were accredited by a committee from each specialty, the RRC (Residency Review Committee). This began to change in the early 1970s when the AMA led in the formation of the CCME, Coordinating Council for Medical Education, with four subcommittees, one for physicians, one for residencies ("graduate medical education"), one for allied health, and one for continuing medical education.

increasingly volatile. As the delay went on and the anti-Washington conversation worsened, I worried that when the Feds arrived, we might end up with a fistfight. Finally, the door swung open and the Feds arrived, in the form of a beautiful young lady about 30 years old, wearing an elegant but tight dress on a shapely body. The good ol' boy doctors were almost falling over each other as they offered the most comfortable chairs with courteous greetings: "Have a seat, Ma'am." "Make yo'self comfortable." It was hilarious.

The visit was not trivial. First, the general practitioners, though immersed in the social environment of the Deep South in Cold War and segregation days, were competent and dedicated servants of their communities, both white and black, and friends of most of their patients. I came to know some from those counties in later years and found them to be excellent physicians.

The conversation that day was polite, but the visitor, Wendy Gobel, was firm that the medical school must help set up and operate a clinic in Hayneville, the largest town in Lowndes County about 100 miles south of Birmingham. We tried to explain that, yes, there were lots of doctors at the medical school, but none were unoccupied. The students were, after all, still students and not legally able to practice medicine, and the faculty was grossly understaffed and already stressed trying to meet their teaching commitments. Most of the residents were already licensed, true, but the accrediting agency would not permit them to leave their residency training at the hospital and still maintain its accreditation.[35] This was a frequent problem in the 1950s and '60s, and even the '70s, as all sorts of organizations, especially prisons and institutions of various sorts (such as "insane asylums," as they were referred to then) pled for medical help, almost always to no avail.

WHEN TINSLEY ARRIVED IN 1950, Birmingham was dominated by U.S. Steel and was nicknamed "the Pittsburgh of the South." The medical center consisted of two rather small city blocks plus one owned by the federal government for a VA hospital, which opened three years later. The only buildings were the Jefferson Hospital, which also included medical school classrooms and teaching laboratories—gross anatomy was taught on the 17th floor. There was also a small five-story student nurses' residence, later named for Roy Kracke, the first dean, adjacent to the hospital. Next to the medical school was a large 50-year-old building housing the auditorium and old clinics of the defunct Birmingham Medical College. These were used for another few years. The dental school was also housed in the 1903 Hillman Hospital building and the 1941 Jefferson Tower.

Across the street from the school and hospital stood a long row of old barracks which had been used during the war (these would be torn down in 1958). There was an old Children's Hospital about seven blocks to the east and not readily accessible to the medical school. A nearby building owned by the county health department housed TB and venereal disease clinics. The groundbreaking for this county health building had been blessed by the attendance

At the dedication of the Lyons-Harrison Building, November 9, 1966. From left, Dr. Joseph F. Volker, Senator Lister Hill, Champ Lyons Jr., Naomi (Mrs. Champ) Lyons, and Tinsley Harrison.

of Governor Jim Folsom and fostered close relations with the medical school. The medical school library was in the basement of the university hospital and was named in honor of Luther Leonidas Hill whose library had been given to the school in 1947.

In 1951 the Monday Morning Football Club, a philanthropic group of local businessmen, opened the six-story, 100-bed Crippled Children's Hospital, meant for the rehabilitation of the many children crippled by poliomyelitis, just to the west across the street from the University Hospital.

By the late 1950s the medical center consisted of several old clinical facilities, older in comparison with the times and trajectory of medicine than necessarily physical age (such as the new polio hospital). Practically nothing was air-conditioned. In fact, even in the University Hospital window units were rare until the late 1950s and 1960s. The newer VA Hospital was not air-conditioned until the 1960s.

The medical school was surrounded by slums. Just a block to the east were houses for prostitutes. To the west were some 60 blocks of low-income housing, with unintentional mixing of poor black and white families, tramps, and drifters. Food was sometimes scarce. At Christmas and Thanksgiving, the Salvation Army delivered free turkeys for dinners to families in the area. Some of the streets were unpaved, and some of the houses had no indoor plumbing or toilets.

36. Many people, including some in the VA or primarily in the school, referred to the VA's research awards as "grants" comparable to the research grants of the NIH. However, the VA support was technically not a grant but in-house support for research of the VA, though the peer review system was similar in the two.

Some married residents rented rooms in the old army barracks or in small frame houses in the area, since they were so cheap. One could rent a fully furnished house with a living room, dining area, kitchen, bedroom, bathroom, and heating paid by the landlord, plus a small garden and tool shed in the little yard, for $65 per month. There were hazards: occasional robberies, shootings by residents when thieves approached, arson by the property owners eager to collect insurance, and other crimes. This was slowly changing, but still a problem at the time.

AS THE SIXTIES MOVED on, there were more concrete changes in Birmingham: the buildings and environment of the emerging new medical school. Tinsley had foreseen and predicted that federal research money would soon increase, with the formation of multiple new institutes at the NIH and rapid growth of voluntary health organizations such as the American Heart Association, American Diabetes Association, and others. He therefore worked to raise money for construction of research space, which resulted in 1960 in the medical school's first real research building, which was promptly named "The Lyons-Harrison Research Building" and displayed the single word "Research" on the side.

The summer of 1966 brought completion of the VA Research Bridge, a five-story span across the street between the VA Hospital and University Hospital, which permitted patients to be wheeled from one to the other on stretchers or in wheelchairs without going outside. The building was funded with research money, and its rooms housed about 20,000 feet of laboratories and a few administrative offices for the VA's research program.[36] There was a grand dedication ceremony at which Tinsley, Volker and others spoke. Although there was a long tunnel connecting the VA with the Shands Hospital in Gainesville, Florida, there had never been a building joining a VA Hospital with the hospital of the adjacent university medical center.

Substantial changes began to occur within society with the civil rights movement of the sixties and with the presidency of Lyndon B. Johnson and his "Great Society Program." Joe Volker, who replaced Robert Berson, M.D., as vice president for the medical center, managed to create a long-range plan for the 60 blocks of slums around the school. He obtained large federal grants to renovate it from HUD, the Department of Housing and Urban Development. In some cities moving numerous largely black households away from the slums and into new housing projects caused resentment and riots. Not so with Volker's projects. He and the city fathers also manipulated funding to complete the new housing projects before moving inhabitants out of their slums, to everybody's advantage. Some of the faculty belittled long-range plans, which they said never worked. But Volker's plan was first of all a physical plan for the area, put forth in graphic form and considerable detail, but without explicit deadlines. It was printed in a large yellow fairly simple paper-bound spiral notebook and was revised at least annually. It really expressed his vision for the future. Most of these changes are captured in the book *Building On a Vision* by Virginia E. Fisher.[37]

IN ADDITION TO THE changes, turmoil, and bloodshed over civil rights, one other event occurred in 1965 to mar the happier events for Tinsley, and to remind him of mortality and change. His friend and colleague Champ Lyons died of a brain tumor. Lyons himself was a giant in building the medical school programs in Birmingham, though his fame was more local than that of Tinsley. Despite occasional real differences, Tinsley and Champ enjoyed each other, respected and trusted each other, and worked well together. Now he also was gone.[38]

Tinsley had been a "councillor" for the Association of American Physicians, the

37. Fisher, *Building.*
38. M. L. Dalton, *Champ Lyons: Surgeon* (Macon, GA: Aequanimitas Medical Books, 2003).

VA Research Bridge Dedication, 1967.

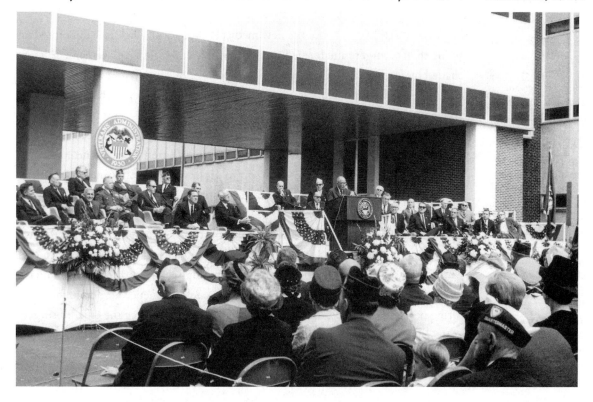

39. The Councillors of these medical organizations functioned as a board of directors.

40. Thorn, personal conversation. By resigning from the line to become AAP president, Harrison moved Thorn ahead a year. Thorn, Harrison's colleague on *Principles of Internal Medicine* since its beginning about 20 years earlier, was scheduled to become AAP president a year or so later anyhow; but Harrison's withdrawal moved him ahead. This is also confirmable from the records of the AAP published in their annual *Transactions* for many years.

41. Frommeyer, trained at Harvard's Thorndike Labs in Boston under W. B. Castle in hematology, was made president of the American College of Physicians as the National Heart Institute (NHI) added blood diseases and became the National Heart, Lung, and Blood Institute (NHLBI).

42. D. C. McGoon, "Foreword" in *Cardiac Surgery: Morphology, Diagnostic Criteria, Natural History, Techniques, Results, and Indications* (New

most prestigious club in academic medicine, from 1959 to 1964.[39] This sequence usually led into the ranks of higher officers and eventually to the presidency, the top honor and a nice one to balance Tinsley's presidency of the Young Turks 30 years earlier. Tinsley did not want the position. He told his colleagues that he wanted simply to return to patient care, teaching, writing, and what little he could do for research at his beloved new medical school.[40] He realized his time was limited, and he wanted to move on.

Lyons's death triggered changes. As things improved and research funding improved, Lyons had created solid foundations on which his department of surgery could build in the years ahead, especially in cardiac work. Not only were the facilities improving, with the new Hill Heart Center, but so were the people, with the recruitment of the likes of the pump-oxygenator engineer Leland Clark and L. M. "Mac" Bargeron, M.D., a pediatrician already specializing in cardiology and cardiac catheterization and angiography useful in defining congenital defects. The cardiovascular surgeon W. Sterling Edwards Jr. had also recently returned from his surgical residency at Harvard's Mass General Hospital.

SHORTLY AFTER LYONS DIED, the new medical school dean Dick Hill appointed an acting chief of surgery and formed a search committee to find a replacement. This was chaired by Joe Reeves, the cardiologist and protege of Tinsley, and included several other leading faculty members, including Walter B. Frommeyer, chief of medicine and recently president of the American College of Physicians.[41] Frommeyer was also a friend of Dr. Hugh "Red" Butt, an internist and gastroenterologist at the Mayo Clinic. Butt was president of the American Society of Internal Medicine, a national organization formed years earlier primarily to protect the economic interests of internists, while the ACP was seen as too academic and too intellectually oriented. By the 1960s the existence of the two somewhat competing organizations of internists was in nobody's best interest, so Frommeyer and Butt worked together to bring the two back into one association. They knew, respected, and trusted each other. Frommeyer had friends at the Mayo Clinic and was known nationally as a respected clinician who understood how the politics of the heart could influence academic medicine hiring decisions. In addition, Hill appointed to the committee the chief of surgery at the McGill medical school in Montreal and Francis D. Moore in Boston, Mosely Professor at Harvard and chief of surgery at the Brigham Hospital. Hill had known Moore well during his years with Thorn, and they also trusted each other.

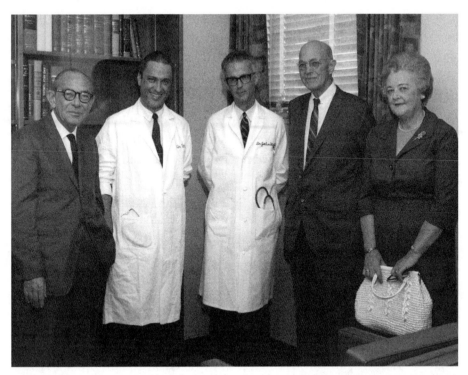

At the dedication of the Champ Lyons House Staff Memorial Library in University Hospital, June 27, 1967. From left, Drs. Tinsley Harrison, Holt A. McDowell, and John W. Kirklin; Mervyn H. Sterne; and Naomi (Mrs. Champ) Lyons.

While the committee was searching, Hill and Reeves had a number of telephone conversations with the surgeon Gurd in Montreal and especially with Moore at Harvard. He learned that John Kirklin of the Mayo Clinic might possibly be recruitable, though it would be a long shot.

Kirklin was one of the leading cardiac surgeons of the day and the originator of the first successful pump oxygenator used for true intracardiac surgery.[42] He had grown up at the Mayo Clinic where his father was chief of radiology and had diagnosed the fatal gastric carcinoma which killed Dr. W. J. Mayo, whom John Kirklin practically worshiped as the best medical administrator he knew.[43] Kirklin was educated at the University of Minnesota in Minneapolis and had helped with the football team, though he was too slight to play himself. He graduated from Harvard Medical School, took a rotating internship in Philadelphia, served as a neurosurgeon in the army, and worked at the Boston Children's Hospital with Dr. Robert Gross, who had made surgical history in 1938 while still a chief resident by being the first to close a patent ductus arteriosus in a child. Kirklin greatly admired Gross, a very neat, well-dressed, dignified man, a bit severe but certainly an important leader in pediatric surgery. Then Kirklin returned to the Mayo staff at Rochester.

York: John Wiley and Sons, 1990). McGoon said then, " . . . [In the early 1950s] Kirklin was just embarking on his unique, pioneering experience with the world's first continuous series of clinical operations using a pump oxygenator."

43. J. W. Kirklin, "Lessons from the History of the Mayo Clinic," *The Reynolds Historical Lectures 1980–1991*, ed. Marion G. McGuinn (Birmingham, AL: The University of Alabama at Birmingham Press, 1993), 118–154.

44. I had dinner at an AAP meeting with Helen Taussig, M.D., of Hopkins, and B. W. Cobbs, M.D., cardiologist at Emory, about 2 weeks before Taussig was killed in an automobile accident. She claimed at that time that she had tried to convince Gross to attempt what later became the Blalock-Taussig operation for relief of patients with Tetralogy of Fallot but that he had refused, saying, "I've just received a lot of praise for surgically *closing* a patent ductus; now you want me to *create* one?"

45. Harold Ellis, *A*

By the early '50s, Tinsley's friend Blalock had also made history at Johns Hopkins with his "blue baby operation" (which Gross had declined to do[44]) for alleviation of the congenital abnormalities of the Tetralogy of Fallot. By 1950 Blalock was one of the most famous and admired surgeons in America. Kirklin realized that the next big advances in surgery were likely to be in the heart, despite the statement by the great European surgeon Theodor Billroth in 1893, "Any surgeon who would attempt an operation on the heart should lose the respect of his colleagues." Others had expressed similar views at the end of the 19th century and the early years of the 20th.

Some surgeons tried anyhow. For example, Harvard's Elliott Cutler in 1923 used a long narrow "tenotome" to insert through a small incision in the heart and cut the scar tissue which was killing patients with mitral stenosis. None of these various attempts was very successful, and all were soon abandoned.

In October 1930, John H. Gibbon, a surgical research fellow with Chief of Surgery Edward D. "Pete" Churchill at the Mass General Hospital in Boston, watched for hours over a patient with a pulmonary embolus waiting for a Trendelenburg operation to remove the clot. As he waited and watched, he thought of how a heart-lung machine which could bypass the thoracic organs might enable dry surgery and save the patient in situations like this. He and his wife worked more than 20 years to perfect a mechanical pump oxygenator which would enable him to safely cut into the thoracic great vessels and remove a pulmonary embolus or cut open the heart and sew closed abnormalities such as holes in the septa. Gibbon managed to make a workable machine and operated successfully on a patient with an atrial septal defect on May 6, 1953. His next patients, however, died and he gave up the field.[45] Gibbon knew of the Mayo work, as well as that of C. Walton Lillihei nearby at the University of Minnesota, and of course they knew of his. In 1954 he published an article in the journal *Minnesota Medicine* titled, "Application of a Mechanical Heart and Lung Apparatus to Cardiac Surgery."[46]

By 1955 Kirklin and his small Mayo Group had a well-functioning machine which they called the "Mayo-Gibbon pump oxygenator" and had used it for a series of open heart procedures, especially atrial and ventricular septal defects, with increasing success.[47] The Mayo-Gibbon Pump-Oxygenator machine became increasingly and exclusively adopted throughout the world, Kirklin's fame as a superb surgeon soared, and well-to-do patients came to the Mayo Clinic from all over the world to have their surgery done by him personally. He was not only imaginative and determined in his pursuit of goals, but he was also a superb technical surgeon (with very small hands).

The Mayo Clinic at its inception in 1914[48] had not owned a hospital but instead, in the early days, used two local hospitals, one Protestant and one Catholic. They trained many doctors of all kinds, but they provided only residency and fellowship post-M.D. training, not medical school itself. As the clamor for increased numbers of physicians in the U.S. increased in the 1950s and especially the 1960s, the trustees decided to launch a medical school in 1964. Kirklin became chief of surgery. The following year he was made a member of the board of governors of the Mayo Clinic as well.

Although some excellent Alabama physicians had worked or trained at the Mayo Clinic, Alabama at that time was considered in Minnesota as an ignorant place, full of indolence, prejudices, and violence. But Lyons was known in surgical circles for his pioneering work on the uses of penicillin in surgery and the natural history of several bacteria, especially Streptococci and Staphylococci, as well as his service for the National Library of Medicine. So Dick Hill wrote Kirklin and requested him to travel to Birmingham to evaluate the current status of the department of surgery and project what would be needed to bring it to the forefront of American surgery—"just as a consultant." Kirklin agreed to make the several day trip.

He arrived, registered at a local hotel, and began meetings with the search committee and other groups and began generally checking around. He wandered into the office of the Dean of Dentistry Charles A. "Scotty" McCallum, D.M.D., M.D., one morning about 5:30 and expressed surprise to find him there so early, and even more surprised to find that this was his usual time of arrival—if not earlier. Hill and Volker were also early risers, though usually not so early as McCallum. Reeves, chair of the search committee, was clearly a highly competent cardiologist and on important NIH and heart association committees. He and Kirklin had some familiarity with each other, not only because of the prominence of each in cardiology circles, but also because Reeves had sent Kirklin a number of patients with aortic valve disease, pointing out that Kirklin's mortality for such operations was "around 2 percent, while the mortality at other centers was about 22 percent or more."[49] Reeves was Director of the medical school's self-designated interdisciplinary CVRTC (Cardiovascular Research and Training Center), the first official "multidisciplinary center," as opposed to a "department," at UAB. This CVRTC was soon to begin receiving more NIH research funding than any other cardiovascular group in the

History of Surgery (London: Greenwich Medical Media Ltd., 2001), 225–227. One of the best brief accounts of the development of intracardiac surgery. C. D. Kay, "John H. Gibbon Jr." in *American National Biography*. This brief biography is far better than a book by Schumacker, which is inaccurate in many places and not a very helpful book, but at least it tells some personal things about Gibbon and his work on heart-lung machines for 23 years and some of the preceding work, e.g., by Charles Lindbergh and Alexis Carrel. H. B. Schumacker Jr., *A Dream of the Heart: The Life of John H. Gibbon Jr., Father of the Heart-Lung Machine* (Santa Barbara, CA: Fithian Press, 1999); G. W. Miller, *King of Hearts: The True Story of the Maverick Who Pioneered Open Heart Surgery* (New York: Times Books/Random House, 2000); Weisse, *Heart*, 93–114. S. Westaby and C. Bosher, *Landmarks in Cardiac Surgery* (Oxford: Isis Medical Media, 1997). This is a superb book by the chief of surgery (Westaby) at the Oxford (UK) Heart Centre, John Radcliffe Hospital, who took a fellowship with Kirklin at UAB in the 1980s. Chapter 2 on the evolution of cardiopulmonary bypass and myocardial protection and the section on Kirklin are especially good.

46. J. H. Gibbon, "Application of a Mechanical Heart and Lung Apparatus to Cardiac Surgery," *Minnesota Medicine* 17 (1954): 171–177.

47. Kirklin, J. W. *Bulletin of the Mayo Clinic*, both 1955 article and 1980 article on 25th anniversary. Also see Ellis, *History*; Westaby, *Landmarks*.

48. The two Mayo brothers had taken in a third associate, Dr. Augustus W. Stinch-field, and formalized their association with a legal partnership in 1905. However, only in 1914 was the partnership formally changed into "The Mayo Clinic." See H. Clapesattle, *The Doctors Mayo* (Min-neapolis: Univ. of Minnesota Press, 1941), 207; Kirklin, "Lessons," 143.

49. T. J. Reeves, per-sonal communication, August 11, 2005.

nation—and probably more than any other in the world at that time. The pediatri-cian Bargeron clearly understood congenital heart problems, was an expert in cardiac angiography in children, and could be a source of major support. Other cardiolo-gists on the faculty seemed outstanding—Harold Dodge, recently recruited from the NIH and doing work at the forefront of cardiac angiography; Lloyd L. Hefner, M.D., a superb clinical cardiologist and physicist interested in echocardiography and computer applications; Richard O. Russell and Charles Rackley, top-level clini-cal cardiologists who later entered practice (Russell) or became leaders in academic medicine (Rackley, chief of medicine at Georgetown Medical School); and others. Of course, the utter integrity and steady hand of the chain-smoking Frommeyer and his famous mentor Tinsley helped the overall favorable medical impression.

Kirklin returned to the Mayo Clinic and dictated a 14-page letter to Hill listing his observations and stating what he thought it would take to accomplish what Hill hoped. Hill reviewed these with colleagues then contacted Kirklin to ask whether he, himself, would consider taking the job. Kirklin wrote back that he found himself in a rather confused state, wondering whether this might be the chance of a lifetime or a wilderness from which he might never emerge. He asked if he could return for a week with his wife and look more carefully, which of course he did.

It is impossible to overstate the dramatic effect Kirklin's move to Birmingham had, both on the medical center and on the surgical world at large, especially at the Mayo Clinic, where they wondered how Kirklin could have so taken leave of his senses. He brought several of his surgical trainees with him, some of whom became world leaders in CV surgery themselves, such as Albert D. Pacifico and Robert Karp, who performed the first heart transplant in the area in 1981. Other Mayo staff soon were following him to Birmingham, such as David Witten, who became chief of radiology, W. N. Tauxe, head of nuclear medicine, and most dramatically the GI surgeon George Hallenbeck. Hallenbeck had been chosen by President Lyndon Johnson to remove his gallbladder (with the famous abdominal scar later published widely), and he had been named chief of surgery to replace Kirklin when the latter moved to Birmingham. Now Hallenbeck was moving to Birmingham!

Patients responded. They came to Birmingham from all over the world, especially western Europe and Latin America. Arrigo Cipriani, owner of the famous Harry's Bar in Venice, Italy, and other enterprises worldwide, had a daughter afflicted with a severe congenital heart defect. She was operated on in Milan, then again in Rome. These were unsuccessful. The doctors and family were giving up on anyplace in

Europe that could do better when someone said, "How about John Kirklin in Birmingham, Alabama?" Cipriani brought her to Kirklin, who corrected the defect so that she grew to become a healthy mother. Professors of medicine from Harvard, Ohio, and other schools came to UAB for surgery.

Kirklin arrived in the summer of 1966, just a year after the Selma-to-Montgomery march and its killings, and not long after the rash of bombings of churches and homes in Birmingham and killings throughout the South. It was also just before the racial intolerance and violence of the North became more vivid in the riots of Washington, Detroit, Newark, and elsewhere in the U.S. as the civil rights laws began to take effect. All this seemed to work to the advantage of Kirklin's and Tinsley's new medical school.

The summer of 1966 saw the admission to the medical school of the first African American students, Richard C. Dale and Samuel W. Sullivan Jr. Dale proceeded to a successful practice of internal medicine and Sullivan to one in obstetrics and gynecology, both in Birmingham. These two also pioneered many changes in medical school policies, practices, and procedures, to the advantage of all minorities in later years.

Consistent with the times, soon after his arrival in Birmingham, Kirklin was heard to ask Tinsley at one of the few cocktail parties he attended, "What are your religious views?"

Tinsley answered that William Osler had the proper answer to that question: "The religion of a physician."

"What is the religion of a physician?"

"A physician does not discuss his personal religion," Tinsley said. He then added that he personally did not adhere to any religious faith other than *medicine* itself. Medicine was enough for him. Kirklin seemed pleased with this answer.[50]

Upon arrival Kirklin had himself named chief of staff of the hospital and to several other important administrative positions from which he set about trying to improve the place. He insisted that all the areas of the department of surgery be kept much cleaner and neater than in the past, especially the conference rooms—no more half-empty Coca-Cola bottles with half-smoked cigarettes in them on the tables or window sills. Some of his aims were unrealistically idealistic: "We must bring the charges for each laboratory test exactly in conformity with the costs" (as if the latter were a scientifically determinable number rather than a matter of opinions!).

One area of major dissatisfaction for Kirklin was the outpatient facilities, which

50. This conversation was witnessed by me in 1966. The family of Tinsley's good friend J. J. Kirschenfeld, M.D., of Montgomery, also said that "Jack's only religion was medicine."

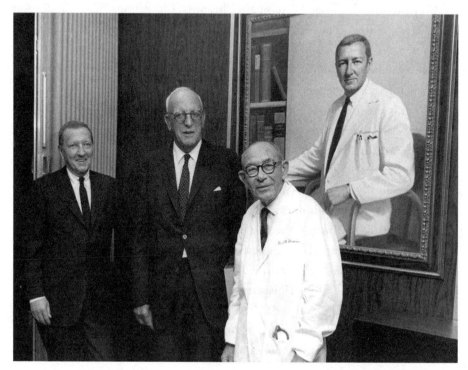

51. I am indebted to
Edward F. McCraw,
M.D. (near Pigeon
Creek) for local details
about Dr. Jernigan,
July 24, 2005.

52. Approximately 12
percent of all residency
positions in the U.S.
were in VA hospitals
and had full salaries
and expenses paid by
the VA.

53. The Bronx VA
Hospital, for example,
was "affiliated" with
five of the New York
City medical schools,
which meant that
none took great

*Dedication of
the Walter B.
Frommeyer
Conference
Room in UAB's
Zeigler Research
Building, 1971.
From left,
Drs. Walter B.
Frommeyer;
William B.
Castle, Veterans
Administration
Distinguished
Physician and
Professor Emeritus
at Harvard; and
Tinsley Harrison*

were in an old discarded office building across the street to the north of the hospital, remodeled into small examining rooms with stretchers. The old outpatient facilities in the original Birmingham Medical College more than 50 years earlier had long since been destroyed. Kirklin often said, "This place was built for research. If you want to examine a patient, you first have to sweep the Erlenmeyer flasks off the top of the lab tables." Only in the later 1970s was the more modern but still inadequate Russell Ambulatory Center constructed based on a large donation from Thomas D. and Julia Russell of Russell Mills in Alexander City, Alabama (a textile center at the time, its factory work was outsourced to another country 40 years later, as was true of many other textile mills of the region).

In 1968, as the technical capacities of the medical school and its staff took large leaps ahead in technology, the clinical capacities of older doctors had not yet disappeared. An excellent internist joined the faculty, T. Albert Farmer, from the town of Wilson, North Carolina, where he had been in private practice. One evening while covering the admissions area of the VA Hospital he was presented with an elderly man sent by a doctor from Pigeon Creek, a rural village south of Montgomery near a river of the same name. Though it was a tiny village in a very rural place, it had a doctor, Robert L. Jernigan, M.D., who had graduated from Vanderbilt early in the century and lived in Pigeon Creek since about 1920. Dr. Jernigan refused to take some of the examinations demanded by the state, with the statement, "I graduated from a good medical school which granted me an M.D. degree and designated me a 'doctor,' and I'm not going to take another examination." He practiced for the rest of his life and apparently gave good care to local citizens. His prescriptions for most drugs and later for antibiotics were honored and filled by the local pharmacists. Narcotics were another matter; permission for them had to be obtained with a separate license from the federal government. But somehow he managed. Dr. Jernigan had cared for many patients with tuberculosis in the past.[51]

The young Dr. Farmer looked at the "See note" the patient had brought (the referral usually written casually on any piece of paper handy) and found that "The patient has a cavity in the left upper lobe and may have TB." When Dr. Farmer questioned as to why he had been sent to Birmingham, the patient responded, "To get my TB taken care of. The doctor told me I have a cavity about the size of a silver dollar at the top of my left lung." Farmer asked if he had brought his X-rays.

"What X-rays?"

"The ones your doctor took."

"He didn't take no X-rays. He just listened to my chest."

Dr. Farmer repeated his physical examination taking special care to percuss the chest and listen to the lungs. After very carefully doing all this and repeating it, including having the patient cough then listening for post-tussive rales, etc., he concluded that the trip might have been unnecessary. He could find no indication of such a cavity, and a silver dollar is pretty small, so the old and probably senile country doctor obviously could not detect a cavity that small by physical exam alone. Farmer sent the patient upstairs for chest X-rays. A few minutes later when the pictures returned, he was amazed to see near the apex of the left lung a small but clear cavity about the size of a silver dollar!

THE U.S. VETERANS ADMINISTRATION medical care system seemed to be doing well in the mid- and late 1960s and had become an integral part of the operations of many medical schools around the United States. Of the approximately 172 VA hospitals, 102 had official "affiliation agreements" with the nearby medical schools, and some, like the Birmingham VA Hospital, were intimately involved. Chiefs of service, that is the chief of medicine, chief of surgery, etc., in the VA were usually

interest in it and the staff did as it wished within the tight federal regulations but had little or no regular support from the schools even though they might have courtesy faculty appointments. VA research support was to its own employees, and the funds were "projects" or "programs," specifically *not* "grants." The VA's peer review, often seen as not so rigorous as that of the NIH, was done by committees sometimes called "study sections," like those of the NIH and resembling NIH study sections, often with the same people on both kinds of research review committees. The VA staff in Washington was often irritated by failure of VA researchers to acknowledge the VA as the source of financial support in publications and presentations; and sometimes the VA administration tried to pull away from associations with the larger community of academic medicine; e.g., the VA had separate annual research meetings in Cincinnati, Ohio, which was the most feasible central U.S. location and economically cheapest for investigators coming from throughout the country. These arrangements were not necessarily to the disadvantage of VA personnel. The "deserted" Bronx VA Hospital spawned the legendary Berson and Yalow of immunoassay fame. The workaholic Solomon A. Berson, M.D., became professor and chief of medicine at the new Mt. Sinai Hospital and medical school and died shortly before his colleague Rosalyn S. Yalow, Ph.D., shared the 1977 Nobel Prize with Andrew Schally, M.D., a full-time VA investigator in New Orleans. See: Eugene Straus, *Rosalyn Yalow, Nobel Laureate, Her Life and Work in Medicine* (Cambridge, MA: Perseus Books, 1998); Nicholas Wade, *The Nobel Duel, Two Scientists' 21-year Race to Win the World's Most Coveted Research Prize* (Garden City, NY: Anchor/Doubleday, 1981).

54. H. Martin Engle, "Press Release from the Veterans Administration," May 6, 1968. Engle was the chief medical director of the VA, and reported to the Administrator of Veterans Affairs, who reported directly to the U.S. President. This terminology was later changed making the administrator "Secretary of Veterans Affairs" and a member of

also full professors in the medical school, nearly all the residents rotated for substantial portions their residencies through the VA,[52] and the VA provided large funding for physician and other healthcare staff as well as research support. Nevertheless, the VA was often looked down on by the pure academics as not quite equal to those whose appointments were completely within the medical school and university. This disdain was probably also largely the result of the fact that the leading medical schools in the Northeast—Harvard, Columbia/Physicians and Surgeons, Cornell, and so on—did not have such close relations between the two institutions.[53]

In 1968 Harold Engle, M.D., who was chief medical director[54] in the VA Central Office in the late 1960s, and had been a hospital director in Chicago, and was thus familiar with medical school relations, implemented a new program to bring leaders prominent in academic medicine into the VA, the "Distinguished Physician Program." The first physician so designated was Harvard's William B. Castle, famous for his work on intrinsic factor and its role in pernicious anemia and for stimulating Linus Pauling's interest in the hemoglobins in 1945.[55] This work of Pauling, directly attributable to Castle's research, led directly to the work paralleling, and perhaps antedating, that of Watson and Crick defining the double helical structure of DNA and the exciting developments in molecular biology during the last three decades of Harrison's life. This historic progress in biology was one of the things that moved medicine beyond Tinsley's beloved bedside approach.

Tinsley's appointment as a VA Distinguished Physician followed soon after Castle's, making him the second among an academically distinguished group, later to include his good friend Paul Beeson. The appointment gave Tinsley a stable base economically and academically for the rest of his life, and it relieved the school of having to provide his salary and support, which would surely have been continued for the last decade of his life.

As a VA-DP Tinsley traveled regularly to the other VA hospitals not only in Alabama but throughout the region and nation, making rounds for patient care and teaching, giving conferences for the medical staffs, and offering suggestions to VA Central Office in Washington for changes. Later chief medical directors of the VA, especially John D. Chase, also a cardiologist, so admired Harrison that they kept him in this position until his death despite his repeated offers to resign and retire completely.

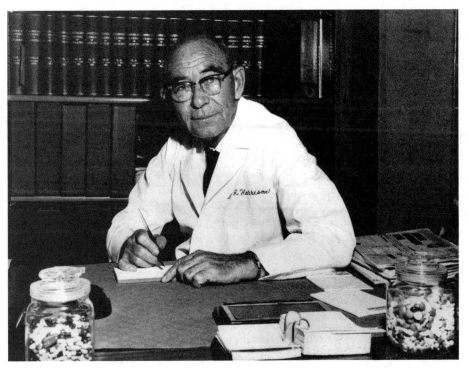

Tinsley at his desk at UAB, about 1970.

the cabinet. At that time the CMD was renamed "Undersecretary for Veterans Health Affairs." Also around this time hospital terminology changed and the VA Hospitals became "VA Medical Centers." Terminology in the civilian sector was also changing the word "hospital" into "medical center." This was not unreasonable, since the hospital complexes often also included outpatient facilities and doctors' office buildings. These changes soon progressed in many private or public hospitals to make them "regional" medical centers, which then added some more elegant designation, like "Northern Alabama Regional Medical Center," in obvious attempts at advertising and expanding turf.

55. A. B. Karnad, *Intrinsic Factors: William Bosworth Castle and the Development of Hematology and Clinical Investigation at the Boston City Hospital* (Boston: Harvard

In the 1970s Tinsley traveled regularly to the VA hospitals in Montgomery and Tuskegee to hold his usual teaching clinics on live patients, make clinical rounds with residents (later from the new Morehouse medical school in Atlanta), and try to help with problem patients.

I was dean of medicine at the medical school in Birmingham at the time, and one evening I received a telephone call from Cornelius P. Hopper, a black neurologist from Wisconsin who was at the time administrator of the private John A. Andrews Hospital in Tuskegee and affiliated with Tuskegee University. I knew him well, having tried to lure him to UAB's Department of Neurology (which he refused; he later became a senior official at the University of California system). Hopper's call was a complaint about Tinsley, who was spending inordinate amounts of time in his lectures and clinics delivering mea culpas for the treatment of blacks in the South for many years (though he always disclaimed having mistreated anybody himself, probably an accurate view[56]). "Ask him to tell us about the heart," Hopper requested, "not about slavery. We know enough about that!" I did mention this to Tinsley, who said he understood and would reform his comments. Otherwise, the people in Tuskegee seemed grateful for his visits.

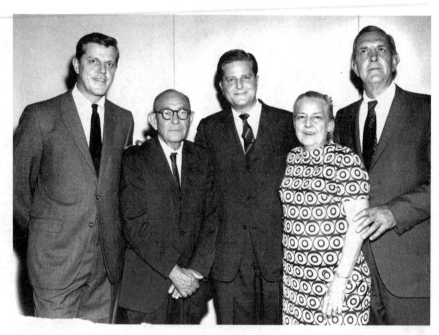

Four deans of the UAB medical school, about 1970. From left, Clifton K. Meador, dean 1968–1973; Tinsley Harrison, acting dean 1950–1951; S. Richardson Hill Jr., dean 1962–1968; Marian Berson; and Robert C. Berson, dean 1955–1962.

University Press, 1997), 173–177.

56. In the last years of his life Harrison had several black medical students who were doing well academically to his apartment for evening discussions about their futures, which they apparently appreciated. Tinsley worked with one such able student to arrange for a program to screen African Americans for hypertension using local black churches as the points of assessment. Medical students helped with the program, and it lasted some years.

As usual, Tinsley had an angle to these trips. As he aged and did not trust his own driving so much, he would ask a medical student to drive his car beginning on a Wednesday or Thursday. He would go to the Montgomery VA Hospital to make rounds, give teaching clinics, have lunch with the staff, and so on, then go to visit his good friend Jack Kirschenfeld, whose struggling UAB-affiliated internal medicine residency program was gaining momentum and recognition. There he would also meet with students and residents (who also affiliated with the local VA hospital and were paid partly from there). Then he and the student would travel to Harrison's lake cabin on the shore of nearby Lake Martin, usually joined by several other students or residents in internal medicine. The following day and weekend would be spent swimming, water skiing, walking around in the woods, and in discussions about medicine or anything else. Occasionally somebody would give a more formal paper, and often other faculty members from Birmingham or other medical schools would join them. One photo from those days shows Tinsley in a hammock with fellow cardiologists Joe Reeves and John Holt, Tinsley holding a long strip of EKG paper. After his heart attack, Tinsley returned to his cabin, "Coronary Seclusion."

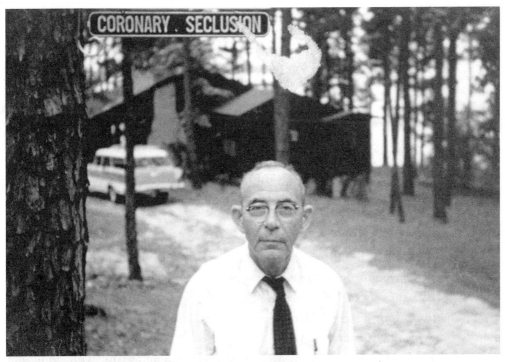

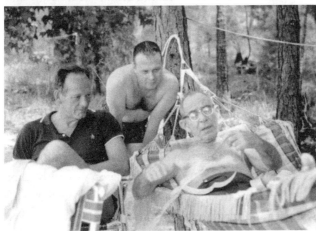

Above, Tinsley at "Coronary Seclusion," his cabin on Lake Martin, about 1970. Left, also at the Lake Martin cabin in the same time period, are, from left Drs. T. Joseph Reeves, John Holt, and Tinsley.

13

The Patient in 1978

Tinsley's Last Days

Tinsley's health was excellent all his life, with two serious exceptions: a myocardial infarct and a broken clavicle. The former was incurred in the summer of 1965 after he had traveled to New Orleans for a weekend of meetings with his good friend George Burch, chief of medicine at Tulane, and other medical friends.

Having returned, he spent Monday at his lake cabin relaxing with family and working. That evening about 11 as he retired, he felt a "slight discomfort in the chest. . . not initially a pain but as a peculiar feeling . . . not unlike the feeling one gets in the retrosternal area and lower neck when one has a craving for a cigarette. . . . [He] deliberately lit a cigarette in order to eliminate the possibility that . . . [such a craving could be the cause]." He carefully assessed whether there was any pain in the back, fearful that despite its mildness it might be the initial symptom of an aortic dissection. He soon realized this was probably the pain of ischemic heart disease and asked his wife to give him an injection of Demerol (meperidine) and call a local physician friend, which she did. Dr. James E. Cameron promptly came and called an ambulance to take them to the nearest hospital, the small Russell Hospital in Alexander City a few miles away, where Tinsley was found to have had a myocardial infarct and was treated by local physicians (and his fellow Birmingham cardiologists and faculty members T. Joseph Reeves and W. B. Jones, who stayed by his side during the remainder of his hospitalization), and did well.

He did not have preceding or subsequent angina pectoris, but the incident did, however, provide another reminder of his own mortality.[1] In 1970, he broke his clavicle in a fall while water skiing, but otherwise he generally enjoyed vigorous

1. Tinsley dictated his own description of the episode within the week, and it was published 13 years later in a local journal just after he died. T. R. Harrison, "The Subjective Aspects of the Case History of TRH as related by TRH," *Alabama J. of Med. Sciences* 15 (1978): 320–325.

physical health throughout his life and even after his heart attack until age eventually caught up with him.

The year and a half before his death were not easy and gave signs that the end was on its way. He faced this period with a doctor's sense of staving off the inevitable. He commented that he thought he might have angina but that the arteries in his legs were so poor he could not exercise enough to learn for certain, because of the pain of intermittent claudication. For a time he gave himself abdominal injections of heparin in attempts to fend off worse blockage somewhere—those he feared most were thrombosis or hemorrhage of a cerebral vessel. Or worse: multiple small strokes or Alzheimer's disease with resulting dementia, perhaps coming on gradually so that the victim was aware of his own deterioration. These things did not really come to pass—he only had a short time of bewilderment brought on by old age.

ABOUT 6 ONE MORNING in late September 1977, Betty phoned me to say that Tinsley had fallen and broken his hip. He was in the UAB hospital, and she asked that I come to provide what help I could. His regular internist was Abraham Russakoff, a superb physician focusing on lung diseases but an excellent general internist.[2]

I arrived to find Tinsley on a stretcher in a hallway, quite cheerful, but complaining that he could not be bothered with having his hip pinned at this time. He was planned to leave the next day on a Carribean cruise accompanied by Ms. Hazel Taylor, a tall and very attractive and able nurse who had been head of nursing on the renal transplant unit. I pointed out that no cruise line would permit him to go with a known broken hip and that he might well have pulmonary emboli on such a trip. He was adamant that Betty did not want to go with him but had no objection to his taking Hazel and that he would indeed go! Further discussion finally dissuaded him.

"All right," he said. "I'll

2. J. Mack Lofton Jr., *Healing Hands, An Alabama Medical Mosaic* (Tuscaloosa: Univ. of Alabama Press, 1995). This excellent local book records firsthand accounts of Alabama phyhsicians from oral histories taken by Lofton. Russakoff is referred to in that book as a "distinguished and exemplary physician," and several vignettes demonstrating this are included.

Tinsley Harrison in his hospital bed in Alexander City, Alabama, 1965.

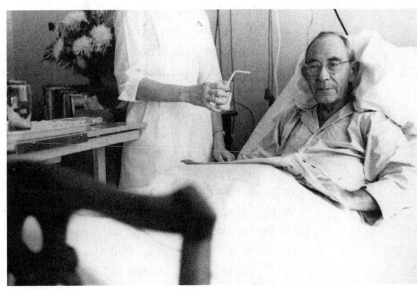

agree to hospitalization, but not in this God-forsaken, medicine-forsaken pseudo-university place. Only in some private hospital where there are real *doctors*!"

He was taken to Baptist Montclair, a private hospital. He again became vociferous and refused hospitalization. By now, his son Randy had arrived, as had Russakoff. Randy disappeared for about an hour then reappeared with commitment papers signed by Russakoff. The papers declared that Tinsley was *non compos mentis* and unable to make his own decisions. Despite his agitated state, this hurt Tinsley. He was furious. He railed at Randy for deserting his elderly and ailing father but saved the real yelling for his old friend Russakoff. "Russ, I *fire* you as my physician and I *fire* you as my friend! You, too, my own physician, have deserted me. You're fired as my physician and as my friend."

"Tinsley, may I make a statement?" Russ asked.

"Yes, but I'm not going to listen." With that he pulled the blanket over his head and apparently pressed the heels of his hands over his ears. Russ proceeded to explain that, in his estimation, all that had been done in the past few hours had been done because they all loved him and wanted to do the very best they could for him. "You can fire me as your physician," he said, "but you can never fire me as your friend."

Tinsley pulled the blanket from his head; he had been listening the whole time. "Well, all right," he said. "You're still my friend, as always. But you're fired as my physician!"

With that he was admitted to the prominent orthopedist Donald Deinlein, who proceeded to pin the hip. He recovered well and was soon more like his old self.

Sometime in 1978 Tinsley was invited to Nashville to hold a live clinic for the internists in town. The invitation came from Clifton K. Meador, M.D., who had known Tinsley since the 1950s. When Meador first applied for a residency in internal medicine, Tinsley advised that in view of his superb record at Vanderbilt medical school and the embryonic nature of the residency in Birmingham, he should aim higher. He did and took his residency training with Robert F. Loeb at the Columbia-Presbyterian Hospital in New York, then returned to Vanderbilt for endocrinology training with Grant W. Liddle, famous for his clinical research on the physiology and pathology of the adrenal glands, especially for having introduced the dexamethasone suppression test for confirmation of the diagnosis of Cushing's syndrome or disease. Liddle asked Meador to remain at Vanderbilt on the faculty, but he entered private practice in Selma where he had grown up. The legendary

Dean of Medicine S. Richardson Hill recruited Meador to endocrinology in Birmingham, where he later became dean himself before returning to private practice at St. Thomas Hospital in Nashville with a clinical appointment as a professor at Vanderbilt. After years of association, Meador's familiar with the popularity of Tinsley's teaching clinics led him to invite Tinsley to teach in Nashville.

Tinsley arrived reasonably dressed, but without shoelaces. When Meador asked if he needed some shoelaces, perhaps because he had forgotten his own, Tinsley commented that at his age he didn't need to be bothered by shoelaces. The next morning Meador became more concerned when he arrived about 6:30 at the motel where Tinsley was staying to pick him up for the first morning conference. He called the room but got no answer, so he went to the door and knocked vigorously several times. Finally there came a barrage of yells, "Don't bother me! Can't you see I'm sleeping? Go away! Get away and leave me alone!" Concerned that he might have the wrong room, Meador returned to the desk, confirmed the room number, and again telephoned, with similar results. After another trip to the room and knocking on the door, he managed to get Tinsley up, shaved, and dressed. But he could see that the old man wasn't right. Meador worried that Tinsley might not be able to handle the clinic without great embarrassment to all. He resolved that if Tinsley seemed confused or otherwise unable to handle the several conferences scheduled for that day, he would simply announce that the famous doctor was sick and the later conferences and teaching clinics would be cancelled.

They drove to the hospital. Tinsley was his usual gracious self with the other doctors at the pre-clinic coffee and doughnuts, and the two patients were presented as usual. Tinsley was again at home in familiar surroundings. He gave a superb clinic in his old style, pointing out sometimes obscure clinical signs and symptoms, citing classical literature on the diseases and their clinical signs and symptoms and his own vast experience. The conference went well.

During the last months, he had several bouts of recalcitrant diarrhea. His old angers resurfaced now that he was a patient instead of a doctor. Convinced that modern university hospitals had deserted personalized bedside medicine and were relying instead on too many technologies and huge impersonal bureaucracies, he refused to go to the University Hospital. Arthur Freeman, the first board-certified gastroenterologist in Alabama and a friend, hospitalized him in the private South Highland Hospital not far from UAB.[3] Under Dr. Freeman's care he recovered. He returned to his usual, if much reduced, schedule.

3. South Highland Hospital later became an orthopedic and rehabilitation hospital, then the base for the HealthSouth Corporation, started by Mr. Richard Scrushy as a network of rehabilitation hospitals around the country. However, early in the next century, after the Enron debacle, HealthSouth and Scrushy were indicted for falsely inflating earnings, the first major federal trial under the new Sarbanes-Oxley Act of 2002; Scrushy was acquitted. In 2005 UAB bought this hospital.

4. The 1977 lecture by John D. Chase, M.D., of the VA, was given July 25, perhaps in anticipation of Harrison's impending departure, though more likely because of Chase's busy schedule.

In the final year of Tinsley's life, his old friend, the hypertension expert George Pickering, M.D., now Sir George of Oxford, gave the annual Tinsley Harrison Lecture. These had been held every year since 1958, always in the fall except for twice, including Pickering's on March 21, 1978.[4]

After the lecture the two old internists made a tour of several VA hospitals and their affiliated medical schools on the west coast, including the San Francisco VA Hospital. The hospital director, Hugh Vickerstaff, later director in Birmingham, assigned himself the duty of chauffeuring his two distinguished guests around town. Late one afternoon Pickering had a separate meeting, leaving Tinsley with a little free time. Tinsley requested that Vickerstaff take him to the shore of San Francisco Bay, drop him off, and pick him up again in 45 minutes or an hour. It was a beautiful afternoon with a spectacular sunset. When Vickerstaff returned he found that Tinsley had taken off his shoes and socks, rolled up his pants, and was wading in the water, occasionally throwing a rock into the sea. Vickerstaff watched a little while, then picked him up and drove him to the next appointment.

On Friday morning, August 4, Betty noticed that Tinsley was giving himself repeated tablets of nitroglycerine and worried that it was his heart again. She called H. Cecil Coghlan, a physician friend and expert cardiologist and professor of medicine from Chile, whom Harrison had met in Santiago in 1956 while becoming an honorary member of the Sociedad Medica de Santiago and lecturing there. At that time Coghlan had been responsible for the simultaneous interpretation from English into Spanish, since the regular interpreters found Harrison's mode of speaking, his strong Southern accent, and the medical terminology beyond them. Coghlan had an English father and Chilean mother. The father had attended medical school in Santiago (where he was a classmate of Salvador Allende Gossens, M.D., the future Marxist president of Chile). Cecil, when speaking English, retained the father's strong British accent. Because Cecil was a top student of medicine as well as having Chilean Spanish as his native tongue, he was tapped to interpret all of Tinsley's Santiago lectures.

Thus did Tinsley come to know him while on that trip and asked him if he was interested in research. When the answer was yes, Harrison suggested they have sandwiches together that evening in Harrison's hotel room. There Coghlan met Betty, then came the discussion with the Chief over sandwiches about what constitutes real research. There was also a rather harsh criticism, as Coghlan remembers it, of what Coghlan was doing as "research" in Santiago. Tinsley thought what they were doing was just rehashing old ideas and work that had been published in Europe decades ago. "You're asking questions that were answered in papers published in 1890!" he said. In Tinsley's opinion, real research required as much study of the literature, including older literature, and as much or more thinking to search out the most critical and basic questions, as actually carrying out the work. Only then could one begin to imagine the best procedures to test possible answers to the important questions. Coghlan was impressed and accepted Harrison's offer of a cardiology fellowship in Birmingham in 1957. Over the years they worked and published together and became fast friends in the father-son relationship Harrison habitually established with his pupils.

That morning in 1978 Coghlan went to Tinsley's apartment where he examined the patient. Coughlan was not surprised to find that classic bulging precordium with every beat of the heart, the very sign Tinsley had taught him about 30 years before as an indication of an anterior myocardial infarct. He told Tinsley that he undoubtedly had a severe MI and should come immediately to the hospital. Tinsley refused. He told Coughlan that he knew very well that he had had an MI, that it was a bad one. He had measured his own blood pressure by the pulse and found it extremely low. He knew that he would die shortly. He did not fear death at this old age and much preferred to die with dignity at home in his own bed rather than at that "den of thieves, the University Hospital."

Coghlan knew Tinsley well and knew that despite his cursings of technology, he really admired the new gadgets and techniques. So he said, "You know, Chief, we now have a machine at UAB where we can actually visualize the infarct and tell you exactly where it is—visually. Let me take you down there long enough to do this test so that I can see it, and let you see it, too. Then, if you want, you can go home again."

"But you'll stick me full of IVs and fill me with all sorts of drugs," Tinsley said.

Coghlan promised there would be no IVs and that he could return to his bed at home when the test was finished.

"Okay," Tinsley said, "but just to see the results of this new test."

An ambulance came and transported him to the hospital. He was admitted to the cardiac intensive care unit. There he was placed in a hospital bed, his head low because of the extremely low blood pressure, despite the danger of acute congestive failure. A technetium-99^{m} scan was obtained. No blood pressure could be obtained even with his head lowered, and he lost consciousness. Coghlan started an IV with a dopamine drip.

Tinsley awakened and said, "Cecil," he said, "you broke your word. You put an IV into my arm."

Coghlan showed him the scan. Because of the massive infarct, the entire left ventricle was dying or dead already.

"Chief," Coghlan said, "that was the only way I could get your blood pressure up and restore your consciousness, and I wanted to do that so you could see that I was keeping my promise to send you home as soon as you had seen the scan. And I'm sending you home now."

With that an ambulance returned him to his small apartment and bedroom, where he was surrounded by his beloved books. Tinsley was made comfortable in his bed. Then Coghlan added morphine to the IV, and Tinsley drifted away.

No final words of wisdom were recorded. But one can think that in his last narcotized state of wandering dreams, he recalled his life:

> Research, Teaching, the Patient.
> The research project,
> The student,
> But above all
> The individual sick person: the *patient*.

THE AUTOPSY WAS NOT unusual. It was done by Tinsley's friend, the pathologist Ricardo Ceballos, originally from Spain and now much admired by students and fellow faculty for his extensive current and historical knowledge of pathology and his enthusiasm for teaching. The gross examination showed the occluded left main anterior descending artery and developing infarct. The brain appeared grossly normal. I was there, watching. I was especially interested in the liver, in view of Tinsley famous love of bourbon whiskey. Upon inspection, there was no evidence of damage or the nodularity of cirrhosis. The liver wall was as smooth as a baby's bottom. The surprise was the wall of his stomach, which was paper thin—probably the result of not only the alcohol but also his prodigious consumption of strong black coffee.

The funeral was held on a drizzly afternoon and was attended by people from around the United States, including Tinsley's former dean Robert Berson, now heading the VA hospital in Baltimore. I telephoned Oxford and invited Sir George

Pickering to fly to Birmingham, attend the funeral, and, while he was there, give some seminars. Pickering's first comment when I told him about Tinsley's death was. "I'm sure Betty is delighted." He then caught himself. He said he was too old himself to attend, but he wrote a letter about how much Tinsley had contributed to the medicine of his times and to the subsequent teaching of internal medicine for years to come.[5] He also remarked that Tinsley's chief characteristic was passion. Tinsley seemed never to be neutral on a subject, especially a medical subject. He held strong opinions, very strongly expressed.

That evening several of us gathered in Tinsley's apartment for some drinks and a few minutes of conversation before dispersing. Outside, there was a thunderstorm and rain. At one point an especially bright flash of lightning occurred almost in the room, accompanied by an extremely loud thunder clap. Sarah Merrill, Tinsley's youngest sister and always the jokester of the family, looked heavenward, her own lit cigarette in one hand and glass of strong bourbon in the other, and said, "Just give him a cigarette and a glass of bourbon, and he'll quiet down."

5. A copy of Pickering's letter is in the UAB Archives.

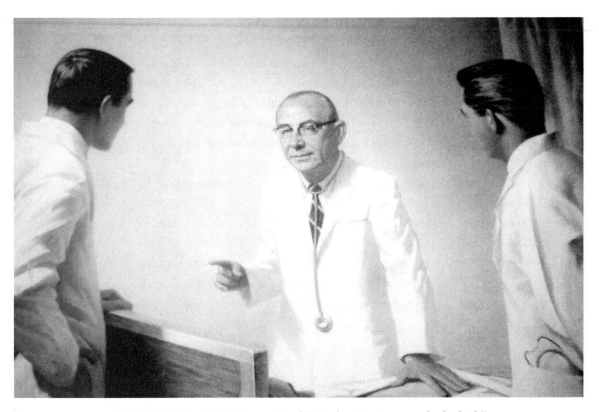

W. W. S. Wilson's 1967 portrait of "Tinsley Harrison at the bedside" that as of 2014 was on display at UAB.

Epilogue

edicine at the end of the 20th century, like everything else, was vastly different from medicine at its beginning. We are attempting to move away from something: disease and disability. But it is less clear what goal medicine is attempting to move toward. Is it eternal life on earth? Perfect health in an eternally youthful body? Do we wish to deny aging and the natural course of events? These are impossible. We cannot escape the natural processes of life. We can only prolong these effects. Improving life and prolonging it in a healthy state seems worthy. Still, some countries are vastly behind in needed medicines and medical care.

An example of the progress made in Tinsley Harrison's century can be seen in the congenital disease now known as cystic fibrosis. It was an unknown disease entity before 1900. In 1910, nearly everyone who contracted this disease died. In the early 1930s, understanding about this disease began to increase. In 1936, it was officially named by Fanconi, a Zurich pediatrician. In 1953,[1] cystic fibrosis care centers began appearing all over the world. In 1981, Alabama's first CF research center opened—the Gregory Fleming James Cystic Fibrosis Research Center at UAB. In 1993, the medicine Pulmozyme Rx for cleaving DNA in CF secretions was approved by the FDA. In 1994, the first gene therapy trials began at Tinsley Harrison's school by Eric Sorscher, who became director of the James Cystic Fibrosis Research Center. In 1996, Howard, Frizzell, and Bedwell demonstrated that aminoglycoside antibiotics restore CFTR function by overcoming premature stop mutations. From 1998 to 2002, the Therapeutics Development Network was established by the CF Foundation to translate laboratory discoveries into improvements in care and longer lives for CF patients. The disease is slowly, methodically, being tracked and defeated. This is the future.

In 1981 the psychotic Hinkley attempted to assassinate President Ronald Reagan,[2] and one shot landed near the heart and great vessels, a wound that a hundred

1. The year the DNA helix was discovered.

2. Benjamin L. Aaron and S. David Rockoff, "*The Attempted Assassination of President Reagan,*" *JAMA* 272, 21 (Dec. 7, 1994): 1689–93. Aaron studied cardiothoracic surgery with John Kirklin at UAB. Stevens, Ralph L., M.D. "*A President's Assassination.*" *JAMA* 246, 15 (Oct 9, 1981): 1673–74. Excellent brief article comparing Reagan's care with Garfield's 100 years earlier. Reagan's wound was life threatening, but he was saved by good doctors, X-rays, blood transfusions and IVs, and prompt surgery with careful attention to asepsis, antibiotics, and avoidance of infection, and good hospital care. Garfield's wound was not life threatening if they had just stabilized

him, kept him clean and sterile, given him good rest, and left him alone.

3. W. B. Fye, "The Delayed Diagnosis of Myocardial Infarction: It Took Half a Century!" *Circulation* 72 (1985): 262–271; Fye, "Cardiovascular Medicine: A Historical Perspective," in *Textbook of Cardiovascular Medicine*, ed. Eric J. Topol (Philadelphia: Lippincott-Raven Publishers, 1998), 10; Fye, "A Historical Perspective on Atherosclerosis and Coronary Artery Disease" in *Arteriosclerosis and Coronary Artery Disease*, eds. V. Fuster, R. Ross, and E. J. Topol. (Philadelphia: Lippincott-Raven, 1996), 1–12.

4. Davenport, *Doctor,* 65–67. The patient discussed was presented March 27, 1908, but Dock had published on coronary disease in 1906. "In the lecture Dock reviewed the history of the recognition of coronary artery disease during life," including the case of John Hunter diagnosed by his younger friend Edward Jenner, or those predicted and verified at post-mortem examinations by Parry.

years earlier would surely have proved fatal, especially with the massive loss of blood.

Other examples abound. The disease that killed Tinsley, myocardial infarction, was not even recognized by clinical medicine generally in 1900[3] (though it was widely suspected by astute clinicians, as seen in the clinical discussions of George Dock at Michigan).[4]

As noted earlier, Tinsley did not recognize the first MI he encountered in 1922 on rounds with Sam Levine. By the middle of the 20th century, coronary artery disease was considered the leading cause of death in the United States. The Western diet of affluence and a high blood cholesterol were blamed.[5] Uncontrolled hypertension also contributed to coronary artery disease and strokes—cerebrovascular accidents. But there was no effective treatment for hypertension until the 1950s and '60s.

When myocardial infarcts were first widely recognized, the attempt was to keep the patient absolutely quiet and in bed for several weeks, on the theory that exertion might cause the unhealed myocardial scar to rupture, an idea promoted by Paul Dudley White. In the early 1950s, an MI patient would be snowed under with sedatives and perhaps narcotics, and given only oxygen by tent or later a nasal catheter. There were arguments over whether more energy was expended having a bowel movement on a bedpan or a bedside commode.

Tinsley was always suspicious of excessive bed rest and thought early ambulation might be beneficial. His ideas prevailed, and the mode gradually moved to more liberal use of early exercise.

None of these changes came about without considerable research and development, some of which occurred in Tinsley's medical school. He loved and respected research, basic and clinical. But the patient always came first. Drs. Richard O. Russell and Charles Rackley had a large grant and several smaller ones to study myocardial infarcts and their treatment. They needed patients to study, and they commandeered every patient possible, within the limits of ethics and the patient's informed consent. The house staff during those days joked, "Don't scratch your chest while you walk down the hall. They'll grab you, shove you into the MIRU (Myocardial Infarct Research Unit), and stick a catheter in your heart before you know it!"

One episode with Tinsley illustrates this atmosphere. A physician-patient had been sent to him from Georgia for examination, treatment, and advice. He had just arrived and was headed for the MIRU. To be courteous to Tinsley, Dr. Russell, a senior physician in cardiology at UAB and former trainee of Tinsley's,[6] mentioned his arrival. They discussed the patient briefly, then Russell said, "Chief, if you don't mind I have to move along now and proceed with the studies of the patient."

"What studies?" Tinsley asked. "Are you going to catheterize him?"

"Well, yes. That's part of the protocol."

"Damn the protocol!" Tinsley exploded. "We're not caring for a *protocol*, we're caring for a *patient!* And this man has already had exercise tests and a good clinical work-up by a competent internist I know in Georgia. Admit him directly to my service, and we'll take care of him."

In the late 1960s, treatment of acute MIs with thrombolytic agents became popular, then, if the thrombus was not lysed, by placement of stents or coronary bypass surgery. One popular professor at Tinsley's school remained in shock despite these procedures and the placement of a counter-pulsing pump in the descending aorta. Finally, a satisfactory donor heart was found, and a heart transplant was performed. He lived many productive years thereafter.

AT THE BEGINNING OF the 20th century medicine had X-rays and electrocardiography, but little else. With the increasing mechanization and computerization in medicine, imaging techniques developed after World War II, with tomograms, then computerized tomography (CAT scans), MRIs (magnetic resonance imaging—originally termed "nuclear magnetic imaging," after the original name of the procedure used by the chemists and physicists, but changed because of fear that "nuclear" would frighten people), "SPECT" (single photon emission computed tomography), PET (positron emission tomography), and others.

Economics intruded increasingly on the adoption of these technologies. They certainly enabled a thorough physical examination of the anatomy, or even some aspects of the physiology, as with the PET scans, which could show some aspects of brain metabolism or the function of certain organs like lymph nodes to distinguish which have been infiltrated by cancers, such as prostatic cancers along the aorta where they generally cannot be examined. But the costs of the machines and of the subsequent examinations to amortize those costs were increasingly difficult to bear.

Yes, some of the new developments from research actually reduce overall costs.[7] But the whole relationship between a doctor and a patient became a financial exchange. The charges[8] on the patient's bill increasingly represent the opening gambit in a game between payer and charger, and increasingly these represent organizations, neither the actual patient or the actual provider of care. When PET scanning was accepted by the federal government centers for Medicare and Medicaid services,

5. Le Fanu, *Rise*, 303–311.

6. Not only had Russell been Harrison's pupil, when the time came for Russell's internship Harrison telephoned the Brigham hospital (perhaps to Sam Levine) to put in a special word for his protege. In addition, Russell had married Harrison's secretary. There was no question that Harrison thought highly of Russell's abilities. Russell later joined a large cardiology group started years before by a pupil of Paul D. White.

7. James A. Pittman Jr., "Research and Health Care Reform." *American J. of Med. Sciences* 309 (1995): 249–251. Discusses how clinical advances such as CT scans may eliminate more invasive procedures, such as the pneumoencephalograms, which involved tapping the cerebral spinal fluid and injecting air into the brain ventricles to visualize brain tumors. The procedure often caused considerable pain and required hospitalization.

8. The numbers on the patient's bill were not the final figure and certainly were not real "costs" any more than

the $10 for an aspirin represented what it cost the hospital to purchase that single pill. The "cost" of that pill came to include more and more ancillary expenses.

9. K. M. Ludmerer, *Time to Heal: American Medical Education from the Turn of the Century to the Era of Managed Care* (Oxford: Oxford University Press, 1999).

10. FASEB included American Physiological Society, American Society for Biochemistry and Molecular Biology, American Society for Pharmacology and Experimental Therapeutics, American Society for Investigative Pathology, American Institute of Nutrition, American Association of Immunologists, American Society for Cell Biology, Biophysical Society, and American Society of Anatomists. See *Directory of Members* published by FASEB, 9650 Rockville Pike, Bethesda, MD 20814. Few cities could accommodate the numbers who attended these meeting, but Atlantic City was one. There were acres of exhibition halls where new scientific instruments were on

the most prominent announcement appeared in a front-page article in the *Wall Street Journal.* The article did not mention the inventor, Dr. Michel Ter-Pogossian, or the Mallinkrodt Institute, the radiology unit at Barnes Hospital/Washington University, where PET scanning was invented. The discussion was totally devoted to the money to be spent and to be made.

As Tinsley departed from life in 20th century medicine, that medicine was also departing. The academic medical centers built structures that were the holy temples of that era. The groups of specialists became ever more massive. Communications became more complex and difficult, in part because of laws such as HIPAA (the federal Health Insurance Portability and Accountability Act). Everything seemed to become more massive, more technical, and less personal. And there were tremendous pressures on *time*, as discussed in Ludmerer's famous book *Time to Heal.*[9]

Tinsley's methods of practice required time and a more leisurely pace than was possible as the century ended, with pressures to process more customers from the masses of people, third parties looking over everybody's shoulders as the accountants looked over theirs, and as the *time* to accomplish things seemed less and less.

The 20th century saw the rise of the great annual meetings of the famous doctors and scientists at the elite great hotels of Washington, Philadelphia, or other grand cities, especially Atlantic City, New Jersey. The practicing doctors tended to cluster at the AMA meetings—the American Medical Association, which had led the way in the 19th century and had risen to great influence in the 20th century. Their recognition and support led to the annual meetings of the rising medical research societies—the AAP, ASCI, and AFCR—as well as the basic scientists of the nation's medical schools, gathered in FASEB (Federation of American Societies for Experimental Biology).[10] Attendance at the FASEB meetings sometimes totaled 20,000, and the exhibits of new instruments and procedures were extensive. But the clinical research meetings of mid-century were also exciting, with such announcements as Macleod's of the discovery of insulin at noon during the meeting of the Old Turks on May 3, 1922.[11] There was high drama at these meetings, as there was in 1922, when one observer, Dr. Rollin T. Woodyatt, said "that [the work of] Macleod 'and his associates' marks the beginning of a new phase in the study and treatment of diabetes. It would be difficult to overestimate the ultimate significance of such a step." The Association tendered a standing vote of appreciation to Macleod and his associates.[12]

The middle of the 20th century was the high point of Tinsley's medicine and perhaps of American medicine in general, although many technical advances and organizational and other changes continued as the new century got underway, including expansion of the offerings of medicine to larger portions of the populace. And there continued to be exciting research advances in medicine and biology. Tinsley and his colleagues and students enjoyed especially the invigorating discussions on the boardwalk of Atlantic City or the restaurants near it. But in 1977, as Tinsley himself was leaving the scene, the presidential address by Robert G. Petersdorf started with the presentation of an aerial photo of the Haddon Hall Hotel and nearby beach and boardwalk, the hotel where many of the world's leading physicians had attended the dinner to commemorate Tinsley's retirement from his last chairmanship of medicine in 1957.[13] Atlantic City had become during the 20th century the most popular place for these meetings. But they would no longer be held there. Atlantic City had changed to a gambling center, "Las Vegas East," for economic reasons. The world Tinsley had lived in was changing and disappearing.[14]

As Tinsley's world of 20th century medicine changed, so did the rest of the world, and Tinsley passed from the scene.

display.

11. Michael Bliss, *The Discovery of Insulin* (Chicago: University of Chicago Press, 1982), 127.

12. Ibid., 127. AAP meetings in the middle part of the century always included the first weekend in May and a formal black-tie dinner with a talk by one of the world's medical leaders.

13. *Transactions of the Association of American Physicians.* Ninetieth Session. Vol. XC. 1. Washington, D.C., April 30 and May 1 and 2, 1977.

14. The big clinical research societies had measured academic success among "academic internists" like Harrison and his friends. Osler and his great English and continental predecessors were the examples to be emulated. The best history of the AAP, most elite, exclusive, and self-congratulatory of all, is by Means. Means, *Association*; Harvey, *Association*. Harvey thought Austin Flint Sr. was the proper paradigm for the AAP; Ellen R. Brainard, "History of the American Society for Clinical Investigation, 1909–1959." *Journal of Clinical*

Investigation, 39. This five-part article included: (1) Origins, (2) The Science of Clinical Medicine; What It Ought to Be and the Men To Uphold It. (Though this "Part 2" was signed by E. Brainard, it is really an essay by the first ASCI president, Samuel J. Meltzer, and well worth a read.) (3) And How It Grew. (4) Space, Time, and Learned Societies. This part starts with Tinsley Harrison's presidential address of 1939, in which he stated his belief that these organizations deteriorate and die because of "institutional arteriosclerosis," the result of failing to select the very best men for membership and leadership. The series concluded with "The Tempering of Traditions." The AFCR was never as exclusive or elite as the other two and didn't help as much academically. But, being less exclusive, it had a larger membership, and later as the AFMR it became the most effective lobby for support of clinical research. The organization started by Harrison's friends, of which he was its first president, was the SSCI, which persists into the 21st century, usually holding its annual meeting in New Orleans, and now with its own journal, *The American Journal of the Medical Sciences,* with Tinsley's portrait prominently displayed in several places.

APPENDICES AND FURTHER READING

EDITOR'S NOTE: Appendices mentioned throughout this volume, along with additional photographs, articles, documents, and letters compiled by Dr. Pittman and contributed by friends, family, and colleagues of both himself and Dr. Harrison are maintained at www.newsouthbooks. com/tinsleyharrison/supplement. Readers interested in submitting their own contributions about the book's subject, its author, or the history of the UAB School of Medicine will find contact information at those sites.

BIBLIOGRAPHY

INTERVIEWS AND CORRESPONDENCE

Audiotape, meeting of medical students of the 1940s in office of George Race, M.D., Ph.D., Southwestern Medical School, January 25, 1993.

Beeson P. B., to James A. Pittman, March 1997. UAB Archives.

Billings, F. T. Oral history transcription for R. H. Kampmeier, 1980. VUMC Archives.

Blalock, Alfred, to Tinsley Harrison, 2 June 1942.

Brooks, Barney, to Canby Robinson, April 23, 1928. VUMC Archives.

Burwell, C. Sidney, to Hugh Morgan, May 17, 1935. VUMC Archives.

——. to T. R. Harrison, August 12, 1941. Dorothy Carpenter Medical Archives, BGSM.

——. to W. S. Leathers, May 14th, 1929. VUMC Archives.

Cabot, Thomas D. Personal communication, July 7 1993.

Carmichael, E. B. Personal communication, 1974.

Carpenter, Coy C., to Dr. Thurman D. Kitchin, February 22, 1944. BGSM Arch.

——. to Tinsley Harrison, July 3, 1941. VUMC Archives.

——. to W. S. Leathers, December 16, 1940. VUMC Archives.

Chapman, C. B. Personal communication, May 1993.

Coghlin, H. C. Personal communication.

Davis, Katherine. Audiotape, April 15, 1993, UAB Archives.

DeGroot, Leslie J., to James A. Pittman, June 13 2003.

Eddleman E. E. Telephone interview. November 17, 2003.

Eisenberg, L. Personal communication, 1997. UAB Archives.

Finney Jr., James O. Personal communication, July 7, 1993.

Friedman, Ben. Interview, 1992. UAB Archives.

Frommeyer, Mrs. Walter B. Interview. November 15, 2003.

Hankins, Joseph B. Audiotape, luncheon discussion, April 15, 1993, Winston-Salem, N.C. UAB Archives.

Harrell, G.H. Personal communication with James A. Pittman, April 24, 1993.

Harrison, Emily, to Tinsley Harrison, Nov. 6, 1944. UAB Archives.

Harrison, Tinsley. Audiotape, 1974. UAB Archives.

——.Interview, 1974. UAB Archives.

——.Interview by James A. Pittman

——.Memorandum. VUMC Archives.

——.to Alfred Blalock, January 19, 1943. BGSM Archives.

——. to Alfred Blalock, March 2, 1944. Chesney Arch., JHMI.

——. to Alfred Blalock, March 8, 1944. Chesney Arch., JHMI.

——. to Alfred Blalock, November 27, 1943. Chesney Arch., JHMI.

——. to Alfred Blalock, October 16, 1943. VUMC Archives.

——. to Archie Woods, November 26, 1940. VUMC Archives.

——. to Coy C. Carpenter, August 1, 1941. Dorothy Carpenter Medical Archives, BGSM.

——. to Coy C. Carpenter, December 8, 1942. Dorothy Carpenter Medical Archives, BGSM.

——. to Coy C. Carpenter, December 10, 1942. Dorothy Carpenter Medical Archives, BGSM.

——. to Coy C. Carpenter, December 11, 1940. Vanderbilt University Medical Center Archives, BGSM.

——. to Coy C. Carpenter, December 14, 1940. VUMC Archives.

——. to Coy C. Carpenter, December 21, 1940. VUMC Archives.

——. to Coy C. Carpenter, July 17, 1942. Dorothy Carpenter Medical Archives, BGSM.

——. to Coy C. Carpenter, May 9, 1943. Dorothy Carpenter Medical Archives, BGSM.

——. to Dr. E. W. Goodpasture, November 25, 1941.

——. to Dr. Rudolph Kampmeier, May 6, 1976. Vanderbilt

University Medical Center Library, Special Collections.

——. to Herbert Wells, 22 October 1940. Dorothy Carpenter Medical Archives, BGSM.

——. to James I. Wendell, 9 January 1944. Chesney Arch., JHMI.

Harrison, Tinsley, Jr. Personal communication, 1993.

Hill, S. Richardson, Jr. Interview. July 2002. UAB Archives.

Hill, Virginia, to James A. Pittman, 1999.

Leathers, W. S., to Coy C. Carpenter, M.D., December 14, 1940. VUMC Archives.

Liang-Cha, Cha. Audiotape of Drs. J. A. and C. S. Pittman, Taipei, Taiwan, May 12, 1981. UAB Archives.

Meads, Manson. Personal communication, August 10, 1993.

Morehead, Robert P. Audiotape. April 15, 1993. UAB Archives.

Pickering, Sir George, to James A. Pittman, August 5 1978. UAB Archives.

Pittman, James A., to S. Schechner, 2003.

Rakel, R. E., to James A. Pittman, December 4, 2001. UAB Archives.

Rasmussen, Howard, M.D. Personal communication.

Reeves, T.J. Personal communication, January 10, 1993.

——.Personal communication, August 11, 2005.

Reichsman, F. Personal communication, April 1993.

Richardson, M. Personal communication, September 22, 2003.

Salter C. L., Interview, 1975. UAB Archives.

Sensenbach, C. W., to Dr. J. R. Williams Jr., January 6, 1944. Dorothy Carpenter Medical Archives, BGSM.

Scoville, Addison, M.D. Interview. VUMC Archives.

Thorn, G. W. Personal conversation, HHMI office, Boston, March 1993.

Toole, Arthur F. Interview. Talladega, AL, June 1993.

Waldrop, Edwin G., M.D. Personal communication, August 9, 1993.

Wyklicky, Helmut, to James A. Pittman, February 26 1997. UAB Archives.

PERIODICALS AND JOURNALS

Aaron, Benjamin L., and S. David Rockoff. "*The Attempted Assassination of President Reagan: Medical Implications and Historical Perspective.*" *JAMA* 272, 21 (Dec 7, 1994.): 1689–1693.

Abeloos, J., N. Barcroft, T. R. Harrison, and J. Sendroy. "The Measurement of the Oxygen Capacity of Hemoglobin." *Am. J. Physiol.*, 66 (1928).

Adams, R. D., and J. M. Foley. "The Neurological Disorder Associated with Liver Disease." *Association for Research in Nervous and Mental Disease 32* (1953): 198–237.

"Advertisement of the E.R. Squibb and Sons Pharmaceutical Company." *N. Carol. Med. J.* 4 (1943): 363.

"Annual Medical Education Number," *JAMA*, 290 (2003): 1119–1268.

Anrep, G. V., A. Blalock, and M. Hammouda, "The Distribution of Blood in the Coronary Vessels," *Am. J. Physiol.* 95 (1930).

Bing, R. J., L. D. Vandam, F. Gregoire, *et al.* "Catheterization of the Coronary Sinus and the Middle Cardiac Vein in Man." *Proc. Soc. Exper. Biol. & Med.* 66 (1947): 239–240.

Braunwald, E. "The pathogenesis of congestive failure: then and now." *Medicine* 70 (1991): 67–81.

Blalock, Alfred. "A Clinical Study of Biliary Tract Disease," *JAMA* 83, no. 26 (1924).

——."The Effects of Changes in Hydrogen Ion Concentration on the Blood Flow of Morphinized Dogs." *J. Clin. Invest.* 1 (1925).

——."The Incidence of Mastoid Disease in the United States." *South. Med. J.* 18 (1925).

——."A Statistical Study of 888 Cases of Biliary Tract Disease," *Johns Hopkins Hosp. Bull.* 35 (1924).

Blalock, Alfred and S. J. Crowe. "The Recurrent Laryngeal Nerves in Dogs." *Arch. Surgery* 12 (1926).

——."Treatment of Chronic Middle Ear Suppuration," *Archives of Otolaryngology* 1, no. 3 (1925).

Blalock, Alfred, Tinsley Harrison, and C. P. Wilson. "Partial Tracheal Obstruction: An Experimental Study in the Effects on the Circulation and Respiration of Morphinized Dogs." *Arch. Surg.* 13 (1925).

Booth, E., K. Willis, T. J. Reeves and T. R. Harrison. "The Right Auricular Electrokymogram of Normal Subjects." *Circulation* 7 (1953).

Brainard, Ellen R. "History of the American Society for Clinical Investigation, 1909–1959." *Journal of Clin. Investi.* 39.

Carmichael, E. B. "Seale Harris—Physician-Scientist-Author." *J. Med. Assn. State of Alabama* 33 (1954): 189–195.

Chabner, B. A., and T. G. Roberts. "Chemotherapy and the War on Cancer." *Nature Reviews/Cancer* 5 (2005): 65–72.

Cournand, A., Bing R. J., Dexter L., Detter C., Katz L. N., Warren J. V., and Wood E. "Report of the Committee on Cardiac Catheterizations and Angiocardiography." *Circulation* 7 (1953).

Crowe, S.J., and A.T. Ward. "Local Use of Sulfadiazine, Tyrothricin, Penicillin and Radon in Otolaryngology." *N. Carol. Med. J.* 4 (1943).

The Daily Times Herald (Dallas), 1942.

Desjardins, A.U. "The Action of Roentgen Rays on Inflammatory Conditions." *Radiology* 38 (1942).

Deutsch, A. "Veterans Hospitals Called Back Waters of Medicine," *PM* (1945).

Dock, William. "Arteriosclerosis." *N. Carol. Med. J.* 4 (1943).

Dock, W., and T. R. Harrison. "The Blood Flow through the Lungs in Experimental Pneumothorax." *American Rev. of Tuberculosis* 10 (1925).

"The Early Years at Bowman Gray." *N. Carol. Med. J.* 44 (1983): 805-6.

Eddleman, E. E. Jr., K. Willis, T. J. Reeves, and T. R. Harrison. "The Kinetocardiogram. I. Method of Recording Precordial Movements." *Circulation* 8 (1953).

Eisenberg J., "Patient Centered Medicine." *AHCPR* (July 1998).

Friedman, B., G. Clark, H. Resnik, and T. R. Harrison. "Effect of Digitalis on the Cardiac Output of Persons with Congestive Heart Failure." *Arch. Int. Med.* 56 (1935).

Friedman, B., H. Resnik, J.A. Calhoun, and T. R. Harrison. "Effect of Diuretics on the Cardiac Output of Patients with Congestive Failure." *Arch. Int. Med.* 56 (1935).

Friedman, B., T. R. Harrison, G. Clark, and H. Resnik. "The Effect of Therapeutic Measures on the Cardiac Output of Patients with Congestive Failure." *Trans. Am. Assoc. Phys.* 69 (1934).

——. "Studies in Congestive Heart Failure. XXII. A Method for Obtaining 'Mixed' Venous Blood by Arterial Puncture." *J. Clin. Invest.* 13 (1934).

Fye, W. B. "The Delayed Diagnosis of Myocardial Infarction: It Took Half a Century!" *Circulation* 72 (1985): 262–271.

Gibbon, J. H. "Application of a Mechanical Heart and Lung Apparatus to Cardiac Surgery." *Minnesota Medicine* 17 (1954): 171–177.

Greve, M. J., E. E. Eddleman Jr., K. Willis, S. Eisenberg and T. R. Harrison. "The Effect of Digitoxin on Sodium Excretion, Creatinine Clearance and Apparent Cardiac Output." *Circulation* 3 (1951).

Grollman, A., B. Friedman, G. Clark, and T. R. Harrison. "Studies in Congestive Heart Failure. XXIII. A Critical Study of Methods for Determining the Cardiac Output in Patients with Cardiac Disease." *J. Clin. Invest.* 12 (1933).

Grollman, A., and C. Rule. "Experimentally Induced Hypertension in Parabiotic Rats." *Am. J. Physiol.* 138 (1943).

Grollman, A. "The Treatment of Hypertension in the Light of Modern Experimental Investigations." *N. Carol. Med. J.* 4 (1943).

"The Gunshot Wounds of Presidents Garfield and Reagan." *JAMA*, 1981.

Harrison, T. R., A. Grollman, and J. R. Williams Jr. "Separation of Various Blood Pressure Producing Fractions of Fenal Extract." *Trans. Assoc. Amer. Physi.* 62 (1942).

Harrison, T. R., B. Friedman, G. Clark, and H. Resnik. "The Cardiac Output in Relation to Cardiac Failure," *Arch. Int. Med.* 54 (1934).

Harrison, T. R., B. Friedman, and H. Resnik. "Mechanism of Acute Experimental Heart Failure." *Arch. Int. Med.* 57 (1936).

Harrison, T. R., C. E. King, J. A. Calhoun, and W. G. Harrison Jr., "Studies in Congestive Heart Failure. XX. Cheyne-Stokes Respiration as the Cause of Paroxysmal Dyspnea at the Onset of Sleep," *Arch. Int. Med.* 53 (1934).

Harrison, T. R., C. P. Wilson, and A. Blalock. "The Effect of Changes in Hydrogen Ion Concentration on the Blood Flow of Morphinized Dogs." *J. Clin. Investi.* 1 (1925): 547–648.

Harrison, T. R., J. A. Calhoun, and W. G. Harrison Jr. "Afferent Impulses as a Cause of Increased Ventilation During Muscular Exercise." *Am. J. Physiol.* 100 (1932).

——. "Congestive Heart Failure. XXI. Observations Concerning the Mechanism of Cardiac Asthma" *Arch. Int. Med.* 53 (1934).

Harrison, T. R., L. Christianson, E. E. Eddleman Jr, R. Pierce, R. Watkins and K. Willis. "Movements of Human Ventricles." *Trans. Assoc. Amer. Physi.* 66 (1953).

Harrison, T. R. and L. Hughes. "Precordial Systolic Bulges During Anginal Attacks." *Trans. Assoc. Amer. Physi.* 71 (1958): 174–185.

Harrison, T. R. "Obstruction of the Coronary Arteries." *Trans. Ala. State Med. Assoc.* (1925).

——. "The Subjective Aspects of the Case History of TRH as

related by TRH." *Alabama J. of Med. Sciences* 15 (1978): 320–325.

Harrison, T. R., and Sam Levine. "Notes on the Regional Distribution of Rheumatic Fever and Rheumatic Heart Disease." *South Med J.* 17 (1924).

Harrison, T. R., S. Harris Jr., and J. A. Calhoun. "Studies in Congestive Heart Failure. XVI. The Clinical Value of the Ventilation Test in the Estimation of Cardiac Function." *Am. Heart J.* 7(1931).

Harrison, T. R. and W. A. Perlzweig. "Alkolosis not Due to Administration of Alkali, Associated with Uremia." *JAMA* 84 (1925): 671–673.

Harrison, T. R., W. Dock, and E. Holman. "Experimental Studies in Arteriovenous Fisulae. Cardiac Output." *Am. Heart J.* 11 (1924).

Harrison, T. R., W. G. Harrison Jr., J. A. Calhoun, and J. P. Marsh, "Congestive Heart Failure. XVII. The Mechanism of Dyspnea on Exertion," *Arch. Int. Med.* 50 (1932).

———. "Studies in Congestive Heart Failure. XIX. Reflext Stimulation of Respiration as the Cause of Evening Dyspnea," *Arch. Int. Med.* 53 (1934).

Harrison, T. R., W. G. Harrison Jr., and J. P. Marsh, "Reflex stimulation of respiration from increase in venous pressure," *Am. J. Physiol.* 100 (1932).

Harrison, W. G., J. A. Calhoun, and T. R. Harrison, "Studies in Congestive Heart Failure. XVIII. Clinical Types of Nocturnal Dyspnea," *Arch. Int. Med.* 53 (1934).

"An Historical Sketch of the Department of Medicine and Surgery of the University of Michigan." *The Medical News*, April 20, 1901.

"In Defense of Mr. McNutt." *N. Carol. Med. J.* 3 (1942): 367.

Jones, T. D. "The Diagnosis of Rheumatic Fever." *JAMA* 126 (1944): 481–484.

Kirklin, J. W. "The Development of Cardiac Surgery at the Mayo Clinic." *Mayo Clinic Proceedings*, 55, no. 5 (1980).

Li, M. C., R. Hertz, and D. M. Bergensal. "Therapy of Choriocarcinoma and Related Trophoblastic Tumors with Folic Acid and Purine Antagonists." *New England J. Med.* 259 (1958): 66–74.

McNutt, Paul V. *JAMA 20, June 1942.*

"Medical Education and The War." *N. Carol. Med. J.* 3 (1942): 366

Morehead, Robert P. "The Contribution of a Great Man to Wake Forest University and its Bowman Gray School

of Medicine—Tinsley R. Harrison, M.D." *North Carol. Med. J.* 44 (1983): 809–811.

New England J. Medicine, Massachusetts Medical Society. (1941–1944).

Palmer, Walter Lincoln. "Chester Morse Jones." Obituary. *Trans. Assn. Amer. Physicians.* 1973.

Pittman, C. S., H. Nakafuji, V. H. Read, and J. B. Chambers Jr. "The Metabolism of 14-C Labeled Thyroxine in Normal Man." *American Thyroid Association: Program of Annual Meeting* (1969), Chicago.

Pittman, C. S., J. B. Chambers Jr., and V. H. Read. "The Extrathyroidal Conversation of Thyroxine (T4) to Triiodothyronine (T3) in Man." *Proc. of the 6th International Thyroid Conference (1970)*, Vienna, Austria.

———. "The Rate of Extrathyroidal Conversion of Thyroxine to Triiodothyronine in Man." *J. Clin. Investi.* 49 (1970): 75–.

Pittman, C. S., V. H. Read, J. B. Chambers, and H. Nakafuji. "The Metabolism of the Ether Linkage of Thyroxine in Normal Man." *J. Clin. Investi.* 48 (1969): 65–.

Pittman, C. S., and W. B. Jones. "Metabolism of Six Specifically Labeled Radiothyroxines in Normal Man and Animals." *J. Clin. Investi.* 47 (1968).

Pittman, James A., and D. M. Miller. "The Southern Society for Clinical Investigation at 50: The End of the Beginning." *Am. J. Med. Sciences* 311 (1996).

Pittman, James A. "Meaning of the M.D. degree from an accredited medical school." *Bulletin of the Federation of American Boards of Medical Examiners* (1994).

———. "Research and Health Care Reform." *Am. J. Med. Sciences* 309 (1995): 249–251.

———. "Service and Significance." *Alabama J. of the Med. Sciences* 24, no. 1 (1987):79–82.

———. "U.S. Academic Community and Foreign Medical Graduates." *The United States Academic Community and the Training of Foreign Medical Graduates for Careers in Asia.* New York: The American Bureau for Medical Advancement in China, Inc., 1983.

———. "Seale Harris." *Oxford's American National Biography.* eds. J. A. Garraty and M. C. Carnes (New York: Oxford Univ. Press, 1999).

Reeves, R. J. "Roentgen Therapy in the Treatment of Certain Inflammatory Conditions." *N. Carol. Med. J.* 4 (1943).

"Report of a Committee Nominated to Investigate the Subject of Myxedema," *Trans. Clin. Soc.* 26 (1888): 298.

Resnik H. and B. Friedman. "Studies on the Mechanism of the Increased Oxygen Consumption in Patients with Cardiac Disease." *J. Clin. Invest.* 14 (1935).

Resnik, H., B. Friedman, and T. R. Harrison. "The Effect of Certain Therapeutic Measures on the Cardiac Output of Patients with Congestive Heart Failure." *Arch. Int. Med.* 56 (1935).

Reuben, Adrian. "Landmarks in Hepatology: There is Nothin' Like a Dame." *Hepatology* 35 (2002): 983–985.

Robinson, G. Canby, and George Draper. "A Study of the Presphygmic Period of the Heart." *Arch Int. Med.* 2, (1910).

Sabiston, C., Jr., "Alfred Blalock." *Annals of Surgery* 188 vol. 3 (1978): 255.

Shakespeare, William. *Twelfth Night.*

Skinner, N. S. Jr., R. S. Liebeskind, H. L. Phillips and T. R. Harrison. "The Effect of Exertion and of Nitrites on the Precordial Movements of Patients with Angina Pectoris." *Amer. Heart J.* 61 (1961): 250–258.

"Special Sunday Section." D*allas Morning News*, May 30, 1943, SWMS Arch.

"Statement of the Origin and Objects of the Society" *Trans. Clin. Soc.* 1 (1868).

"Ueber die Beziehungen des Nervus vagus zum Atmungsmechanismus." *Zeit. fur Die Gesellschaft Exper. Med.*, 31(1928).

Viar W. N., B. B. Oliver, S. Eisenberg, T. A. Lombardo, K. Willis, and T. R. Harrison. "The Effect of Posture and of Compression of the Neck on the Excretion of Electrolytes and on Glomerular Filtration: Further Studies." *Circulation* 3 (1951): 105–115.

Victor, M., and R. D. Adams. "The Effect of Alcohol on the Nervous System." *Association for Research in Nervous and Mental Disease 32* (1953): 526–573.

Willis, Hurst J. "James Edgar Paullin: Internist to Franklin Delano Roosevelt, Oslerian, and Forgotten Leader of American Medicine." *Annals of Int. Med.* 134 (2001).

Wilson, C.P., T. R. Harrison, and C. Pilcher. "The Action of Drugs on Cardiac Output. IV. The Effects of Camphor and Strychnine on the Cardiac Output of Intact Unnarcotized Dogs." *Arch. Int. Med.* 40 (1927).

DOCUMENTS, SPEECHES, UNPUBLISHED WORKS

Advisory Council Minutes, 27 December 1943. Dorothy Carpenter Medical Archives.

Announcements. "Special Collections." Vanderbilt Univ. Medical Center Library.

Annual Reports of the Department of Preventive Medicine and Public Health. VUMA Archives.

Burwell, C. S. "Methods and objectives in the organization of the outpatient department of a teaching hospital." J. Amer. Med. Coll. 1935.

——."Report of the Department of Medicine for the Year 1930–3." VUMC Archives.

Carpenter, Coy C. Manuscript in private holdings of Dr. Manson Meads, BGSM.

Carpenter, Coy C. Memorandum to Advisory Council, December 31, 1943. Dorothy Carpenter Medical Archives, BGSM.

"Centenary Anniversary of Harrison's Birth." Video. Birmingham, UAB Archives, 2000.

Department of Medicine Annual Reports, 1929–1935. VUMC Archives.

Engle, H. Martin. "Press Release from the Veterans Administration." May 6, 1968.

Harrison, Tinsley R. Curriculum Vitae. UAB Archives.

——.Department of Medicine Annual Report, 1941–42. Dorothy Carpenter Medical Archives, BGSM.

——.*The Medical School of the University of Alabama: Some Reminiscenses. Manuscript.* UAB Archives.

——.Presidential address, 1939. *J. Clin. Invest.*

——."Some thoughts about medical education." Address, Opening of the Medical School, University of Michigan, September 30, 1940. VUMC Archives.

Harrison Sr., W. G. "Memoirs" UAB Archives.

H.R. 4717, Public Law 293, 79th Congress, 1st Session.

Francis, K. "A Textbook Case of Medical Innovation: Austin Flint's *Principles and Practice of Medicine* and the Germ Theory of Disease." in *American Association for the History of Medicine*, Abstracts of the 73rd Annual Meeting, Bethesda, MD, 2000.

Minutes of Advisory Council Meeting, January 6, 1944. Dorothy Carpenter Medical Archives, BGSM.

Minutes of the Advisory Committee meeting of June 2, 1943.

Dorothy Carpenter Medical Archives, BGSM.

Minutes of Advisory Council Meetings, March 5, 1943 through 1944. Dorothy Carpenter Medical Archives, BGSM.

Minutes of Advisory Council Meeting of March 31, 1943. Dorothy Carpenter Medical Archives, BGSM.

Morgan, Hugh J. Department of Medicine Annual Report, 1939–40. VUMC Archives.

Pittman, James A. "Prominent Textbooks of Internal Medicine in the 20th Century." Paper presentation, International Society for the History of Medicine, Galveston, Texas, 2000.

President's Annual Report. University of Michigan, 17. 1893.

Schulze, C. "What Happened During 1943–1968." Dallas, Texas, 1971. Archives of University of Texas Southwestern Medical School, Dallas.

U.S. Veterans Administration. Policy Memorandum No. 2. "Policy in Association of Veterans' Hospitals With Medical Schools." Washington DC. January 30, 1946.

"Variety Shade Landowners of Virginia Association" meeting. Audiotape. Lake Martin, Alabama, June 18–20, 1993.

Weller, Thomas. Harvard Medical School course in Tropical Medicine (1949).

Wilson, JD. *Memories of Tinsley Harrison at Dallas.* Video. 2000. Birmingham. UAB Archives.

WEB PAGES

Oyez. *U.S. Supreme Court Multimedia*, ThisNation.com. American Government & Politics Online, October 4, 2005.

SONGS

Lehrer, Tom. "Take Me Back to Alabamy." *The Remains of Tom Lehrer.* CD. Los Angeles, CA: Warner Brothers Records, Inc. and Rhino Entertainment Co.

BOOKS

Adkins, R. *To Care for Him Who Shall Have Borne the Battle.* Washington, DC: House Committee on Veterans Affairs, U.S. Gov. Printing Office, 1967.

Barger C., S. Bennison, and Elin Wolf. *Walter B. Cannon, A Life.* Cambridge: Harvard-Belknap Press, 1998.

Bates, Ralph S. *Scientific Societies in the United States.* Cambridge: M.I.T. Press, 1965.

Beecher H. K. and M. D. Altschule. *Medicine at Harvard: The First 300 Years.* Hanover, NH: The University Press of New England, 1977.

Benison, Saul, A. Clifford Barger, and Elin L. Wolfe. *Walter B. Cannon, the Life and Times of a Young Scientist.* Cambridge: Harvard University Press, 1987.

Bennett, M. J. *When Dreams Came True: The GI Bill and the Making of Modern America.* Washington: Brassey's, 1996.

Berg, A. S. *Lindbergh.* New York: Berkley Books, 1998

Billings, J. S. and E. H. Clarke. A *Century of American Medicine 1776–1876.* Philadelphia: Lea Publications, 1876.

Bliss, Michael. *The Discovery of Insulin.* Chicago: University of Chicago Press, 1982.

Burch, George E. and N. P. DePasquale. *A History of Electrocardiography.* 1964. Reprinted. San Francisco: Norman Publishing, 1990.

Bynum, W. F., and R. Porter, eds. *Brunonianism in Britain and Europe.* London: Wellcome Institute for the History of Medicine, 1988.

Carpenter, Coy C. *The Story of Medicine at Wake Forest University.* Chapel Hill: The University of North Carolina Press, 1970.

Cecil, Russell L., ed. *Textbook of Internal Medicine.* Philadelphia: W.B. Saunders Co., 1927

Chapman, Carleton. *Order Out of Chaos: John Shaw Billings and America's Coming of Age.* Boston: The Boston Medical Library in the Countway Library, Harvard Medical School, 1994.

Chapman, John S. *The University of Texas Southwestern Medical School. Medical Education in Dallas 1900–1975.* Dallas: Southern Methodist Univ. Press, 1976.

Chesney, Alan M. *The Johns Hopkins Hospital and The Johns Hopkins University School of Medicine: A Chronicle. Vol. III. 1905–1914.* Baltimore: The Johns Hopkins Press, 1963.

Clapesattle, H. *The Doctors Mayo.* Minneapolis: Univ. of Minnesota Press, 1941.

Conkin, P. K., H. L. Swint and P.S. Miletich: *Gone With the Ivy: A Biography of Vanderbilt University.* Knoxville: The University of Tennessee Press, 1985.

Corner, George W. *A History of the Rockefeller Institute 1901–1953, Origins and Growth.* New York: The Rockefeller Institute Press, 1964.

Cushing, Harvey. *The Life of Sir William Osler*, vol. I. London: Oxford Univ. Press, 1941.

Daniel, C., ed. *Chronicle of the 20th Century*. Mt. Kisco, N.Y.: Chronicle Publications, 1987.

Dalton, M. L. *Champ Lyons: Surgeon*. Macon, GA: Aequanimitas Medical Books, 2003.

Davenport, Horace W. *Doctor Dock. Teaching and Learning Medicine at the Turn of the Century*. New Brunswick and London: Rutgers University Press, 1987.

Davison, W.C. *The Duke University Medical Center (1892–1960)*. Durham: Duke University Medical School, 1960.

Dietrick, John E., and Robert C. Berson. *Medical Schools in the United States at Mid-Century* (New York: McGraw-Hill, 1953).

Djerassi, Carl. *The Pill, Pygmy Chimps, and Degas' Horse*. New York: Basic Books, 1992.

Drake, Daniel. *Diseases of the Interior Valley of North America*, 1854. Reprinted. New York: The Classics of Medicine, 1990.

Durr, Virginia Foster. *Outside the Magic Circle: The Autobiography of Virginia*. Edited by Foster Durr and Hollinger F. Barnard. Tuscaloosa: The University of Alabama Press, 1990.

Ellis, Harold. *A History of Surgery*. London: Greenwich Medical Media Ltd., 2001.

English, P. C. *Rheumatic Fever in America and Britain*. New Brunswick: NJ, Rutgers University Press, 1999.

Ettling, John. *The Germ of Laziness: Rockefeller Philanthropy and Public Health in the New South*. Cambridge, Harvard Univ. Press, 1981.

Faden, Beauchamp, and King. *A History of Informed Consent*. New York: Oxford Univ. Press, 1986.

Ferrell, R. H. *The Dying President: Franklin D. Roosevelt 1944–45*. Columbia: University of Missouri Press, 1998.

Finland, Maxwell. *The Harvard Medical Unit at the Boston City Hospital*. Boston: Harvard Medical School, 1983.

Fishbein, Morris. *A History of the American Medical Association 1847 to 1947*. Philadelphia: W. B. Saunders Co., 1947.

Fisher, V. E. *Building On A Vision: A Fifty-Year Retrospective of UAB's Academic Health Center*. Birmingham: University of Alabama at Birmingham, 1995.

Fleming, Donald. *William Welch and the Rise of Modern Medicine*. 1954. Reprinted. Baltimore: The Johns Hopkins University Press, 1987.

Flexner, Abraham. *Medical Education in the United States and Canada*. New York: Carnegie Foundation of the Advancement of Teaching, 1910.

Flynt, Wyane. *Poor But Proud: Alabama's Poor Whites*. Tuscaloosa: The University of Alabama Press, 1989.

Fogel, R. W. and S. L. Engerman. *Time on the Cross: The Economics of American Negro Slavery* 1. Boston: Little, Brown and Co., 1974.

Fosdick, Raymond B. *The Story of the Rockefeller Foundation*. New York: Harper and Brothers, Publishers, 1952.

Fredrickson, D. S. "Science and the Culture Warp" in *Emerging Policies for Biomedical Research*. Edited by W. N. Kelly, M. Osterweis, and E. R. Rubin. Washington, DC: Association of Academic Health Centers, 1993.

Fye, W. B. "Cardiovascular Medicine: A Historical Perspective." in *Textbook of Cardiovascular Medicine*, Edited by Eric J. Topol. Philadelphia: Lippincott-Raven Publishers, 1998.

——. "A Historical Perspective on Atherosclerosis and Coronary Artery Disease" in *Arteriosclerosis and Coronary Artery Disease*, Edited by V. Fuster, R. Ross, and E. J. Topol. Philadelphia: Lippincott-Raven Publishers, 1996.

Garraty, J. A. and M. C. Carnes, eds. *Oxford's American National Biography*. New York: Oxford University Press, 1999.

Geiser, Samuel Wood. *Medical Education in Dallas 1900–1910*. Dallas: Southern Methodist Univ. Press, 1952.

Hamer, Philip M., ed. *Centennial History of the Tenessee Medical Association, 1830–1930*. Nashville: Tennessee State Medical Association, 1930. Quoted in Randolph H. Kampmeier, et. al. *Vanderbilt University School of Medicine. The Story in Pictures from Its Beginning to 1963*. Nashville: Vanderbilt University School of Medicine, 1990.

Hamilton, Virginia Van Der Veer. *Alabama, A Bicentennial History*. New York: W. W. Norton Company, 1977.

——. *Lister Hill: Statesman from the South* (Chapel Hill, NC: University of North Carolina Press, 1987).

Harden, Victoria. *The National Institutes of Health: A History Since 1937*, forthcoming.

Harvey, A. M., G. H. Brieger, S. L. Abrams, and Victor McKusick. *A Model of Its Kind: A Centennial History of Medicine at Johns Hopkins, Volume I*, 29. Baltimore & London: Johns Hopkins Press, 1989.

Harvey, A. M. *The Association of American Physicians*

1886–1986: A Century of Progress in Medical Science. Baltimore, MD: Waverley Press, Inc., 1986.

——.*Science at the Bedside, Clinical Research in American Medicine 1905–1945.* (New York: The Johns Hopkins University Press, 1981).

Harvey, A. M. and Victor McKusick. *Introduction to Osler's Textbook of Medicine Revisited.* Birmingham, Alabama: Gryphon Editions, Ltd., 1978.

Harvey, A. M., Victor McKusick, and John Stubo. *Osler's Legacy: The Department of Medicine at Johns Hopkins 1889–1989.* Baltimore: The Johns Hopkins University Press, 1990.

Hecht, J. *City of Light: The Story of Fiber Optics.* New York: Oxford University Press, 1999.

History of Alabama and *Dictionary of Alabama Biography.* Chicago: The S. J. Clarke Publishing Company, 1921.

Hobby, Gladys L. *Penicillin, Meeting the Challenge.* New Haven: Yale Univ. Press, 1985.

Holley, H. L. "Highlights in the History of Medicine in Alabama (fourth Reynolds Historical Lecture)" in *The Reynolds Historical Lectures 1980–1991.* Edited by Marion G. McGuinn. Birmingham, AL: The University of Alabama at Birmingham Press, 1993. 66–99.

——.*A History of Medicine in Alabama.* Birmingham: University of Alabama School of Medicine, 1982.

Holmes, J. D. L. *A History of the University of Alabama Hospitals.* Birmingham: University of Alabama in Birmingham Print Shop, 1974.

Honan, J. H. *Honan's Handbook to Medical Europe: A Ready Reference Book to the Universities, Hospitals, Clinics, Laboratories and General Medical Work of the Principal Cities of Europe.* Philadelphia: P. Blakiston's Son and Co., 1912.

Kampmeier, Randolph H. Mary Teloh, Robert M. Vantrease, and William J. Darby. *Vanderbilt University School of Medicine: The Story in Pictures from Its Beginning to 1963.* Nashville: Vanderbilt University Medical Center, 1990.

Kampmeier, Rudolph H. *Recollections: The Department of Medicine, Vanderbilt University School of Medicine 1925–1959.* Nashville: Vanderbilt University Press, 1980.

Karnad, A. B. *Intrinsic Factors: William Bosworth Castle and the Development of Hematology and Clinical Investigation at the Boston City Hospital.* Boston: Harvard University Press, 1997.

Kaufmann, S. R., *The Healer's Tale: Transforming Medicine and Culture.* Madison: University of Wisconsin Press, 1993.

Kirklin, J. W. "Lessons from the History of the Mayo Clinic." in *The Reynolds Historical Lectures 1980–1991.* Edited by Marion G. McGuinn. Birmingham, AL: The University of Alabama at Birmingham Press, 1993.

Kirschenfeld, J. J. *No Greater Privilege.* Montgomery, AL: Black Belt Press, 1992.

Laszlo, J. *The Cure of Childhood Leukemia: Into the Age of Miracles.* New Brunswick, NJ, 1995.

Lederberg J., R. E. Shope, and S. C. Oaks Jr., eds. *Emerging Infections: Microbial Threats to Health in the United States.* Washington, D.C.: National Academy Press, 1992.

Le Fanu J., *The Rise and Fall of Modern Medicine.* New York: Carroll & Graf Publishers, 2000.

Lesky, Erna. *Die Wiener Medizinische Schule im 19. Jahrhundert 1908.* Trans. by L. Williams and I. S. Levij. *The Vienna Medical School of the 19th Century.* Baltimore: Johns Hopkins University Press, 1976.

Lewis, Benjamin. *VA Medical Program in Relation to Medical Schools.* Washington, D.C.: Committee on Veterans Affairs, U.S. Gov. Printing Office, 1970.

Lineback, N. G., ed. *Atlas of Alabama.* Tuscaloosa: The University of Alabama Press, 1973.

Lofton, J. Mack, Jr. *Healing Hands: An Alabama Medical Mosaic.* Tuscaloosa: Univ. of Alabama Press, 1995.

Longmire Jr., W. P. *Alfred Blalock: His Life and Times.* Los Angeles: W. P. Longmire, 1991.

Ludmerer, K., *Learning to Heal: The Development of American Medical Education.* New York, Basic Books, Inc., 1985.

——.*Time to Heal: American Medical Education from the Turn of the Century to the Era of Managed Care.* Oxford: Oxford University Press, 1999.

Magnuson, P. G. *Ring the Night Bell: The Autobiography of a Surgeon.* Boston: Little, Brown & Co., 1960. Reprinted by UAB, Birmingham, AL, 1986.

Maisel, A. O. *The Hormone Quest: The Story of the Century's Most Exciting Advance in Health and Human Welfare.* New York: Random House, 1965.

Marwick, A. *The Sixties: Cultural Revolution in Britain, France, Italy, and the United States, c.1958—c.1974.* Oxford-New York: Oxford University Press, 1998.

McGoon, D. C. "Foreword" in *Cardiac Surgery: Morphology, Diagnostic Criteria, Natural History, Techniques, Results, and Indications.* New York: John Wiley and Sons, 1990.

Means, J.H. *The Association of American Physicians: Its First Seventy-five Years*. New York: The Blakiston Division, McGraw-Hill Book Company, Inc., 1961.

Meads, Manson. *The Miracle on Hawthorne Hill: A History of the Medical Center of The Bowman Gray School of Medicine of Wake Forest University and the North Carolina Baptist Hospital*. Winston-Salem: Wake Forest University, 1988.

Miller, G. W. *King of Hearts: The True Story of the Maverick Who Pioneered Open Heart Surgery*. New York: Times Books/Random House, 2000.

Mooney, B. *More than Armies: The Story of Edward H. Cary, M.D.* Dallas: Mathis, Van Nort & Company, 1948.

Moursund, Walter H., Sr. *A History of Baylor University College of Medicine 1900–1953*. Houston: Gulf Printing Co., 1956.

Nevins A. "Irving Stone." *Book of the Month Club News*. Reprinted in "Foreword." *The Origin, A Biographical Novel of Charles Darwin*. New York: New American Library,1980.

Novick Peter. *That Noble Dream—The "Objectivity Question" and the American Historical Profession*. Cambridge: Cambridge University Press, 1988.

Nuland, Sherwin B. *Doctors, the Biography of Medicine*. New York: Vintage Books, 1989.

Oglesby, Paul. *Take Heart, the Life and Prescription for Living of Dr. Paul Dudley White*. Boston: The Francis A. Countway Library of Medicine, 1986.

Paschal, G. W. *History of Wake Forest College*, vol. III. Wake Forest: Wake Forest College, 1943.

Postel-Vinay, Nicolas, ed. *A Century of Arterial Hypertension 1896–1996*. New York: John Wiley & Sons/Imhotep, 1996.

Read, Nicholas Cabell and Dallas Read. *Deep Family*. Montgomery: NewSouth Books, 2005.

Reiser Stanley, *Medicine and the Reign of Technology*. Cambridge: Cambridge University Press, 1981.

Riven, Samuel S. *Worthy Lives*. Nashville: Vanderbilt University Medical Center, 1993.

Robins, Natalie. *The Girl Who Died Twice: Every Patient's Nightmare—The Libby Zion Case and the Hidden Hazards of Hospitals*. New York: Delacorte Press, 1995.

Robinson, G. Canby: *Adventures in Medical Education: A Personal Narrative of the Great Advance of American Medicine*. Cambridge, MA: Harvard University Press, 1957.

Rosdick, Raymond B. *The Story of the Rockefeller Foundation*. New York: Harper and Brothers, 1952.

Sellers, Charles. *The Market Revolution—Jacksonian America 1815–1846*. New York/Oxford: Oxford Univ. Press, 1991.

Scheidlower, J. *The F Word*. New York: Random House, 1999.

Schumacker, H. B., Jr. *A Dream of the Heart: The Life of John H. Gibbon Jr., Father of the Heart-Lung Machine*. Santa Barbara, CA: Fithian Press, 1999.

Smith, Anita. *The Intimate Story of Lurleen Wallace, Her Crusade of Courage*. Montgomery, AL: Communications Unlimited Inc., 1969.

Stover, John F. *The Railroads of the South, 1865–1900*. Chapel Hill, 1955.

Straus, Eugene. *Rosalyn Yalow, Nobel Laureate, Her Life and Work in Medicine*. Cambridge, MA: Perseus Books, 1998.

Thomas, Vivien T. *Pioneering Research in Surgical Shock and Cardiovascular Surgery: Vivien Thomas and His Work with Alfred Blalock*. Philadelphia: University of Pennsylvania Press, 1985.

Wade, Nicholas. *The Nobel Duel, Two Scientists' 21-year Race to Win the World's Most Coveted Research Prize*. Garden City, NY: Anchor/Doubleday, 1981.

Weatherall, D. J., J. G. G. Ledingham, and D. A. Warrell, eds. "The Role of Medicine." *Oxford Textbook of Medicine* 1, 1996.

Weisse, A. B. *Heart to Heart*. New Brunswick, NJ: Rutgers University Press, 2002.

Westaby, S. and C. Bosher. *Landmarks in Cardiac Surgery*. Oxford: Isis Medical Media, 1997.

Wilson, J. D., et al. *Harrison's Principles of Internal Medicine*, 9th ed. New York: McGraw-Hill, Inc. 1980.

Wu, J. G., C. S. Pittman, R. H. Lindsay, S. D. Sweeney, and C. H. Choe. "Identification of Thyroxine 5'-deiodinase Among Purified Proteins by Affinity Label with a Radiosubstrate After Equilibrium and Heating" in *Progress in Thyroid Research*, edited by A. Gordon, J. Gross, and G. Hennemann (Rotterdam: A. A. Balkema, 1991).

Zachary, G. P. *Endless Frontier: Vannevar Bush, Engineer of the American Century*. New York: Free Press, 1997.

INDEX